THE CHILDHOOD EMOTIONAL PATTERN AND MATURITY

BOOKS BY LEON J. SAUL, M.D.

Emotional Maturity

Bases of Human Behavior

Technic and Practice of Psychoanalysis

The Hostile Mind

Fidelity and Infidelity

Dependence in Man (with H. Parens)

Psychodynamically Based Psychotherapy

Psychodynamics of Hostility

The Childhood Emotional Pattern: The Key to Personality, Its Disorders
and Therapy

The Childhood Emotional Pattern and Corey Jones

The Childhood Emotional Pattern in Marriage

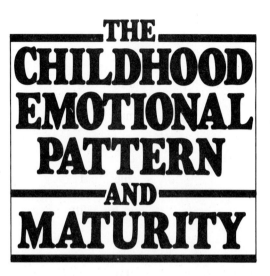

THE CHILDHOOD EMOTIONAL PATTERN AND MATURITY

Leon J. Saul, M.D.

Emeritus Professor of Psychiatry
Medical School of the University of Pennsylvania

Honorary Staff, Institute of the Pennsylvania Hospital

Emeritus Training Analyst
Philadelphia Psychoanalytic Institute

Emeritus Chief Psychiatric Consultant
Swarthmore College

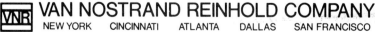 VAN NOSTRAND REINHOLD COMPANY
NEW YORK   CINCINNATI   ATLANTA   DALLAS   SAN FRANCISCO
LONDON   TORONTO   MELBOURNE

Van Nostrand Reinhold Company Regional Offices:
New York   Cincinnati   Chicago   Millbrae   Dallas

Van Nostrand Reinhold Company International Offices:
London   Toronto   Melbourne

Manufactured in the United States of America

Published by Van Nostrand Reinhold Company
135 West 50th Street, New York, N.Y. 10020

Published simultaneously in Canada by Van Nostrand Reinhold Ltd.

15 14 13 12 11 10 9 8 7 6 5 4 3 2 1

Library of Congress Cataloging in Publication Data

Saul, Leon Joseph, 1901–
    The childhood emotional pattern and maturity.

    Includes bibliographical references and index.
    1. Emotional maturity.   2. Personality.   3. Neuroses.
I. Title.
BF710.S28   155.4'18   78-26075
ISBN 0-442-27356-8
ISBN 0-442-27357-5 pbk.

*To my wife and children
and
grandchildren*

Acknowledgments

It is a pleasure to thank my super-secretary and editorial assistant, Susan (Mrs. Vernon) Bender, who did all the typing and correcting and acted as personal bosun, running errands, driving me hither and yon in mid-winter during a period of easy exhaustibility, and who made invaluable suggestions for the manuscript itself; June (Mrs. Walter) Strickland, librarian of the Institute of the Pennsylvania Hospital, who so willingly and conscientiously furnished needed references; my wife for her patience and support; and my patients in treatment, who have kept me alert to the psychological realities and to their unconscious patterns which needed to be worked out analytically.

Introduction

A glance at the newborn babies in any hospital nursery will immediately remind one that each of these neonates is unique in size, shape, weight, restlessness or placidity, tension or relaxation, motility and other characteristics. They are all born with individual potentials and *talents* that will not appear until later, such as the musical gift of a Mozart, the insight and language of a Shakespeare, the coordination in sports of a Jim Thorpe. There are also differences in *temperament,* in emotional make-up and reactions. Whether or not these emotional differences may be pathological, innate disorders, is not yet a settled question scientifically. Available evidence * based mostly upon the study of twins suggests that extremes of psychosis such as severe schizophrenia might be innate, yet this is hard to prove because one cannot know with certainty what influences—physical and emotional—affected the fetus before birth, nor how each baby was treated in the first hours, days and weeks of its life. Even loving parents can cause trauma to a baby without realizing it during those early days when "imprinting" occurs, i.e., the ability to form attachments, first to the mother and then to other humans. Konrad Lorenz † showed that newly-hatched ducklings with no mother present attached themselves to Lorenz's shoes, as he walked, and then continued that attachment when the shoes were still. Harry Harlow ‡ observed

* Kety, S., and Rosenthal, D., eds. (1968): *The Transmission of Schizophrenia,* Proceedings of the Second Research Conference of the Foundations' Fund for Research in Psychiatry. New York: Pergamon Press.

† Lorenz, K. (1952): *King Solomon's Ring.* New York: Crowell.

‡ Harlow, H. (1964): Primary affectional patterns in primates, in: *Contributions to Modern Psychology.* New York: Oxford University Press, pp. 274–284.

_____ (1965): Sexual behavior in the rhesus monkey, in: *Sex and Behavior* by F. Beach. New York: Wiley.

_____ and M. K. Harlow (1966): The effect of rearing conditions on behavior, in: *The Causes of Behavior* by Rosenblith, J., and Allinsmith, W. Boston: Allyn & Bacon, pp. 134–139.

that in the absence of a mother, the infant monkeys attached to a substitute made of terrycloth stretched over wire, to which they clung.

Without question the newborn are enormously malleable, hugely conditionable, and remain so for at least six years. Reduced to the essential, we may say that their temperaments and latent talents *interact* with how they are treated physically and emotionally by their parents and others close to them and responsible for them— whether they are treated with love, acceptance, patience, tolerance and respect for their personalities, or with rejection, hostility, ruthless authority and other aberrations of childrearing. Obviously a baby of warm, responsive, cuddly temperament is much easier for some parents ro raise lovingly than a so-called "hyperactive," "hyperkinetic," tense, unresponsive one. However, other parents, because of their *own* make-ups, may be uncomfortable with a warm, cuddly baby. In any event, the interaction with those who are responsible for it does shape and condition the baby and child during its most formative years, from birth to approximately the age of six or seven.* The parents' reaction to their child is usually not determined by the tiny, feeble, helpless child's temperament but overwhelmingly by their own personalities; a truly loving parent will love his child regardless of the child's temperament.

These interactions between the child and its relatively "omnipotent" parents build certain emotional patterns: the child reacts lovingly if the parents treat it with love, it reacts with fear if the parents are inconsiderate or cruel. This is *"object"* interest. But the small child, in its helplessness and efforts to reach an adjustment, also *identifies* with his † parents, tending to be like them, to feel, react and behave as they do.

There are two striking facts about these *childhood emotional patterns:*

First, they do not remain confined to the parents. Once formed

---

* Even today there exist some unbelievably naive ideas to the effect that the child is not affected by what is done to him before six or seven because he is not yet sufficiently aware. The exact opposite is true: the less awareness, language and thought processes he has to comprehend his experiences and to express his reactions to and feelings about these experiences, the more traumatic they are.

† For simplicity of style, the words "his," "him," or "he" will be used throughout, but will indicate both sexes.

they "spread" and are "transferred" to other persons. If the mother was too critical and controlling from birth, the child is insecure in all human relations, especially with women; criticism and control are all the child knew during its formative years from the omnipotent, controlling woman in his life. So the child expects this from all women, and often from all adults, including men.

Secondly, childhood emotional patterns, once formed, persist for the individual's entire life. How strong, deep, rigid, unalterable they are depends upon how *early* in life they were impressed upon the child, how unrelievedly, insistently and consistently they were impressed, how balanced they were by a tolerant loving father, aunt or other person. The mixture varies from person to person. But the basic truth remains, quantitatively: as the twig is bent, so is the tree inclined.

These fateful, inexorable patterns, developed during the earliest hours, days, weeks, months and years, from reactions to and identifications with parents and others reponsible for it, can facilitate the development of the child to emotional maturity, or can block and warp his emotional growth. This is of vital importance for our world—every human being, with his inferiorities, frustrations and hostilities, seems basically to be striving for the inner peace which comes only from emotional maturity.

How he can reach such maturity, how the psychodynamics of the childhood emotional patterns can either help or warp the normal growth of the individual, is the subject of this book and the key to relieving man's suffering and probably also is the key to his survival on this planet as a species.

The fundamental of Freud's explorations of the human mind is his discovery of "the dynamic unconscious," that interplay of instincts and basic reactions that we experience, when they are conscious, as "emotional forces." The interplay of mature and mostly conscious forces with those emotional patterns formed in childhood which are usually mostly unconscious, dictates our lives. When a pathological childhood pattern dominates the mature and realistic it produces all manner of neurotic and psychotic symptoms and pathologically hostile behavior. Many philosophers, religious leaders and creative writers with gifted insight had glimpsed parts of "the dynamic unconscious," but Freud was the first to explore it in detail, and through free associations plus dream interpretation, actually to go there. *The Interpretation of Dreams* * should be studied rather than read; it is scientifically exciting and most rewarding. One of the most intuitive of the early psychoanalysts, Gregory Zilboorg, once told me he re-read this book every two years.

In exploring this new internal territory, Freud seems to have tried, like most explorers, to map its main features. He wrote of "complexes" such as the oedipus complex, the castration complex, etc. These are combinations of individual emotional forces. In this book, except for the fight-flight reaction which is a physiological response, we shall focus upon the *individual emotional forces* that combine in different ways and degrees to constitute the complexes.

As Robert Waelder † wrote a few years ago, we must fear that knowledge of the dynamic unconscious and the role in it of the childhood emotional pattern may be lost to the world by again being repressed. If this occurs, we would lose along with it our hard-won knowledge of human nature and also hope of making a better life for violence-prone, suffering humanity. Orthodox members of organized psychoanalysis are becoming more dictatorial as to how analysts should be trained, what analysts should read and how they should think. This dictatorial attitude naturally provokes rebellion. Such absurd political contention threatens a sound, open-minded devotion to scientific truth, and threatens the grasp of psychic reality that Freud himself so intrepidly explored.

The promise of dynamic psychiatry lies in the fact that in the last 50 years it has learned to deal scientifically with the human spirit itself. Until recently its interest focused on the extremes of breakdown, and its history had been largely the recognition that mental disorders have natural causes, the story of a long struggle to make the custody of the insane more humane, and the emergence of a system of classification. But about 50 years ago there were discovered technical, psychological procedures which opened the human mind, even in its depths, to scientific observation and study. Van

---

* (1900) *Standard Edition* 4.

NOTE: All references to the works of Sigmund Freud in this book will be to the Standard Edition (S.E.).

† (1976) *Psychoanalysis: Observation, Theory, Application.* New York: International Universities Press, p. 1.

Leeuwenhoek, by inventing the microscope, had made possible the founding of microscopic anatomy and of bacteriology—and so of modern medicine. Freud, by discovering psychoanalysis, provided a psychological microscope to observe the mind and so made possible the new science of psychodynamics, the basis of modern psychiatry.

The primary interest of modern psychiatry is no longer the "insane." The "insane" or psychotic represent only the extremes of breakdown, and are a drop in the bucket compared with the neurotics.* For the neuroses result from faulty childrearing combined with the emotional tensions of living from which no one is entirely free. To understand the neuroses is to understand the average person with all his expressed and secret loves and hates and fears and desires, to understand motivations and feelings within him which he himself may sense but dimly, if at all. It is to understand men's drives and men's motives as they appear in life and literature.

It is through just these desires, drives and motivations that men and women and children make for each other their highest happiness—and their most profound suffering. From these come the loftiest achievements and the most unutterable degradations and cruelties. From these come mental turmoil and madness—or inner peace. From these come wars and, in the atomic age, the threat of total destruction. In the light of the achievements of the physical sciences in medicine and industry we may hope that this new science of motivation will yet enable people to realize and enjoy their full constructive potentialities and experience their lives as richly satisfying rather than as blind and anxious struggles in a vale of tears.

"We remain on the surface so long as we treat only of memories and ideas. The only valuable things in the psychic life are, rather, the emotions. All psychic powers are significant only through their fitness to awaken emotions. Ideas are repressed only because they are connected with liberations of emotions which are not come to light." †

Knowledge of human emotions is fundamental to insight not only

---

* Recent statistics indicate the psychiatric hospital population has fallen from a high of 650,000 in 1955 to 190,000 in 1976; this has been largely attributed to the use of psychotropic drugs.

† Freud, S. (1907): Delusions and dreams in Jensen's *Gradiva, S.E.* 9.

into the disturbances of mood, thought and behavior as seen in the neuroses, the functional psychoses and criminality but also into those disturbances of physiology which are caused at least in part by emotional tensions (psychosomatic symptoms), such as ordinary headaches, nervous stomach, certain cases of ulcer, of asthma and perhaps of high blood pressure, some allergies, etc. Such knowledge is also basic to the understanding of man's behavior toward man. It is therefore hoped that this book will prove of some use not only to psychiatrists and to physicians in other specialties who are interested in the scientific basis of the art of medicine, but also to those in other fields such as law, religion, industry, social work, government—to all who deal with people and strive to make human life more livable.*

Although the national and world scenes have shifted since the late sixties, man's basic motivations and how they are influenced remain unchanged. Yet new forms of disturbance become prominent and recognizable. Today neurotic hostile acting out (as seen in the still climbing crime rate) is becoming increasingly prominent— the most fateful form for society. Neurotic characters, addiction and other behavior disorders have long been recognized as pathological, but irrational hostile acting out is usually less obviously an emotional disorder when it appears frankly as crime or rationalized as political action. The central underlying motivation within the individual is the predisposition toward neurotic hostility, anger, destructiveness, cruelty and violence. "Neurotic" means arising primarily from frustrations deep within the personality and only secondarily in reaction to external circumstances, which the individual uses both as excuses and rationalizations for his internally motivated behavior.

There is no longer doubt that emotional illness, in almost every case, is a continuance of patterns of response to some sort of mistreatment or mistraining or both over long periods during early childhood; it is a disorder in the feelings toward others. Those with similarity in their disorders tend to form groups which express these, and which attract other like individuals.

---

* This is not a book based on the existing literature, but the author uses this literature only to help him understand what he sees. Therefore, the discussion of combat fatigue is based entirely upon the author's first-hand observations while in charge of such units on active duty in the Naval Reserve during World War II.

Of course the psychodynamics of human nature and behavior are also the result of biological and sociological factors, but these are not described in detail in this book.

Many American psychiatrists enlisted in the armed forces after Pearl Harbor. It was, I believe, their experiences in World War II which increased precipitously their awareness of "emotional forces" and the personal interactions of these, and brought into prominence the term "psychodynamics." Psychiatry became "dynamic psychiatry," and these men, returning to civilian life, took over the leadership of the American Psychiatric Association and also created the Group for the Advancement of Psychiatry.

A comprehensive introduction to this new and still developing science of psychodynamics is needed within a single textbook. However, the following four volumes might constitute such an introduction. These are interrelated, but each stands on its own in dealing with a particular aspect of psychodynamics:

The Childhood Emotional Pattern: The Key to Personality, Its Disorders and Therapy
The Childhood Emotional Pattern and Corey Jones
The Childhood Emotional Pattern in Marriage
The Childhood Emotional Pattern and Maturity

Because I am temperamentally a clinician and not a theoretician, no effort has been made in this book to supplement the clinical observations with a review of the vast literature relative to all subjects within this volume, especially as each subject has statistical, sociological, ethological aspects as well as the analytic psychodynamic ones which are our primary concern.

List of Figures

Contents

THE CHILDHOOD EMOTIONAL PATTERN AND MATURITY

PART ONE

The Achievement
of Maturity

1 | Emotional Development and Preventive Psychiatry

GOALS—MATURITY

The end goal of medicine is prevention. For psychiatry this means the prevention of all kinds of emotional disorders. Emotional disorders cause not only neurosis but many other sorts of behavior that result in man-made misery. The first step in prevention must be the clarification of objectives. Then working toward them becomes primarily a practical matter. The psychiatrist has nothing so simple to offer as vaccination. But dynamic psychiatry is now far enough advanced to describe in some detail man's course of development to maturity and so to discern what facilitates it and what obstructs it. Psychiatry discerns also the incidence and the consequences of the achievement of maturity, as well as some of the implications and the applications of this concept.

It was in the late twenties that Freud once remarked that psychoanalysis had been operating in the Mediterranean Sea of the neuroses but would emerge soon into the broad Atlantic of the total personality. This emergence has now been realized, and neurosis can be viewed from the wider perspectives of our increasing knowledge, which has been extended still further by the war experience.

Neurosis signifies a failure in adaptation in which the personality partially relinquishes mature reactions and regresses to childish ones or fails to outgrow childish reactions upon reaching physical maturity. *Neurosis is the excessive predominance of disordered childhood emotional patterns* caused usually, if not invariably, by faults in upbringing. The internal disposition to neurosis is determined by specific factors in the individual's emotional development.

The emotional development of some persons has been so faulty

3

that their functioning is always highly precarious, even under the most favorable circumstances. Others react with neurotic symptoms only when under severe and prolonged duress. Many of these "reactive" cases are seen in civil life, especially by the social agencies; but the most clear-cut and extensive experimental situation for the production of such cases was the state of widespread stress seen in this country in World War II and later in the Korean and Vietnam conflicts. This showed that each person has one or more *specific emotional vulnerabilities,* and reacts violently when stresses strike these.

Despite the many complications and variations, the essence of neurotic reactions boils down to this: A variety of external and internal factors, both physical (danger, exposure, disease, etc.) and psychological (separation from home, morale, relationship to leaders and groups, etc.), exerts stresses on the organism which cause: (1) *general* weakening and sensitization, (2) reactions resulting from *specific* emotional vulnerabilities, and (3) the weakening and the impairment of the *powers of control.*

Once a person is threatened by increasing pain, frustration, anxiety and weakening forces of control, he reacts, as does every animal organism, by physiological and psychological mobilization for fight or flight. This mobilization is felt subjectively as anger and/or fear. The fight impulses manifest themselves, so far as they are directed outward, by tendencies to hostile-aggressive behavior, irritability and belligerency; so far as the fight impulses are repressed, they probably always generate anxiety and combine with flight reactions, to cause all kinds of psychological and somatic symptoms from anxiety, paranoid trends and nightmares to palpitations of the heart and many other physiological symptoms. The flight impulses, so far as they are expressed outwardly, lead to actual fleeing from the unbearable situation or to a conscious attempt to withdraw in some other way. When repressed, they may unconsciously motivate misbehavior, produce physiological symptoms which offer a means of escape, or they may cause flight in the form of physiological and psychological regression, that is, an unconscious partial return to childish and infantile reactions, which may result in eating disorders, difficulties in walking, loss of capacity for responsibilities, alcoholism, drug abuse and so on.

Impulses to fight and to flight, the hostile aggressive and the regressive reactions, combine to produce a variety of impulses, tensions and symptoms, which activate childhood patterns and cause neurosis if they are not handled maturely.

The role of the fight-flight reaction in neurosis has not been fully appreciated and deserves further study and emphasis. Of course, aggression and regression have been studied intensively, but their interplay and their specific relation to the fight-flight reaction have not been worked out in detail. For example, in many depressions, the flight reaction in the form of biological withdrawal seems to be as important as the fight reaction of aggression, repressed and turned inward. In the field of psychosomatic medicine it is common to see an individual under emotional pressure whose constantly aroused fight reaction influences his hypertension, while his flight reaction, in the form or oral regression, causes gastric symptoms. More accurately, every neurosis, and possibly even every neurotic symptom, is motivated, in part, at least, by a combination of both fight and flight impulses in various proportions. Freud stated long ago that someday our psychological understanding would rest on a physiological basis. Our understanding of hostile aggression and regression and their interplay is furthered by the recognition of their relationships to the fight-flight reaction.

Once a person is under stresses that cause mounting tension, he, or more precisely, his ego, struggles to master the tension and in doing so usually contributes further to certain other symptoms such as fatigue.

As we have said, the study of war neuroses has clarified and rendered somewhat more precise our understanding of the reactive neuroses and, indeed, of the nature of neurosis in general. From it, we can conclude that if the emotional development of the individual is relatively complete, his adaptability is high, his regressive tendencies low, and his vulnerabilities minimal. Susceptibility to neurosis (the internal factor as opposed to the external stress) thus appears to be due to disturbances in one's development toward emotional maturity, disturbances which cause specific vulnerabilities to stress and impairment of adaptability. Presumably, a fully mature individual is in general less vulnerable and more adaptable than a less mature one, and therefore is less prone to relinquish mature handling of reality in favor of neurotic, that is, regressive, childish or infantile reactions. But of what, more precisely, does this maturity consist?

Although most psychoanalytic work has an implicit bearing upon this question, the concept of maturity has not received a great deal of explicit attention in the literature. Delineation of libidinal development has yielded the important formulation of the "genital level" and "object interest" (Freud, 1924) and recent emphasis on the conflict between the regressive, dependent, versus the progressive, productive forces in the personality has directed interest toward the more detailed nature of maturity. Meanwhile, growing knowledge of the ego and of the total personality contributes much of importance to this problem (Allee, 1951; A. Freud, 1937; Freud, 1924; Kardiner, 1939; Laughlin, 1970; Marmor, 1968; Saul, 1945). We shall approach the subject in terms of the major forces that motivate us.

NATURE OF MATURITY

If, in the light of modern psychodynamics, we review our therapeutic experience by listing the patients treated intensively over a ten-year period, we see that each patient has a more or less specific emotional problem; that this usually arises from defects in his emotional development; and that, if these defects can be partially resolved, his development is reopened, and adaptation is improved. He comes to see the nature of his defects, the course of his development as it would have been if it had not been obstructed, and also the kind of person he would have become if his development had been unimpeded. The result of full, unimpaired development must be full maturity. By simple extrapolation, we visualize a condition which, hopefully for correctable reasons, is rarely achieved in reality. Let us enumerate some of its characteristics. A guide to these must be the attitudes and the feelings of the parent toward the child in contrast with those of the child toward the parent.

1. One of the most obvious pathways of development, long emphasized by Sigmund Freud and Franz Alexander, is from the parasitic dependence of the fetus to the relative independence of the parent, with parental capacity for responsibility for spouse and child. Reviewed from this angle, biological development consists in

the achievement of the capacity to live independently of the parental organisms and to take for others such responsibility as was taken for oneself during childhood. The fetus is parasitic; the suckling is nearly so. With walking, talking, improved coordination, a grasp of reality and development of thought comes increasing independence from the parents. Attending nursery school is a big step in this direction. Grade school is another. With adolescence the organism achieves its full size. The energies no longer needed for its own growth form a surplus, now available for expenditure. They can be put out in the form of mating, sexual productivity, responsibility for spouse and children and responsible work. The animals ensure independence from the parents by pushing out their young as soon as they are mature, but in human beings this independence is not achieved so readily.

Long years of childhood leave a taste for the pleasures of childhood, the freedom from responsibilities and the dependence on parents. This reflects a counterforce, a "regressive" tendency. Humans are children for so long that they never get over it. Much of the struggle of adolescence results from the conflict between the developmental drives to be free and independent and the regressive attraction to the protection and the dependence on the parents so long enjoyed throughout childhood. All too many parents play upon this clinging to childhood and try to hold their children. Others are anxious about them and try to continue to protect them, even after they are working and married. Others force children prematurely into work and responsibility and produce similar effects in this opposite way. The adult then continues to long for dependence, whether because as a child he missed it too much or had too much of it. Either way, his normal development to the full emotional independence and self-reliance of the mature adult is impaired.

Some people never overcome this dependence sufficiently to make much of a go of life. Others get through life with all sorts of supports from friends, relatives and others. Higher on the scale are those who operate with reasonable independence until some hardship throws them back, and then, by way of classic neurosis, alcoholism or neurotic behavior, they partially regress. Still higher on the scale are those who stand their ground and repress their desires for retreat and help, only to have these repressions generate inner tensions which cause a variety of long-standing symptoms. At the top of the scale the more fully independent individual would maintain his functioning even in the face of great frustration.

All this should be common knowledge. In a vague way it is, but it is not sufficiently articulated. It is the task of psychiatry to clarify, formulate and make known this aspect of emotional development as well as others.

For what are the results of excessive dependence? It can cause not only neurosis but also crime and misery. A wife "runs to mother" at the first squalls and responsibilities of marriage. A man's pride is hurt by feeling this underlying dependence and he drives himself to deny it until he develops a gastric ulcer. A boy feels it as a weakness and in his rage because of this, and to prove his strength, he takes to gangsterism. Others, because of their underlying dependence, feel unable to cope with life on their own and drift to the fringe of society, many of them clay for demagogues. No prevention of neurosis or crime, no stable marriages, no steadiness and enjoyment of work, no healthy nation is possible if children are not permitted to develop fully to emotional independence and self-reliance.

2. Intimately bound up with the organism's development from parasitism on the mother to relative independence from the parents is its increased capacity for responsibility and productivity and its decreased receptive needs. The fetus must be given *everything;* the infant can take in air and food for itself, but obviously throughout childhood what the child contributes is negligible in proportion to what it gets. What it gets comes from its parents; when it matures it can *be* a parent and enjoy *giving,* whether to its mate, to its own children or to society in the production of what is useful. It still gets, and should remain able to receive freely, but the give-get balance is grossly altered.

If the child is deprived emotionally or overindulged emotionally, it tends to cling too strongly to the *getting* and does not develop sufficient capacity for, or enjoyment of, *giving.* It is doomed to frustration and hence to anger; emotional frustration spells unhappiness, leads to fight-flight, anger, repressed or overt, and can become the basis for depressions and other neurotic reactions—for alcoholism, for unrest and for antisocial behavior. Children learn to control their hostilities, their sexuality and other impulses, and to develop the orientations of maturity, largely through the incentive of being loved. If they feel unloved they care little about controlling themselves, and hence socialization and smooth emotional growth are disturbed. Being loved is the emotional assurance of security, of satisfaction of the core of the dependent needs, and thereby of survival for the helpless child. Hence the need for love, the guarantee of survival, is the overriding craving to which well nigh all else is subject and will be sacrificed.

The capacity to enjoy a well-proportioned amount of play, dependence, receiving, and other respite from independence, responsibility and giving is a normal component of maturity. This is part of the meaning of a "well-balanced" life. In recreation we balance the enjoyment of the activities of maturity with the enjoyment of the playtime of childhood. In sleep we normally regress deeply and return refreshed. *To love and be loved, to give and to receive, to work and to play and rest*—these are the bases of the emotional life.

To delineate the normal course of development from getting to giving and the limits of normality for the give-get balance in adult life and to disseminate this knowledge, are fundamental steps for understanding and for prevention.

Social ideologies sometimes reflect an unhygienic unbalance. For example, an exaggerated puritanism of all work and no play is as certain to generate inner frictions as is a cavalier ideal of all play and no work. Both attitudes make Jack many worse things than a dull boy. We must not take any ideologies for granted, however widespread they are—they may themselves reflect neurotic trends in the group. We must measure them against our scientific knowledge of the normal course of emotional development and of what mature functioning is.

3. A third characteristic of maturity is relative freedom from the well-known constellation of inferiority feelings, egotism and competitiveness. Much of the child persists in every adult, and it is this sense of being partially a child which is a primary source of mankind's pervasive feelings of inferiority. The adult unconsciously repeats, especially toward those in superior positions, many of his childhood feelings toward his parents, such as the dependent and receptive desires just mentioned; but with the childhood desires go the child's feelings of weakness, inadequacy and inferiority in

comparison with his more independent, more giving parents. This hurts the child's self-love, which is normally greater during this period when its energies must go into its own growth and cultivation and when, too, it is usually encouraged in self-love by the parents. The wounded self-esteem generates envy of parents and siblings and the tendency to want to compete with them. This constellation persists in adult life: the unconscious desires of childhood with respect to others, the hurt pride, the envy and the competition, and consequently hostility and guilt, which in turn produce anxiety, inferiority and further feelings of insecurity. Tortured by the sense of anxious, impotent childishness, man strives to be god and remains beast. His real and achievable goal is to mature as a human being.

Much of the social scene is apparently motivated by this constellation. The universal sense of inferiority which torments mankind and generates the mad struggle for prestige and power is largely the adult's feeling of being infantile and his frustrated urgency to identify with the parent and not with the child. He is inexorably driven by the developmental forces within him toward this goal, which he has as yet been unable to define or achieve. He fights to demonstrate his strength and, at the same time, although usually unconsciously, to satisfy his childish impulses. This constellation is also evident in man's tendency to form organizations and in influencing the kinds of organizations and social and economic forms that human beings have developed throughout history.

The fully mature individual would not feel inferior; he would derive his major satisfaction from the enjoyment of the responsible, relatively independent productive use of his powers and would be basically parental, that is, kind, responsible and cooperative rather than competitive and hostile toward others. With modern technology, the difficulties of life now lie primarily in the "human element," which we are beginning to discern as the specifically childish part of human nature. Even physical handicaps cannot hinder productive work or cause serious feelings of inferiority if the basic emotional development is mature.

Various authors have pointed out how common this emotional constellation is in our culture. In the mental life all is quantitative—normal or abnormal is a matter of degree. Competition is a normal phase in which the child tests itself against others.

Competition, to a degree, is normal and advantageous in the adult. But when too strong, it defeats its own purpose and causes guilt, anxiety and strain, which preclude enjoyment even in the successful. It is not an end in itself. Intense competition belongs to childhood, to the time of weakness and insecurity, when one's life itself depends on others. But when the adult lord of creation competes excessively, he blocks himself and shows that he has not out-grown his childhood. *Independently to live and let live, to enjoy one's own productive activity, to love one's own, and to achieve brotherly cooperation—this is the orientation of the parent, the adult. It is not only the ethical and religious but also the mature ideal.* Again and again, in practice, one sees how freeing a patient's energies from his egotistic competitiveness relieves his anxieties and leads him to increased capacity for, and enjoyment of, work and love and recreation, and so to greater achievement and inner satisfaction. This we know, and the time is ripe to formulate it explicitly and to utilize it in the proper rearing of children and also in the shaping of healthy cultural ideologies.

4. Another aspect of maturity consists in the conditioning and the training necessary for socialization and domestication. This results in standards, ideals and conscience which, once formed, operate unconsciously and automatically and often against the wishes of the individual. The conscience, lauded as part of man's higher nature, is also often looked upon as a necessary evil which, as Shakespeare phrased it, "fills a man full of obstacles"; but, in actual fact, proper upbringing should facilitate the emotional development toward maturity. The core on which the conscience is developed is probably the innate tendency to cooperation which is seen throughout the animal kingdom—the cooperation which seems to be an extension to other members of the species of the loving cooperation which is seen in mating and care of the young. Proper upbringing should, among other things, form a conscience which is not only a negative, restraining force but furthers the innate tendencies of growth toward independence, responsibility, productivity and cooperation. This is perhaps the essence of the psychological contribution of Christianity and other great religions, quintessentially expressed as "love thy neighbor as thyself"—that is, to set as the goal, beyond a negating superego to check anti-social behavior, the psychological maturing to what Freud de-

scribed as "object interest." At this level the major pleasure in life derives not from the satisfaction of infantile, egocentric tendencies but from the exercise of the adult capacity for productivity and loving. Religion and ethics reflect mankind's long struggle throughout the ages to handle its instincts and to grow up—the same struggle and the same course of development that we see in the growing child.

The mature adult, then, would be in harmony with his conscience, and this conscience would be integrated with and would support his biological development toward parental and socially cooperative attitudes.

Even if we know clearly the goals of development, the task of helping children to achieve them is awesome. We must know not only the *goals* but also the *rate* and the *course* of the emotional development. Of course, a certain amount of training is necessary, and we must know how to do this, how much to expect of the child and at what ages and stages. Because of too little or too lax training, we see infantile, impulse-ridden adults; because of too much, too early or too harsh training, we see anxious, inhibited individuals overburdened by pathological consciences; because of inconsistent training, we see indecision and confusion. Here we have far to go indeed, for general ignorance of this phase of child rearing is vast and profound. The training is so often dominated by the convenience of the parents or by misguided notions rather than any sound knowledge. To formulate such sound and detailed knowledge is a primary task of psychiatry. When such knowledge is widely available, perhaps we shall see fewer mothers, however neurotic, beating six-months-old babies to enforce eating, and year-old ones because they are not fully toilet-trained, trying to make girls into boys and vice versa, and, in general, trying to force the youngsters into preconceived molds instead of tending with tolerance and patience the unfolding of their emotional development.

The conscious and unconscious emotional reactions of parents cause them to behave in certain ways toward their children and often interfere with their own best judgment. Besides this, children acquire their standards not only from training but even more through love and identification. They tend to do not so much as the parents *say* but as they *do*. This wish to be *like* the parents, this *identification* with them, is a potent force toward development. But it also brings us to what is perhaps the crucial difficulty in educational and preventive programs: the lack of maturity in the parents which exerts its effects emotionally in spite of reason and knowledge; how can such infantile parents learn to raise their children to proper maturity? Hence, the formulation and the dissemination of the essential knowledge cannot be expected to produce quick or dramatic results, but it is the necessary first step, the *sine qua non*, of any rational program at all.

But more than reason is on our side. If we seek to liberate man's full capacity for development, this developmental force is in itself a powerful ally. The ideals and conscience should be allies also, facilitating and not inhibiting development. It is not always recognized that ideals and conscience do not result only from the training and the conditioning imposed from without, but that, like the basic goals of religion, ethics and morality, they reflect a striving for maturity from within. Here science fuses in its goals with morals, ethics and religion. Facilitating the human emotional development to maturity is the procedure of science for the achievement of the moral goal of brotherhood. Man's suffering on this earth is caused predominantly by man himself and is a manifestation of his emotional immaturity. As such it is a soluble psychological problem.

5. Well-known psychoanalytic studies have traced the libidinal development in detail through the infantile stages to the "genital level" with its mature capacity for "object interest" in people and things outside oneself and the capacity for love and productivity, both social and sexual. The sexual feelings are an important part of the total emotional development. To help children achieve mature sexual attitudes when they reach adult life, we must see clearly what these attitudes are and how they develop.

The onset of full sexual feelings, power and ability to reproduce comes only as the individual approximates his own limits of growth. Genital sexuality, evident from infancy on, has a twofold relationship to the process of emotional development. In the first place, it is a powerful force in itself, and one which acts in the direction of emotional development. Secondly, it is an expression of the individual's particular make-up and degree of development, and a channel for the drainage of all kinds of feelings and impulses. As a force in itself, it is, in essence, a part of the tendency toward mating and reproduction. As such, it leads the young away from dependence on the parents toward independence and the responsibility of loving, supporting and caring for a family. Thus it is a powerful, constant stimulus toward mature attitudes. Hence, if the sexuality does not evolve properly, the whole process of emotional growth can be influenced. Too great repression of sex tends to impair the freedom and the ease of functioning as an adult and may prevent mating and even sexual satisfaction. However, too great sexual freedom in childhood may prevent its integration with the rest of the development and its channeling into the capacity for falling in love and mating, so that it remains too childish in nature, a matter of play and personal pleasure but never a proper part of the adult function of mating.

In the converse relationship, the sexuality usually cannot itself mature properly or function smoothly in the adult if the rest of the personality is not well developed emotionally. For then it is used by the individual, consciously or unconsciously, in many different and often childish and infantile ways which may be remote from its mature biological and psychological intent. For example, a Don Juan uses it to bolster his prestige and a gold digger to pad her purse; it may express loneliness or drain hate and anger; and so on in the many variations we see and read of daily. Divorce and separation rates reflect the degree to which the infantile components have not been overcome.

Sex education must not merely teach a few facts of physiology but must be a true education in the emotional orientations which are basic to mature sexual attitudes. The mature attitude toward sexuality seems to be little different from a mature attitude toward work or toward social living. When the sexuality and the rest of the personality mature together, the two are integrated in a proper balancing of the needs for love, the self-love and the self-interest with a high degree of enjoyment of the loving, the activity, the interest and the responsibility involved in the relationship to lover, work and friends (Saul, 1979).

6. Hostile aggressiveness, using the term to include all sorts of anger, hate, cruelty and belligerency, is always a sign of emotional irritation or threat. This, as all emotional disorders show and as the war neuroses so clearly emphasized, is because any and every threat, frustration or irritation, external or internal, arouses the

primitive defense reaction of all animals: mobilization for *fight or flight*. This irritation or threat is, as we have seen, determined not only by external pressures but also by the individual's emotional vulnerability; and this, in turn, is, in general, a result of deficiencies in his emotional development. Therefore, *human hostility,* more fateful than the atom bomb and the *central problem of mankind, appears as symptomatic of a childishness which has not been outgrown.* However mistakenly regarded by some individuals and some ideologies as strength, hostility is usually a sign of weakness, fear and frustration. As the saying goes, "Only the strong can be gentle."

That children should be quick to fear, anger and tears is readily understandable. As a necessary part of their training and domestication, they are frustrated almost constantly in some degree, if only by the fact that they are children, that in reality they are weak, dependent and insecure.

But what of the adult who has bent the elemental forces of the universe to his command? Why should he be so chronically hostile that humanity is ravished by wars, crime, violence and unrest, so that man's greatest danger is man himself? Studying adults, one finds that such exaggerated or chronic hostility regularly stems from unresolved emotional problems of childhood which impair adult adaptation. Childish hates and rages, never outgrown, persist in the adult and form an inner source of irritation and hostile aggression which can continue for a lifetime. Revenge for mistreatment as a child, feelings of weakness from being driven into submissiveness and every other type of unresolved childhood problem can warp the development and cause permanent irritation and hostile aggressiveness. Where hate and violence are glorified in a whole ideology, then on the scale of maturity, the ideology is itself immature.

Displaceability is a most fateful characteristic of hostility. Generated toward parent or sibling, it can be taken out on animals and playmates in childhood and, following the childhood pattern, on any victims it can find throughout life. Often it is taken out on the person himself ("masochism"), thus torturing him with neurosis and with a mismanaged life. In addition to the sources of the hostility, another point to consider is how it is handled—whether vented freely or tempered by judgment, sublimation and control.

The mature adult is parental and creative and is not destructive toward himself or others. His hostile aggression is available, but normally it serves, not old, infantile, sadistic and masochistic patterns but constructive, productive ones. Most parents have little idea of how to avoid generating unnecessary hostility in children or of how to handle their children's hostilities once they are generated; often, they have as little idea of how to handle their own hostilities toward their children. No preventive step is more important than formulating our knowledge of hostile aggression in the interests of diminishing this central threat to mankind. The author attempted this in *Psychodynamics of Hostility* (1976).

In every psychoanalysis, insofar as development is reopened, with childish tendencies outgrown or overcome and adjustment improved, hostility decreases. The most dread danger to man, namely man's own cruelty, thus appears as essentially a neurotic symptom and "pathologically hostile acting out" becomes a potentially soluble therapeutic problem.

7. Another important attribute of maturity is a firm sense of reality. This is not merely a matter of intelligence but also of emotional outlook, of a feeling for reality. This is shown by contrasting the familiar figure of the brilliant but impractical and unworldly professor with the equally familiar realism of even a relatively dull but practical peasant.

The sense of reality, especially of psychological reality, evolves gradually through a long course of development and experience. Disturbances in development impair and warp it. The schizoid individual remains remote from reality, living too egocentrically in his own fantasies. The overprotected child whose mother has been his eyes and ears never learns to use his own. The "oral character," intent on the infantile goal of getting something for nothing, is termed a "sucker." The overly loved and favored child tends to be unduly optimistic, while the internally frustrated person takes a depressed and gloomy view of life. The guilty person tends to feel threatened and put upon by others. Thus, each man tends to color reality in accordance with his own feelings, and these in turn represent the results of childhood reactions which have not been overcome—in other words, disturbances in the achievement of maturity.

The practical significance of this is obvious. A distorted sense of reality impairs the effectiveness and the enjoyment of work and life. It makes it difficult for people to understand one another. It creates a sense of insecurity and inferiority and leads to frustration, fear and hate. Yet not much has been written on the development of the sense of reality; and certainly most parents are not over-conscientious in preserving the superb intelligence of the growing child by keeping it close to the truth it seeks and shunning deceit and illusion. Much can be done in gradually acquainting children, adolescents and young adults with the realities of life, chiefly, that is, the nature of people and what one can expect from others in life. This is hard enough to grasp even with experience and without internal difficulties in addition. It should not be left to the back alleys, hard knocks and chance. Small wonder that people find such difficulty in understanding one another and in cooperating when each sees the world through different lenses which tend to warp it to fit unconscious childish needs. Education to emotional reality stands out as one of the great needs and goals for our schools at all levels.

8. Another characteristic of maturity is flexibility and adaptability. A child learns what to expect of other persons from its early experiences with those who reared it. The personality, that is, the accustomed method of functioning, is of course shaped and colored by the emotional influences of childhood. But in some people the childhood emotional patterns do more than this—they are so powerful and fixed that they dominate the behavior. Then the normal enjoyment of loving and working, giving and creating is impaired by a fixed pattern of repeating over and over throughout life reactions which were appropriate to traumatic situations of childhood. An overindulgent mother may cause in her son a life-long tendency to become attached to older women. Undue displacement by a sibling may cause exaggerated competitiveness toward colleagues in adult life. A cruel father may generate resentment and fear of all men, even of all authority.

Children who remain too long in too intense emotional situations in childhood form fixed patterns and fail to discriminate between the father or the mother or siblings of childhood, who caused the particular emotional reactions, and other persons later in life whose only similarity may be sex, age or position. The tendency to reestablish in adult life toward one's marital family, friends, professional and even national and international groups the patterns of childhood is universal; but when it is warped and overly strong, that is, when the individual has not sufficiently outgrown these emotional patterns, the behavior in life becomes proportionately rigid, prejudices flourish, and the normal discrimination, flexibility and adaptability are impaired. For proper maturation children need what young plants need: to be given the proper conditions of warmth, light, nourishment and protection, and then to be allowed to unfold in their own way with only such interference as is really necessary. Keeping them in states of intense emotion warps the development and causes feelings and patterns of childhood to dominate the adult. Many parents do not understand this and feel that their role is to force their wills upon the children. For the parent tends to repeat, often with uncanny accuracy, toward his children and frequently toward his spouse the treatment which he himself received at the hands of his own parents.

THEORETICAL AND THERAPEUTIC IMPLICATIONS

We have mentioned eight of the major aspects of the emotional development of human beings and some of the characteristics of maturity to which each leads. This list is not exhaustive; these aspects are interrelated and are not all on the same level. But we have tried to discern some of the forces in the personality which are basic and from which the many other attributes of maturity are derived. We have seen that when the development is fulfilled the adult is *predominantly* independent and responsible, with little need to regress, and also is giving and productive, although still able to relax and to receive normally; he is cooperative rather than egotistical and competitive; he is in relative harmony with his conscience, which easily integrates with his mature feelings and behavior; his sexuality is free and integrated with mating and responsible productive activity, both sexual and social; his hostility toward others and toward himself is minimal but is freely available for defense and constructive use; his grasp of reality is clear and unimpaired by the emotional astigmatisms of childhood; and freed from childhood emotional patterns, he is discriminating and highly adaptable. Among the many results of such development, his anxiety is at a minimum.

It cannot be emphasized too strongly that maturity means not merely the *capacity* for such attitudes and functioning but also the ability to *enjoy* them fully. It means that the individual now derives pleasure from the exercise of his adult powers and not only from his infantile demands. In the neuroses there is typically a protest against the adult productive, responsible activities and guilt and shame over the childish impulses; each vitiates the other. Normally, they are in such proportion and relationship that both are enjoyed.

Few adults achieve such maturity. These characteristics represent an ideal, and even this ideal must, of course, be a relative matter. We know that in the mental and emotional life all is quantitative. And we know that in its psychological and historical aspects (not in its deeper physiological ones) the unconscious is essentially the persistence in the adult of the infantile emotional patterns. We know from psychoanalytic experience the impressive extent to which the unconscious can be reclaimed and unconsciously motivated symptoms can be ameliorated, but how much can be corrected and how much might have been prevented? Certainly we cannot imagine a human being without an unconscious and without persisting infantile impulses. However, this means only that the infantile, more particularly the *traumatic* infantile, if not too warped and pathological, can be outgrown *sufficiently* and to such degree that the mature attitudes *predominate*, and the remaining infantile impulses can be integrated with the mature drives and can be handled maturely.

For the child, with all its childish impulses, is not normally unduly hostile. It becomes so only under traumatic treatment and influences. "There are no problem children, only problem parents." Without these traumatic influences, the child matures normally, and the childish impulses which persist in later life form a source not of evil but of play, color, freshness and pleasure. The mature adult is in harmony with these persisting normal infantile impulses in himself, and they contribute, directly and in their sublimations, to his constructive activities as well as to his capacity for fun, zest and recreation. He *enjoys both* play and responsible activities and keeps them in proper balance.

The formulation of the major characteristics of maturity and the course of development in achieving these is of both practical and theoretical importance. In the field of psychotherapy, it tells something about at least one of the goals of psychodynamic therapy. One effect of such treatment is to reopen the individual's emotional development. This is a regular result of analytic treatment, whether employing the classic technique or psychoanalytically based causal therapy, and distinguishes it from palliative methods. Technically, knowing clearly the path and the goals of development, much time can be saved for the patient by indicating these to him. Typically, the patient sees only two or three choices, each of which is neurotic, that is, childish, and does not see the attitudes which lead out of the conflict and toward maturity and a workable and enjoyable adjustment (provided, of course, that the life situation is not so bad as to prevent this). For example, a patient may feel that he can only be dependent and feel inferior or else indulge his prestige-seeking narcissism, competitiveness and belligerency—yet as an adult he needs none of these attitudes but can enjoy exercising his powers in the direction of constructive interests in persons and pursuits. Merely to point out such a conflict does not necessarily result in its resolution or in any secure therapeutic result unless the patient is given some idea of what mature attitudes are. Without this, he may long rage because of his feelings of inferiority and his inability to achieve maturity, the nature of which he does not understand.

The qualities of maturity also indicate those attributes which are not only desirable but also necessary in psychotherapists and especially in analysts. There is no other field in which the personality of the therapist is so fundamental to his activity. The training analysis presumes that the patient cannot be properly freed from the unresolved trends and conflicts of his childhood and thereby helped toward the goal of full emotional development if the analyst himself has not solved these problems in himself. The analysis reopens the emotional development and the capacity to learn new attitudes through correcting the faults in upbringing and the traumatic emotional influences of childhood, not by insight alone, which is a necessary first step, but through the *deconditioning and the reconditioning effected by the transference and then by life*. (This view has received substantiation from experimental work with animals, an excellent brief statement of which is Liddell's *Emotional*

Hazards in Animals and Man, 1956.) The patient becomes highly suggestible toward the analyst, and not only takes over his tolerant attitudes but also tends to solve his own problems by imitating the analyst and identifying with him, for, to the patient, the analyst represents maturity. The transference repeats the childhood patterns toward the parents, including the tendency to do as they do rather than only as they say. Hence, if these powerful forces are to be truly in the direction of maturity, the analyst must understand the goal clearly and be well on the way himself. Only a few succeed in doing this.

The use of a formulation of maturity is not only for therapy but, above all, for *prevention.* In the negative sense we are helped to see what interferes with the normal course of development to maturity and the ubiquitous results of such interference in neurosis, crime and social problems. We see the misery which is caused in later life, even under the best external circumstances, by overprotection, deprivation, vanity, harshness, hostility and all the other forces to which children are subjected wittingly or unwittingly, which warp their development. Presumably, the unavoidable jealousies, rivalries and frustrations of childhood, involving siblings or parents, are soluble problems when these traumatic forces do not supervene to prevent their resolution. Any program of prevention must see clearly the course and the goal of the human emotional development in order to distinguish and combat all those forces which impair and warp it. These forces are the true causes of neurosis, crime and war.

A definition of maturity indicates what people would be like if they achieved full emotional development. As we have said, these characteristics represent an ideal. Nevertheless, this ideal is based upon sound clinical experience, for in every case we see what the patient would be if his development were fully released from the inhibiting and warping effects of traumatic childhood emotional influences. Therefore, it is not unduly optimistic to picture this ideal as the normal mental and emotional state of man. It is not normal in the sense that it is not average; but it was not average to be free of pockmarks in India, nor was it average for the upper class women of old China to have feet that were not deformed by binding. So the normal, *full,* emotional development may be rare in our culture or in the world, and yet this may be because we all have psychological pockmarks due to errors in upbringing.

PREVENTION OF HOSTILITY AND VIOLENCE

This leads inevitably to an unexpectedly optimistic conclusion, namely, that the crime, the wars, the abysmal selfishness and the cruelty which form the scene in human history are essentially *child-ish* qualities, the reactions of children to mistreatment during their early years. These should be outgrown normally and could be if children were reared properly from birth.

This provides a scientific basis for morality—it reveals the *evil* in man as the *persisting traumatic infantile,* the result of impaired emotional development, and it shows that the *true good* is not submissiveness to a code but rather an expression of the *strength of maturity.*

The goal of human brotherhood thus reflects man's striving not only for peace and the capacity to live together in societies but also for maturity—mankind's struggle to grow up.

The price of social peace is inner peace; and the only path to inner peace is the path to maturity.

Only if we see clearly the course and the goal of development are we in a position to find effective means of facilitating it. The task is enormously difficult but herein lies the only hope of preventing neurosis, crime and war. People in general, because of atrocious upbringing, have failed to reach full maturity. If, through proper prevention, this could be achieved on a wide scale, a new dawn would yet break for humanity.

If we now view the world scene in the light of the foregoing considerations, we see that *humanity is composed mostly of* partially neurotic or otherwise immature individuals, i.e., *persons dominated by disordered infantile patterns* of feeling, thinking and behavior; and the therapeutic problem is no different in its nature from that observed in private and clinical practice despite the colossal quantitative and practical differences. In history, as well as in the individual, we see man's attempts to grow up and to solve his problems in a mature fashion—and also the counterforce toward the maintenance and the gratification of infantile impulses and emotional patterns. It is a sinister fact that these are usually vented more frankly in groups, especially national groups, largely because of the sanction an the support given by the leader and the group and because of what the individual permits himself in the name of the group.

We treat reactive neuroses in the first place by removing the traumatic external pressures. On the world scene, this is the task of government and other leadership or governing agencies—to alleviate overpopulation, hunger, lack of shelter, insecurity, excessive demands and hardships, inadequate satisfaction and other threats and pressures to which people eventually react with desperate regression or hostile aggression.

Clinically, we try at the same time while treating the condition, whether it is reactive or not, to control the symptoms when this is indicated. In dealing with groups there is little difference. Government uses supportive measures, moral persuasion and educational efforts. If these are ineffectual, then just as guardianship or commitment may be necessary for individuals, so forceful policing may be unavoidable. This is the one fully legitimate and morally justified use of force—namely, to suppress selfish hostile aggression for the sake of the common good.

LONG-RANGE SOLUTION TO HOSTILITY

But the machinery of government, including a world government, which is of such urgency as to be a matter of life and death for most of the world, fulfills only a short-range program. It aims at the palliation and the suppression of symptoms but not at the treatment of their ultimate causes. There are always *two* factors—the life situation and the emotional make-up of the individual who reacts to it. There is crying need to relieve the terrible external hardships and dangers which engulf many and threaten more, and provoke desperation and violence. But, in the long run, this will not keep men from one another's blood so long as the internal irritants, the residues of childhood, the traumatic pathological childhood emotional patterns, torment them from within. This is the great central lesson not only of modern analytic psychiatry but also of all human history. This is the great central blazing fact of human life, reflected in religion, in literature, in all human history, missed by many recondite studies and consistently ignored, although glaringly obvious, in a way always known yet rarely comprehended. Yet if it is directly and goal-consciously faced, though vastly difficult, it is not unsolvable.

For unrest, cruelty and hostile aggression are by no means always reactive to current external hardships. They are even frankly extolled as pleasure and virtue, as by some primitive tribes, and by some political groups. Often the hardships are merely utilized as excuses to justify the hostility to which the members of the group are impelled by immature impulses. Hence, alleviating external pressures and exerting moral, educational or physical force are only palliative and must be quite ineffectual unless the population is sufficiently mature to respond to them. Otherwise the population will handle both its external problems and its inner urges in childish ways.

RESPONSIBILITY OF PSYCHIATRY

In clinical practice, the only secure and lasting therapeutic result in the treatment of any type of emotional or personality problem, reactive or internal, depends on reaching and correcting the *causes*. If only the external stresses are relieved but the infantile reactions remain, the patient, left to himself, will soon be in another predicament. Only if he matures emotionally can we expect a secure adjustment. If all the world's problems were magically solved, we can be sure that they would mushroom again so long as men are dominated by infantile motivations. Living and working conditions must be such that adults can function pleasurably—but conditions must also be such that children, now so ignorantly and cruelly mishandled, can develop normally and fully.

The problem is no different in essence when we deal with millions instead of single individuals. Obviously, the percentage of persons who can be treated causally is utterly insignificant—but the true goal of all medicine is not treatment but prevention. Obviously, faulty upbringing of children should be prevented and not left to attempts at correction when the children are grown. This defines the social responsibility and the task of psychiatry—to contribute to the long-range program of preventing emotional disorders by facilitating the emotional development of children, in order to assure a society of predominantly mature adults and the kind of society in which mature adults can function enjoyably. Only such a society can provide any secure basis for a life which is more than sweat, blood and tears.

Despite the immense practical difficulties, material improvement can be expected from the serious application of modern scientific knowledge. This includes all the social sciences, but the basic knowledge is that possessed by modern dynamic psychiatry, which deals explicitly, directly and goal-consciously with human motivations and their development. The task is, in part, short-range; but the greater task is long-range—to delineate clearly the characteristics of maturity, the paths of development toward it and the means of facilitating this development and of preventing obstacles to it. If the scientific basis is laid, if the goals are clear, the ways and the means eventually can be found.

The prevention of man-made misery is the prevention of emotional disorder. But is not this goal of preventive psychiatry the goal of church and state, the proper goal of management and labor, and of all men? The psychological atom, the disorders of the childhood emotional patterns, is the traumatic infantile core in human nature. To split it is to free at last man's potential constructive and cooperative energies. This is the "research magnificent."

REFERENCES

Allee, W. (1951): *Cooperation Between Animals*. New York: Abelard.

Freud, A. (1937): *Ego and Mechanisms of Defence*. London: Hogarth Press.

Freud, S. (1924): Heredity and the etiology of neuroses. *S.E.* 3.

Kardiner, A. (1939): *The Individual and His Society*. New York: Columbia University Press.

Laughlin, H. (1970): *The Ego and Its Defenses*. New York: Appleton-Century-Crofts.

Liddell, H. (1956): *Emotional Hazards in Animals and Man*. Springfield, Illinois: Thomas.

Marmor, J. (1968): *Modern Psychoanalysis*. New York: Basic Books.

Saul, L. J. (1945): Psychological factors in combat fatigue, with special reference to hostility and the nightmares, *Psychomatic Medicine* 7(5).

———— (1976): *Psychodynamics of Hostility*. New York: Jason Aronson.

———— (1979): *The Childhood Emotional Pattern in Marriage*. New York: Van Nostrand Reinhold.

PART TWO

Emotional Forces in the Development of Personality

2 | Independence and Dependence

GENERAL FORMULATION

In the previous chapter, eight emotional forces involved in the development to maturity have been surveyed. Now we devote a chapter to each individual force and the most common combinations.

1. From Conception to Independence

All life begins as a single cell, formed and passed on by the parent organisms. In man, and in the other higher forms, this egg-cell forms the new individual by dividing again and again, and during the whole process is utterly dependent on the maternal organism. (We are speaking of life as it is, and not of experimental laboratory conditions.) Certainly man and the other mammals are completely dependent on the mother during this fetal stage—for protection, warmth, nutrition, respiration, circulation, everything. In this view, the unborn child is indeed parasitic. Birth has been acclaimed the first great trauma, and the cry of the newborn is its protestation at being forced from the warm, dark, soft, fluid protection and nutriment of the womb, where every need is met, into the necessity for being an independent being, an individual, in a strange, new world. The newborn infant must now breathe for himself, and quickly. (Later in life, in situations of fear and other strong emotion, he will catch his breath and otherwise respond with altered respiration—sometimes even with asthma.) The aperture in the septum of his heart must close, and his heart must pump the blood through an altered course, independent of the mother's circulation. (Later in life, when in rage or fear, his heart action and blood pressure will again increase and alter.) His skin flushes (as it will later to strong emotion). He must now take in nourishment himself and excrete the wastes (and his eating and bowel action will always be sensitive to emotion). This great step toward independence from the mother is only partial. The whole first year is a period fraught with danger to the still delicate, highly dependent being. Although breathing for himself and taking food for himself, at first he must imbibe only a food prefabricated by the mother or by a substitute for her, namely, milk. His temperature-regulating mechanism is not yet functioning, so he must be kept warm. He requires constant care and protection. Gradually his wondrous physiological mechanisms take form. His sucking reflex is established. Soon his eyes will begin to coordinate—and his movements also. His teeth come in, and he can be weaned—another step toward independence. Soon the crawling mechanism makes possible independent locomotion. He begins to show curiosity—to be able to communicate, to toddle, to walk, to talk, to help himself in simple ways—to begin to comprehend something of the outside world, something beyond himself and his own immediate needs (Gesell, 1940; 1972).* His development leads him toward an increasing grasp of reality, an increasing curiosity and interest in the world outside himself, an increasing strength and capacity to make his way independently in this world. And to do this he must not only learn about his physical surroundings, and the relatively simple, fixed, dependable qualities of objects, gravity, heat and cold. He must also sustain the vicissitudes of training, and he learns something of the infinitely more complex and bewildering behavior and feelings of other persons. And in some way or other he must learn to handle the emotional influences to which he is exposed—love, sternness, jealousy, criticism, expectations and so many other forces—and the many

---

* Freud repeatedly pointed out that the child's long period of dependence on its parents is basic in the genesis of emotional problems and in shaping the whole life of the mind. He saw it as one source of need for belief in an all-wise, all-powerful God. (Freud, S., 1927.) He remarked its importance for the Oedipus complex, which term, incidentally, he sometimes used broadly to signify the child's interrelationships with the members of its family; but Freud never devoted a separate study to dependence. Hence, its fundamental significance has not been appreciated in the psychoanalytic literature. It has been forced into the libido theory as a subdivision of the oral phase. Here the tail wags the dog. Fairbairn deserves great credit for courageously proposing that the libido theory should be so revised as to rest upon this solid, broad observational base of the child's long dependence and its development from it. Dependence is becoming better recognized.

This recognition is now reflected in Parens, H., and Saul, L., *Dependence in Man,* New York, International Universities Press, 1971. This book summarizes the scattered psychoanalytic observations on this subject up to 1970.

emotional problems of his relations to the other members of his immediate family. He must learn to manage and domesticate his own animal impulses and emotional reactions.

In general, adults greatly underestimate the intellectual capacities of the child, its powers of observation and the depth of its feelings, while at the same time they overestimate its powers of emotional control. No doubt, this is in large part for the general reason that adults themselves are too much engrossed in their own problems and feelings to be good observers of others except in matters which concern themselves.

School is the great step toward independence from the family. Long before this the child is taking increasing responsibility for himself, learning to eat, take care of his eliminations, wash, dress, retire, and so on with less and less help. He even begins to do simple chores about the house—fetching articles, clearing the table and similar minor, but nevertheless real, contributions. The schoolage child shows an appreciable degree of independence. Still a child, dependent for physical and emotional support on his parents, or substitutes for them, in fact, dependent on them for his very existence, he has become capable of life in school apart from them, with all the problems that school entails. With school comes not only the new step of intellectual tasks to be performed alone and interests to be developed in new things, persons, ideas, events and amusements but also the partial actual separation from the family. Still sheltered at home, the child is much less protected in the average school, and while going and coming he is apt to be entirely on his own. He is partially forced out of the protected dependence on the parents. He must accomplish the work and satisfy the teachers; he must face the emotional interplay with other children away from home; and while coming and going, he must deal with situations without help or direct protection from either home or school. This emotional interplay will not be new to the child. He has already encountered it in intense form in his intimate family—the love, the rivalry, the rebellion, the self-assertion and all the undercurrents and crosscurrents which are inevitable in every family, as they are inevitable in any close human relationship. But at school the experiences are on a wider scale and are with strangers. For the child of a secure, reasonably harmonious family, school may be the first experience with the ways of the wide outside world and with its evils. Here he meets children of all types, friendly and hostile; here he finds comradeship but also fights, intrigues, gangs, violence, cruelty. And little help will he get from parents or teachers—for his pride itself tells him that he must face these problems alone, and even if he tells his troubles, what protection school or home can give is limited. He has partly grown out of the shelter of the family, and there is no help for it. He is on his way to the independence, the self-reliance and the consequent solitariness of the adult.

No longer can he scurry to mother like the baby monkey which, as can be seen at any zoo, at the first hint of alarm, clings to its mother's breast to be carried about by her.

Birth and the completion of infancy have enabled the child to develop beyond the close physical, parasitic dependence on the body of the mother. The school child is achieving the capacity to emerge from the family circle. Puberty is the next great biological push toward full growth and strength, which gives the maturing individual the equipment, and forces him with its urgency, to face alone the problems and collisions of life, fully out of the family and in the great world of reality. With adolescence come powerful sexual and ambitious urges, heightened competitiveness with adults and increased turning toward adult goals. The intensified process of development now drives the organism toward independence, self-reliance, marriage, reproduction and family. The energies which have gone into the growth of the still immature individual now become available for productivity, both social and sexual. The child, once dependent on his own parents, now becomes an independent being, i.e., an adult, interdependent with other adults, socially and sexually productive, standing alone, making his own way in the world with children dependent on him. After an adult life, lived in the fullness of his powers and accomplishments, man comes to the inevitable decline of age and then to the prospect of a second childhood, with strength diminishing until it becomes inadequate longer to maintain animate life, and the cycle of earthly existence is completed. Life has been likened to a cup * into which,

---

* Alexander, quoting Shaw's *Heartbreak House*. The reader who is not acquainted with the works of Franz Alexander will now find his major articles available as *The Scope of Psychoanalysis,* New York, Basic Books, 1961. These studies, like his books, are distinguished by a depth of insight combined with a down-to-earth practical grasp of psychic reality and human nature rare among psychoanalysts.

during childhood, one receives from others; in maturity it over-flows and can fill other vessels; in the declining years it dries up again. From such observations, Alexander (1942) has developed his principle of the surplus—the energies of growth overflow after puberty sexually into reproduction and socially into responsible, productive work.

2. Development and Regression

A. The Biological Base. Let us pause for a few comments on these facts of growth and development. In the first place, it appears that in essence development is biological. The period of pregnancy, the rate of growth, the phenomena of teething, puberty, sexuality, menopause, death—the whole cycle and the approximate time rela-tionships are internally determined for man, as for each of the animals. Probably the higher the functions—feeling, thought, idea-tion, speech and ways of dealing with the emotions—the more they are influenced by environmental and cultural factors. But however influenced, we deal with fundamental biological forces. Depen-dence, for example, may be variously handled in different cultures and times, but whether extolled or despised, indulged or reacted against, it is still a basic biological force. *For understanding human beings, all these forces, the biological, the intimate interpersonal, the cultural and the impersonal environmental are not mutually exclusive but interacting and complementary. The biological forces of growth and development are facilitated or hindered or warped by various physical and psychological experiences and in-fluences.*

B. Variability in Development. Let us note secondly that develop-ment proceeds irregularly. Our description has been greatly over-simplified. The developmental forces are not homogeneous. De-velopment consists of many elements, and the proportions between them and the vigor and the rate of maturation of each vary from individual to individual, to a large extent on what seems to be an almost purely hereditary basis. Thus, one child walks precociously at nine months but has no teeth at that age, while another child has teethed precociously at nine months but does not walk until nearly 20 months, even though there is no noticeable difference between the two children as to diet or general management. Similarly, one child's intellectual development outstrips his physical and emotional development, while in another child the reverse occurs. The development of the various psychological and emotional characteristics is also uneven, and many separate traits are easily distinguished. A child may be very dependent in some respects, very willful in others. The outcome of these various component forces depends on the congenital strength of each and on the emotional influences to which the child is subjected. Perhaps some individuals never reach intellectual or emotional maturity, no matter how favorable their upbringing. Perhaps others achieve it in high degree in spite of adverse influences. Parents usually encourage and facilitate, and sometimes overstimulate, development along certain lines, and hinder or distort it along others. This they often do unwittingly. To give the child the proper soil and atmosphere for his development, without interference but with adequate training and socialization, is no easy task. But if in reality the child is basically loved and secure in the parents' affection, and if he is allowed to develop without undue interference, and if he grows up with relatively well-balanced parents as models, then, barring specific disabilities or defects, normal development into an essentially stable, well-balanced adult can be assumed to be assured, in spite of numerous transient periods which at the time seem to be cause for concern. This is not the place to elaborate on these general remarks with examples. We must pass on to a third and most important point concerning the course of development—the problem of maturity.

C. Maturing and Regressing Forces. Since the normal course of development seems to lead so clearly to realistic, constructive, kindly, giving, life-preserving, parental attitudes, why do we not all achieve them naturally?

The answer seems to lie, at least in part, in the fact that growth and development do not take place unopposed but progress against a counter-current in the personality, a powerful tendency to maintain and to return to earlier attitudes, reactions and stages of development. A simple example of such retrograde or regressive tendencies, latent in the personality and aroused in certain circumstances, is easily observable in children. A three- or four-year-old is well trained and socialized, but along comes a new little brother or sister, with its infant behavior, its needs for training and its infantile demands upon the parents. The older child now shows a recurrence of its own infantile reactions, which presumably have been outgrown and overcome. It wants a bottle again, sometimes even a suck at the breast, it wets its pants and its bed and even sometimes soils; it frequently crawls again and repeatedly demands to be picked up and carried; it wants to be fed, and so on. These reactions are extremely common but are not always so simple, for the progressive, developmental parts of the child's make-up, its adulthood-looking vanity, its wishes to be grown up, are hurt by this infantile behavior and may cause reactions against it. When this occurs, one sees clearly the conflict between the progressive and the regressive forces and the importance of this interplay for the establishment of patterns of reaction and for the development of the personality. The absolute and relative strengths of both the progressive and regressive forces are powerfully affected by the early upbringing.

3. Some Salient Conclusions

A. The Balance of Responsibility and Recreation. The formulations we have made in this chapter thus far lead to some revealing conclusions. First, let us recall that a cardinal feature of childhood is freedom from adult responsibilities and having the necessaries of life provided. The child has many demands and activities. It can play with the greatest energy, but it is in reality dependent. But even the strongest, most stable adult can tolerate only a certain amount of responsible, productive effort. "All work and no play make Jack a dull boy." The perfectly normal adult finds his relief from the requirements, the burdens and the strains of life in ordinary forms of recreation, amusement and relaxation. He forgets his responsibilities and cares and plays again, as in childhood. The play now takes an adult, often a highly sophisticated, form, but its essential quality, freedom from independent responsibility, remains. Mark Twain said: "Work is what you have to do." Baseball is recreation and play to the fans, but a profession to the players, whose livelihoods depend on their contributions to their teams. Fortunate the man who retains or achieves in his serious, breadwinning work a feeling of the joy of play as well as the adult satisfaction in productive accomplishment.

B. Quantitative—a Matter of Degree. In the emotions, all is quantitative. The fundamental importance of this fact for the understanding of mental phenomena can hardly be exaggerated. The cinema, for example, is to the relatively normal person a harmless, if not always edifying, form of entertainment which admirably satisfies his passive, dependent needs. Seated comfortably in darkness and warmth, lulled by music, secure for a few hours from the harsh world outside, he moves in fantasy among the demigods on the screen, enjoying, without moving a muscle, delights of the mind and of the flesh. But this form of enjoyment, which the normal person uses sparingly as relaxation and escape from the demands of real life, can be used as too much of an escape. Excessive attendance at the movies, like prolonged absorption in television, can even signify an early symptom of schizophrenia—a condition which is marked by deep regression from occupation with real life to excessive preoccupation with fantasy.

It is correct to call normal recreation "regressive" and not only when it is obviously excessive and overly escapist. It maintains an essential and well-established unity to do so. For the interplay between the responsible, productive, independent (RPI), adult trends and the regressive needs for relief from them (passive, receptive, dependent PRD) is present in everyone and is important in the configuration of every personality. Therefore, it is simpler and more nearly correct to consider that some tendency to regression is in everyone, and that, in certain degrees, and satisfied in certain ways, it is within normal limits. Beyond these it becomes a problem, not because it has changed its character of being regressive, but because of its form or its intensity. Watching television, seeing movies and reading books are normal relaxations—but doing nothing else, and for no purpose, can be pathological. Occasional drinking is a common form of relaxation—too much is alcoholism. As we shall see, neuroses and even psychoses can arise from regressive tendencies which are too strong. It was one of Freud's most important discoveries that the often peculiar and even apparently senseless behavior in neurosis and psychosis becomes intelligible in terms of the reactions of the child to a certain situation. Perhaps the most important of Alexander's contributions has been his expansion and clarification of these observations, particularly in relation to infantile passive dependence versus mature independence and productivity.

C. Persistence of Childhood Desires. The concept of regression includes the persistence of, or return to, earlier reactions of all kinds. Even in the relatively normal person, relief from the efforts and the responsibilities of productive adult activities does not consist only in the negative satisfaction of escape or in the fun of play. One of the most important characteristics of the life of the child is his emotional dependence on the members of his family and the satisfaction that he gets from being cared for. Like all attitudes which have brought pleasure, this one persists in some degree, however unobtrusive and unnoticed. Hence, even the essentially normal person, no matter how independent, strong and self-reliant, besides the escape and fun of recreation, derives positive satisfaction from the emotional support which he receives, often unconsciously, from parental family, friends, business associations, spouse and even children.

Although the adult requires much less interest, attention, esteem, approval (that is, emotional support, or, in the broad sense of the term, love) than the child, yet no adult fully outgrows these needs. Again, it is a matter of degree, a shift in the balance of the emotional metabolism. As the adult matures, he requires less and can give more than the child, but he will never be completely giving and will never derive all his satisfaction from this role. The well-balanced life includes a workable balance of satisfactions, the enjoyment of adult activities and also, within normal limits, of the persisting childhood ones. To receive love and emotional support remains a deep need and a deep gratification. When these desires are too strong, they lead to feelings of insecurity and frustration and to all forms of neurotic symptoms. Even hardened criminals are found to be little children underneath, trying neurotically to escape from feeling rejected and unloved, or taking a misplaced revenge for lack of love in their childhood. The loose but convenient phrase "passive-receptive-dependent" has come into use to describe all these needs for love, care and support required by the child.

D. Regressive Needs. Man can stand only so much of reality at a time. An obviously normal escape which can be interpreted psychologically and biologically as regression is sleep. Numerous authors have remarked on its similarity to fetal life; many sleepers even assume the position of the child in the womb. After birth, the newborn sleep almost constantly, and only gradually does this need diminish.

Another feature of sleep bears the stamp of childhood—the dream. Freud showed how the dream was formed and related it to the whole gamut of normal and abnormal psychological phenomena. The essence of his discovery is that the major emotions which form the dream are traceable to childhood, that "the child with all its impulses survives in the dream." Whatever adult reactions are aroused in a person by the events and the pressures of the day, there are also aroused those of his feelings which persist from childhood and were never fully outgrown, although they may be pushed aside and given little attention. These childhood feelings, hard for the adult to accept or admit even to himself, find expression in the dreams, along with every other impulse that seeks satisfaction and threatens sleep. (Of course, these statements do not imply that the more mature the person the less sleep and the fewer dreams, since many factors determine smooth functioning in these respects.)

As an example, a successful, energetic, hard-working businessman who feels tense and suffers from headaches and stomach trouble dreams repeatedly that he is a little boy at home, being taken care of by his mother. Then something interrupts this scene, and he must run or climb or do something of the sort. It turns out that this man had a hard childhood. For a period he was indulged and protected by his mother, and it is of this period that he dreams. He was soon forced to sell newspapers and earn money for the family, and his father shamed him out of his dependence on his mother. Since then he has been deeply ashamed of any dependence and has always made a great point of his independence and self-reliance. Others are dependent on *him*—he shows no such weakness. But he is tense, nervous, unhappy, even a little depressed, and he has his headaches and his stomach trouble. It soon appears that his adult, giving, independent, productive accomplishments do not all stem from the strength and maturity of his development. In large part, he feels forced to them by shame for being otherwise. And although his pride at first will not let him admit it, underneath part of him craves to be otherwise, to relinquish the burden of independence, effort and responsibility and to be again, what he was all too briefly in his childhood, the one who is dependent and cared for. He is driven by his conditioning to live beyond his emotional means, driven to do more than he can normally enjoy or tolerate, and because of this his wish to escape the strain and the burden and to regress to the happier time of childhood is proportionately intensified. But he cannot escape, and this wish, unsatisfied in life, causes his feelings of unhappiness, his headaches and his stomach trouble—and it also forms his dreams. The dream shows both sides of the conflict—the desire for the dependent situation and the inability to accept it—he must leave his mother and strive and climb. The dream is the patient's creation. The frustration in it must arise from the patient himself, as we know it does.

4. Recapitulation

Our discussion of development and regression has now led us to an understanding of the fundamentals of normal and abnormal emotional psychology. Let us review these. We have seen that no one matures completely, no one fully outgrows the many long years of dependence on the parents, so much longer for man than for any other animal. Childhood cravings, reactions, attitudes and patterns persist in everyone, and there is always a tendency to return to them. Scratch the adult and one finds the child. The more mature the adult, the stronger, the more stable, the more resistant is he. The more the child persists, the greater the tendency toward childhood reactions and behavior.

These childish reactions and the tendencies to return to them are usually pushed aside, disregarded and rejected (repressed) by the adult, for they conflict with his trends to maturity, his training and standards and his pride and vanity. He cannot admit his childish reactions fully even to himself. They thus form an unconscious part of his mind. And in childhood they were "put out of mind" or "forgotten" as a way of controlling and shunning them. Some of them are more or less conscious, although their force and significance may not be realized, while others are truly unconscious, particularly certain mental mechanisms, such as the steps by which the depression or the stomach trouble developed in the example given. They are nonetheless alive and powerful in motivation and feeling. In fact, they are like steam under pressure—the more repressed the more powerful. They cause inner emotional tension, and this causes disturbances of thought, feelings, behavior and physiology, that is, neurotic symptoms. These same tensions also come to expression in the dreams. If they are too intense and are not relieved by the dream, the sleep is disturbed and the person may waken. We thus find in the childhood tendencies, in their relationship to the developmental forces and processes, a key to unconscious motivation, to dreams, to normal functioning and to neurotic symptoms.

ILLUSTRATIONS WITH SOME DYNAMIC CONNECTIONS

Finally, then, we come to the sources of these observations, formulations and conclusions—human life and the operation of the human mind, be it in sleep or waking, in its highest or its most primitive functions, in action or in fantasy.

The plan of each chapter of this section is to present at the outset a general description of the emotional forces therein discussed and then to follow this statement with a variety of illustrations. These illustrations are meant to show the operation of the forces in many areas of life and also to bring out by way of example a few of their significant psychodynamic connections. The examples are selected to illustrate not only the particular motivations but also some of their connections with other forces in the mind. Being fundamental, the forces discussed in these eight chapters can be observed in animals and in children as well as in adults, in neuroses and psychoses, in human productions such as art and literature, and throughout the social scene.

1. Literature

The conflict between forces of development toward independence and responsibility and those tending in the opposite direction has been represented by Shakespeare in *Henry IV*. This is discussed in a short and interesting paper by Alexander, "A Note on Falstaff" (1961). As the king lies dying, Prince Hal cannot resist trying on the crown just to feel how it fits. But as he does so, he realizes that its assumption involves far more than personal satisfaction and prestige. It means assuming with it an interest in the realm and the heavy responsibilities entailed therein, which he alone and independently must bear. It means relinquishing the irresponsible playtime he has had with Falstaff and their cronies, the epitomes of carefree self-indulgence. Prince Hal decides to assume his father's responsibilities, but he banishes Falstaff, for he knows him to be a temptation and so must put him far away. Thus he seeks to "repress" these desires in himself which would tempt him away from the adult, "father" position of responsibility and would struggle to drag him back to the "son" position of carefree play.

2. Institutionalized Persons

This type of conflict is seen repeatedly in patients; indeed, to some extent it probably takes place in everyone. Clinical material lends itself to arrangement on a scale, grading from persons who are so passive, receptive and dependent that they never really got started in adult life, through those who manage their lives successfully by repressing their regressive tendencies, which then cause symptoms, to those persons who have achieved a relatively normal, workable balance. The best example of the first group, the ones who have never really gotten started as adults, is the classic "simple schizophrenic." This term designates a subgroup of schizophrenia characterized by extreme passivity and emotional shallowness. The depth of the regression is considered to be a feature of all schizophrenia. Such persons may be seen at state hospitals. I once wanted to talk to one, who was lying quietly on the floor. He finally answered, bored and logical, without stirring, "I leave you alone, why don't you leave me alone?" This is what he wanted—to lie on the floor, totally effortless, totally uninterested in anything outside himself and his thoughts, fed and housed by others, totally dependent, and all this with very little even in the way of face-saving. Other patients often try to excuse their extreme passivity and helplessness and their wish to be cared for in the hospital by insisting that they have an incapacitating illness or that they are forced by others to stay in the hospital against their own wishes or for some other rationalization.

Another example is an adolescent girl who, on one pretext or another, finally managed to spend all her time in bed, where she got her mother to care for her like an infant—feed her, bathe her and so on.

Consciously or unconsciously, very many patients love the hospital because, whatever its disadvantages, it reestablishes a childhood situation of interest, care and dependence and is a haven of escape from the burdens of our complex life, which demands so much energy, initiative, independence, responsibility and social productivity. Once, incidental to a research study, the reactions of about 50 state hospital patients to the proposal that they leave the hospital were elicited. A very large percentage resisted this strongly, and some became panicky at the prospect. Among these were patients who previously had claimed that they were kept there against their wills. Of course, there were other reasons too, but this wish for passive, receptive, dependent care was a central one for their finding all sorts of reasons why they should not be discharged from the protected hospital environment into all the struggles of independent life in the outside world.

This reaction is observable in general hospitals also, in different forms. Not infrequently one sees a person who kept going in life only with difficulty until the occurrence of some organic illness, either purely fortuitously or in some part brought on by himself unconsciously. This illness and the consequent helplessness and nursing care then stimulate the tendency to relinquish the struggle of life and regress, to such an extent that it is extremely difficult for the patient to recover and return to his former position in life.

In the Middle Ages, a variety of crude treatments for mental patients were sometimes employed. Patients were flogged, spun on stools until they bled or dropped by trap doors into icy streams (Saul et al., 1956; Alexander and Selesnick, 1966). Good results have been reported with patients who have spent years in institutions and have relapsed into almost complete passivity by simply ordering them in no uncertain tones to simple activities ("total push") (Saul, 1972). Possibly, in these treatments, whether the old, crude, physical ones or the modern psychological ones, effects resulted in some part from spanking, pushing or luring (Rosen,

1968) the patient out of his passivity, dependence and preoccupation with his own fantasies and problems and forcing him back to increased contact with reality. Possibly this is one factor, among others, in modern shock treatment. Certainly, long before modern psychiatry learned that much of the behavior of mental patients is intelligible when viewed as a fight against regression to the reactions of children and infants, many psychiatrists reacted unconsciously to these patients as though they were naughty, preoccupied children who could be helped in their own efforts to get well by a good spanking. This, the feeling was, should bring them to their senses, that is, help them face reality.

It is interesting and important that one of the disadvantages of hospitalization, in spite of the food, shelter, care, interest and companionship it provides, is that it demands the relinquishment of sexual relationships. This is quite like the childhood situation—all is provided so long as sexuality is not evinced or indulged. The sexual urge is generally but not always toward freedom, initiative and development and counter to the regressive tendencies to be childishly dependent. In some, it even expresses the latter.

If, at first glance, it seems surprising that many patients in mental hospitals are in part attracted to this existence, then it may seem even more surprising that many convicts, in parts of their personalities, should be attracted to jails. Yet this is what has been found (Alexander and Healy, 1935; Alexander and Saul, 1937). To many criminals, despite their protests, jail is a refuge. Some actually had unconsciously behaved in such a way as to get themselves apprehended so that they might return to it. Of course, as always, other motives than passive dependence enter, for example, guilt and its relief by punishment. But here we are focusing on the one aspect—dependence. The jail satisfies the regressive tendencies, while at the same time saving face, in a certain respect, since a jail sentence is commonly regarded as a mark of toughness, despite the social stigma. In many cases, the attraction to the jail is quite conscious, and it is well known that some of the older men in particular are apt to do whatever they can to extend their stay. One young man contested his parole before Christmas—he wanted to have his Christmas dinner in jail, where his attachments had formed.

Two points emerge from these remarks which require special

emphasis—overdetermination and the heterogeneity of the personality. No personality is homogeneous and perfectly integrated. On the contrary, it is composed of many conflicting forces (e.g., love, hate, pride, modesty, ambition, guilt, and so on). Therefore, we must speak, as we have, of a person partly objecting strenuously to incarceration, while at the same time another part of his personality accepts and even desires it. An appreciation of, and watchfulness for, such countercurrents are indispensable to an understanding of the mental and emotional life. Equally indispensable is a realization that probably every psychic act represents a "final common path," to use a neurological expression. This means that a mixture of (many) impulses pulling in all directions, some reenforcing one another, others conflicting, all strive for expression and eventuate in the particular feeling, thought or act as a "final common path." This is but natural, for all the impulses which motivate us strive for expression and satisfaction, and very many of them, possibly all, must enter into our every feeling, thought and act, now some predominating, now others. At any rate, we must guard against accepting any single motive as an explanation, for usually there are several. This multiplicity of motivations of a single psychic act is called "overdetermination."

3. Neurotic Reactions

The two simple schizophrenic patients mentioned above are examples of individuals who never really got started in adult life. Examples of those who start, but very inadequately, are not difficult to seek. It is not unusual to see candidates for university degrees develop anxieties shortly before coming up for their examinations or shortly after receiving their degrees. One important factor in these cases, sometimes the central one, is often the inner fear and protest aroused by the prospect of stepping out from the sequestered academic walls, leaving the alma mater, the foster mother, to face the dangers and the responsibilities of life as an independent adult. And in organizations of all kinds, business or professional, men sometimes develop symptoms or even breakdowns when they are promoted and must carry new and increased responsibilities. (Another motive in this type of case is often the "wrecked by success" reaction of guilt.)

Extreme cases often reveal these mental mechanisms most clearly. A young man, A. C., some months before his examinations, became anxious and so neglectful of his work that he decided to postpone taking them. He then managed to postpone them repeatedly in spite of his adequate intelligence and ample time for preparation. He was the son of an overprotective and indulgent mother. He had married, but now his wife was working to support them both until he got his degree. He became relatively stabilized in this adjustment of neglecting his work, postponing his examinations and living on his allowance and on his wife's earnings. As always, there were other motivations, but a central one was his deep emotional dependence, which impaired his ability to make his way on his own. He repeatedly dreamed of being away from all responsibilities, off in the country alone with his mother, who supported and took care of him. Because of his overdependence on his mother, his father had had little respect for him even as a child. He, in turn, felt his father's disapprobation and reacted with resentment and further withdrawal to the mother. A common vicious circle was thus established. The whole situation was not helped by the fact that the father was a rather cold person, immersed in his own interests, without much energy or warmth for his family, which he left entirely to his wife. This, in turn, was one reason why she turned to the patient in an overclose relationship, to compensate her for those emotional desires which her husband did not satisfy adequately. The patient reacted to the father's disapproval in a regressive fashion. Instead of feeling spurred to win the father's esteem by independence and accomplishment, he felt that his father did not respect him and never would, so what was the use of trying and struggling, why not accept what his mother, and now his wife, gave him? Of course, this was by no means all a conscious process. He sensed it vaguely but did not realize its power in arresting his emotional development to mature attitudes and in undermining his marital and professional life. These reactions operated automatically within him, ruining his life as he struggled to salvage it. He sensed that forces within himself were the source of his problems. He even sensed their nature and origin but could not grasp their real portent or their processes of operation. He felt that he was wrestling in the dark and came for help to bring these forces and problems into the light. This is characteristic of the "unconscious." Like an iceberg, five-sixths of which is submerged, one can see some of one's own motivations, reactions and emotional processes fully, clearly and consciously; and one may look further and sense the deeper contours; but the core, the intermediate process and the details that make each personality what it is, these can rarely if ever be grasped by introspection alone. There is much that is unknown in us all. The study of just what these forces are and how they operate is the new science of *psychodynamics, the basic emotional psychology.* The diagnostic label (e.g., phobia, compulsion, paranoia) is only descriptive of a symptom, secondary to understanding what is going on in the patient. This understanding is always paramount for diagnosis, prognosis and treatment, and it will often be found that some people with psychotic symptoms respond better to treatment than do some with only neurotic symptoms, depending on the balance of forces.

Another young man, P. D., presented a similar problem, but in him the developmental forces were much stronger. The balance between these and regression to dependence was nearer to normal. He was much higher on our scale and needed only a little insight and help to be able to get on well. He, too, had become the perennial student. Greatly overprotected by his mother during his childhood, he nevertheless succeeded, against her opposition, in marrying the girl of his choice. However, he soon managed to repeat this relationship with his wife. He had decided to return to school, and now in his thirties he was still working for a degree, while his wife went to work to support him. Just as his mother had done, she would get him up for school in the morning, prepare his breakfast and then go to work herself. Evenings she would prepare dinner, and he would help her with the dishes and housecleaning, just as he had helped his mother. But he felt that something was wrong. This was one of those cases in which the dependence impaired the sexuality. He came for treatment, and as soon as he began to understand his dependence and to realize what he was doing, he reacted against it. Thereby his development was reopened and could continue. He rapidly got his degree and then a good position and was soon supporting his wife; his sexual life with her also improved. He might still have problems, but his development was reopened. Henceforth, he was on the way *out,* toward the adult adjustment that he wanted, and not on the way *in,* toward a deepening dependence and conflict—a neurosis (i.e., a childhood emotional pattern) which he could not understand. He finally got started in life, but only with help and with some difficulty.

Next on the scale one sees young men who get started and manage to get on, but weakly. One such young man was an only child whose parents wanted him to enter the father's business. But he fought his dependence on his parents, went through engineering school and obtained a position in this field. Although personable and capable, after some years while the other young men in his office advanced, he dragged along in the lowest position in the firm at the same salary he had started with. Although nearing 30, he had not really completed his adolescence psychologically. He had not fully accepted an independent career. He struggled constantly with the problem of giving up engineering and going into his father's business as his parents wished. Every weekend he made the trip home. He was not quite free of his dependence on his parents— emotionally or financially. His allowance still nearly equaled his salary. The same conflict was evident in the sexual sphere. Just as his dependence on his parents impaired the free giving of his interest and efforts to his professional work, so it interfered with his free, independent, responsible sexual mating interest in a girl. He held his position but wavered over the temptation to return home and enter his father's business. And in the same pattern, he became engaged to a girl but could not quite make up his mind to marry her. Moreover, typically for such an emotional conflict, he felt that he was not fully potent. He lacked confidence in the sphere of sex as well as in the professional sphere. As he gradually progressed through analytic help from a first intellectual insight to a real emotional appreciation of his problem, he began to do well, although for a while it was a considerable struggle. But here, too, the balance of emotional forces was favorable for a resumption of his development as he came to realize the nature of the forces which were holding him back.

Psychological processes are so complex and so individual, and writers in this field are so readily misunderstood, that another brief digression is necessary. Misunderstandings often arise from regarding as generalizations what were never so intended. For example, to the patient we have just considered, entering the father's business meant chiefly (and even then not entirely) yielding to tendencies to avoid an independent life. But in other cases it might have the opposite meaning. One sees young men who fear to enter the world of business and for whom a profession is the opposite of an assertion of independence; for these men a profession represents an escape from the more hurly-burly world of business and from a pursuit in which the individual feels himself to be inadequate and unable to hold his own. In still other cases, the problem revolves around competition with the father, or submission to him, and so on. Hence, the fact that choosing a profession instead of entering his father's business meant an effort toward independence on the part of the patient just discussed does not imply that such a choice has the same meaning in other cases. The situation may even be precisely the reverse.

A young man who had been overprotected by his parents lost the private income which he had inherited from them. He only partly regretted this. Within him he felt a certain exhilaration, for now he felt that he would be forced by necessity to make his own way and by so doing would achieve the independence, strength, maturity and fellowship with other men which he had always lacked, and which caused painful feelings of inferiority. As things turned out, he went through a terrible struggle trying to make his way in this hard, hostile, selfish world after knowing only softness and protection. That is why he came for help, but with it he achieved a reasonable degree of maturity and inner harmony. His financial misfortune turned out to be the salvation of his soul.

Another young man reacted to every forward step in his career with anxiety. He had anxiety attacks when he was graduated from college, when he was graduated from law school, when he left his clerkship and also when he married. He was an overprotected only child. Through childhood he had led a sheltered and comfortable existence. He assumed that everyone would treat him as his fond parents did, and this assumption was not without some justification, for, as is so often the case with loved children, his personality, accustomed to receiving affection and to responding with affection, stimulated others to like him. He knew unconsciously and automatically how to win the love and the acceptance which he felt to be his right, which his nature demanded in such purity and abundance. He, too, sensed that something was wrong, although he had no idea what it was. He occasionally suffered a relative impotence. He felt some difference between other, more mature persons and himself, although he could not define it. He especially could not comprehend what their attitudes were which enabled them to do their jobs on their own. It soon became clear that the patient's central longing was to remain ensconced as the favorite child in the bosom of his family. Every new responsibility and obligation raised in him his lack of self-confidence, his fear of standing alone and a great protest and resentment against so doing—a protest so angry that he developed anxiety. He became enraged at leaving the easier, more dependent situation and at being pushed further and further out of the position of dependent favored child into the requirements of adult life. For his personality operated automatically to win love and support and not to discharge responsibilities. And because of his passive, dependent orientation, he felt insecure at every step away from the protection of his home. The progress of his career, marriage and sexual life represented such advances. Because of his ambition, he was eager for big cases in his law practice. Yet when they came, at first he would be thrilled, then immediately angry and anxious and strongly resistant against accepting them. And with each case he would want to call in help in order to be relieved of carrying the responsibility alone, although at the same time his pride rebelled against doing so.

Anxiety is felt whenever one is threatened in any way, by external dangers or by one's own impulses. When he felt pushed out and forced into responsibilities, this not only frightened him, because he was not oriented to them emotionally, but it also enraged him, just as it would a child. Rage which is repressed is one of the commonest causes of acute neurotic anxiety. The relationship of hostility and fear is very close. Let us recall that the physiological mobilization of the body, in man and animals, is the same whether for fight or flight, aggression or fear (Cannon, 1929). And in practical psychiatric work, in cases of acute neurotic anxiety, one must always look for a possible part played by repressed, angry, hostile feelings.

We have thus far discussed problems of transition from the childhood to the adult orientation toward life. We have come up the scale (see Fig. 1) from persons who have been too infantile to get along outside an institution to those who have managed to get started in life but only with help and after considerable difficulty. Other persons get on well in an adult role until some special difficulties or temptations throw them back to the childhood attitudes. This is "regression" in the true technical sense of the term. Hitherto they may have seemed quite mature and stable, but now the other side of their natures, the tendency to be passive, dependent little children, so long hidden, repressed, latent, comes out and shows its power, often by disrupting their lives and sometimes even their entire personality organization, so that they become incapacitated and develop severe mental symptoms.

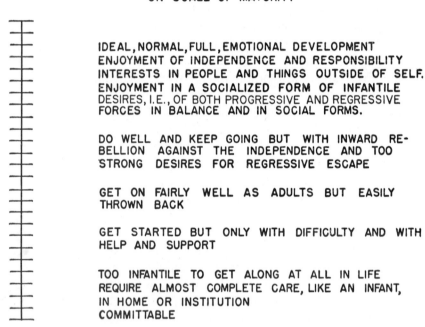

INDEPENDENCE - DEPENDENCE

ON SCALE OF MATURITY

IDEAL, NORMAL, FULL, EMOTIONAL DEVELOPMENT
ENJOYMENT OF INDEPENDENCE AND RESPONSIBILITY
INTERESTS IN PEOPLE AND THINGS OUTSIDE OF SELF.
ENJOYMENT IN A SOCIALIZED FORM OF INFANTILE
DESIRES, I.E., OF BOTH PROGRESSIVE AND REGRESSIVE
FORCES IN BALANCE AND IN SOCIAL FORMS.

DO WELL AND KEEP GOING BUT WITH INWARD RE-
BELLION AGAINST THE INDEPENDENCE AND TOO
STRONG DESIRES FOR REGRESSIVE ESCAPE

GET ON FAIRLY WELL AS ADULTS BUT EASILY
THROWN BACK

GET STARTED BUT ONLY WITH DIFFICULTY AND WITH
HELP AND SUPPORT

TOO INFANTILE TO GET ALONG AT ALL IN LIFE
REQUIRE ALMOST COMPLETE CARE, LIKE AN INFANT,
IN HOME OR INSTITUTION
COMMITTABLE

Figure 1

How temptation can cause such regression is illustrated by a man who rose to prominence in a large business concern. For years he was respected in his community and was apparently well adjusted in his work, his marriage and his social life. Only a slight tendency to drink a little more than he should gave any indication that all was not so perfect beneath as it appeared on the surface. Then, unexpectedly, his wife came into a considerable inheritance. Thereupon, the man felt that he could use some of his wife's money to improve his business connections through joining clubs, traveling and the like. At first this seemed entirely realistic and legitimate, but it soon became apparent that these steps, and other similar ones, had quite the opposite effect. They were pleasant, time-consuming diversions and excuses for *not* working. They were not additional business efforts—they were flights. He unconsciously and with ample rationalizations so handled his affairs that he lost his excellent position, his business connections became little more than a fiction, and he was no longer supporting himself or his wife but was living on her money. She wanted a husband and not just another son, so serious marital trouble arose. To escape his problems he took to drinking a little too much—and alcoholism is an excellent method, both directly and indirectly, of achieving (in destructive fashion) escape, passivity, irresponsibility and dependence. His wife's apparent good fortune in coming into the money disrupted the marriage and undermined his self-confidence and his security rather than increasing it, as it would have if he had reacted with the mature rather than the childish parts of his personality.

Another step up the scale are those who remain self-reliant and maintain a strong adult life but inwardly rebel, sometimes violently, against the lack of satisfaction they feel and the demands made upon them. Often they do not consciously realize their problem but develop symptoms. They may feel the strain, they may be tense, worried and anxious, their hair may turn gray, often they develop stomach trouble, even ulcers, or different psychosomatic or other disorders; still, despite the price, they do not give up the struggle but maintain their adult level of orientation and functioning. A man with high blood pressure held his adult position and carried his responsibilities, but only at the cost of great suffering, and it seemed that his elevated blood pressure was part of the price. Already in his poverty-stricken childhood he had been forced prematurely into responsibilities and breadwinning efforts and he yearned underneath for the indulgence, the rest and the play which he never had had. But this temptation to throw up the whole effort meant, of course, a threat to his business and his financial and social position, as well as to his mental health. And so he fought bitterly, automatically and unconsciously against this vaguely apprehended danger.

This fight against a tendency to give up adult orientation and regress to the passivity, the receptivity and the dependence of the child can cause all kinds of symptoms. The temptation is a threat. And the organism reacts to any threat with arousal for fight or flight. What this usually amounts to psychologically, at least in part, is an inner rage, which is a reaction to and also a defense against the temptation to regress, which in these cases is threatening the life adjustment and the whole personality organization. In the cases lower on our scale, the position of the young child is accepted with but little conflict, but in these more mature personalities it is intolerable and causes intense struggle. Unfortunately, this rage and the aggressiveness thus aroused can cause all kinds of psychological and physiological disturbances and symptoms. If this rage is "projected," that is, felt as being in others and directed toward the patient, true paranoia may develop. We have already noted that even criminality can arise on this basis. In such cases, the symptoms, even psychotic symptoms, like paranoia, signify a fight against the deeper threat of regression, an effort to keep going, an attempt at cure. A less mature personality would give in, sink to a low level, where the individual might reach some sort of adjustment and so spare himself such a psychosis. The paranoid would be the superior person from the point of view of development. This is an important point when one thinks of neurosis, psychosis and adjustment. The balance between development and regression is the key to many problems and a touchstone for human values.

Not long ago I was introduced to a softish, well-dressed man of about 50, who began to speak of his present illness, which consisted of headache, weakness and weeping. Exhaustive studies had revealed no organic cause. At first, he only recounted the details of his symptoms, but then, with considerable emotion, he said: "And it came on suddenly just when I was going to support my wife. All these years she has worked too, and a wonderful worker she is, strong, beautiful and never gets tired, but now I thought she should stop and I would support her. And just then this happens so I cannot, and she must continue working and help support me." Anyone who knows the reality and the power of these forces, anyone who has digested the central idea of this chapter, will certainly raise the query whether this was mere coincidence or whether this man's anticipated emotional shift to full support of his wife did not have something to do with precipitating his symptoms.

We have used men for our examples because of the clarity of this developmental-regressive conflict in these cases. But this conflict is, of course, not confined to men. In women it is sometimes less clear because in our culture, the dependent tendencies may be part of the feminine attitudes and interwoven with them, or, at any rate, not in such sharp contrast with them as they usually are with our masculine ideals of self-reliance and independence. For cultural and economic reasons, if not for biological reasons also, we accept the man as the supporter and the defender of his wife and children. Rather than give further examples of cases of women suffering from this conflict, which we have already illustrated extensively, it will suffice to mention that it is often the central motivation of the "back to mother" reaction which occurs when the wife is confronted with the problems, the demands and the responsibilities of marriage and finds that her husband, home and children are a full-time job, and that her husband is only a husband and not an adequate substitute for her parents. This dependence is central in "momism," so called. Of course it is also seen in working wives and single women, increasingly as more and more women, married and single, join the work force.

All individuals have dependent, regressive tendencies in some degree, but, of course, they vary in different persons in strength, importance, the extent to which they are indulged or repressed, and the balance they reach with the forces of development and maturity. Hence, they cause conflict and symptoms only in certain cases, such as those we have been reviewing. In the relatively normal individual they are adequately satisfied by the personal emotional relationships and by all sorts of recreation, and they are not sufficiently an issue to impair the enjoyment of the responsibilities, the efforts and the demands which are imposed by life—these being felt as a challenge and a source of enjoyable activity. But when any person encounters difficulties in life, whether only the ordinary demands and responsibilities or special pressures or harrowing blows of fate, there is a tendency to seek help, to give up the struggle, to "regress" to the role of the child who runs to his parents with his troubles. The extent to which an individual stands his ground in the face of trials depends not only on the intensity of the stress and its specific nature in relation to the man's vulnerable emotional spots, but also, in large part, on the relative strength of the forces of development and of regression within him. As World War II showed us, and Korea and Vietnam confirmed, under sufficient stress, and stress which strikes a vulnerable emotional spot, even the strongest man breaks, loses his adult functioning and partially regresses.

All regression is partial; even in the most extreme psychoses some little fragment of the personality usually holds to reality and to adult understanding. The personality is a complex, dynamic, nonhomogeneous organization and mixture of impulses of all sorts. It does not develop evenly, and conversely it does not regress fully or evenly to the reactions of earlier states.

SOCIOLOGICAL IMPLICATIONS

It seems correct to state that, in general, overly passive-receptive-dependent persons are at a disadvantage in life, although there are situations to which they may be able to adapt better than more mature persons. Often they do not know what an interested, responsible adult is and strive for maturity without comprehending its nature, which, indeed, they are not taught in school, important though it is for their lives.

Persons who are very dependent have been referred to as "passive characters," and this has come to be a useful auxiliary diagnostic term. Sociologically, they have difficulties in adjusting to a highly competitive, individualistic position in society. Many get on reasonably well so long as life provides them with a rather protected niche, and they fit well into certain jobs, but they also contribute considerably to the army of unemployables. If we can judge from experience in the clinics and in military selection, their number must be very large. If so, it should be recognized that this segment of the population cannot be expected to adjust unless these individuals are provided with a relatively simple, sheltered existence.

There is a type of person who is represented in cartoons as a penniless but happy tramp. The idea is that such a person does not try to hide his passive receptivity with shame but extols it as a way of life. Perhaps there is some sociological justification for this. It has been pointed out that, sociologically, some criminals represent the "cultural lag" of the frontier, one way of endeavoring to cling to the old life and ideals of adventure, self-reliance, freedom, individualism and daring in a mechanized society in which so many men are but tiny cogs in vast organizations and are doomed to unimaginative, repetitive routine work. So perhaps this type also represents a rebellion against exaggerated drive and the sometimes frenzied competition, effort and activity which our civilization often demands—and, ironically, demands increasingly almost in proportion to the production of labor-saving devices.

Far more complicating than technological developments has been the change from a gradual rise in population to its explosion since World War II. One result is that by 1970 half of our total national population was age 25 and under. Thus youth preponderates, like joins like in groups large and small, and television's instant communication reports and catalyzes. The hippies were another expression of passive dependence, insofar as the goal is to withdraw from responsible effort, to enjoy life without the labor it requires of all but the wealthy to survive. Some extol such passivity and dependence—the drugs, lounging, sex without responsibility, neglect of personal care and cleanliness, and the like, all so reminiscent of the behavior of children. Many infantile personalities and schizophrenics of various degrees find companionship and personal closeness with others like themselves who gravitate to this subculture.

In general, "youth" is a time when the feelings of the childhood emotional pattern are still strong and have not been completely left behind. As youth steps into adulthood, the childhood emotional forces are at a maximum. Experience in living with oneself and others is usually minimal and weak. But despite this inexperience, young persons must deal with powerful feelings and major forces: in most cases a career must be chosen, and this requires a degree of independence and responsibility which most individuals do not possess. The sex drive is at its height and must be handled in some way—why not indulge it freely, especially now that the "pill" has been introduced? Youth feels a pressure for money, financial security, status or power: how to satisfy these needs when one is young and inexperienced? If morality stands in the way of one's egoistic self-interest, is morality wrong, and should it be discarded? There is much truth in the old saying: "If you are not a socialist when young, you have no heart; if you are still a socialist at maturity, you have no head."

Growing up means that one escapes the dependence upon parents and their control; much current behavior in society reflects this "rebellion." Faced with difficult external decisions, even though they are coming of age in a time of relative peace, driven by powerful internal drives and feelings, the young people of today get into real difficulties in life, with permanent after-effects; venereal disease is again almost epidemic and illegitimate pregnancies are too common for the good of the children; many seek escape because they cannot cope, and flee to communes, drugs, and religious freakouts. When these escapes do not work, this occasionally means involuntary breakdown into psychosis, frequently involving murder and suicide.

Can blame for the mental and emotional disorders of young people today be laid at the doorstep of society? Are young people rebelling realistically and with supersensitivity to the defects of "the system"? This book cannot answer that question—its goal is to illustrate the emotional forces and reactions which are fundamental in all human beings. These forces are universal; only differences in degree make up the endless variety of human personalities. Neurosis, psychosis and health are quantitative variations in the balance of emotional forces.

If the development out of the dependence of childhood to the relative independence and interdependence of maturity does not progress smoothly because the dependence has been in some ways pathological, then the adolescent may react to it with hurt pride, envy and anger, even with a proneness to violence. Thus, much of the "generation gap" and of adolescent rebellion and militancy is caused by a neurotic, displaced protest and battle against an inner dependence.

To make virtues of necessities and even of vices is part of human adaptability and of the human capacity to make the best of any bargain. Throughout history we find all sorts of infantile desires extolled and socially accepted by certain groups—cruelty, parasitism and all kinds of fads and fancies. This is the nature of certain cults, groups of people with similar emotional needs, who are drawn together and make the satisfaction of these needs directly or indirectly a socially desirable goal (Groddeck, 1928). *What emerges from the study of human emotional development is a stable, scientifically based scale of moral, ethical and social values which takes cognizance of the nature of mature adjustment.* This holds even if life is thought of purely mechanistically, as a sort of chemical accident; for with atomic power at its disposal, other than mature behavior probably will result in *homo sapiens* destroying himself and bringing down most other species with him—like Samson slaying more in his own death than during his life.

Strongly dependent behavior may be scorned in one society and extolled in another. It is generally scorned in this country and was even more so in the frontier days. But it was made a virtue in certain strata of prewar Europe, where a man would be ashamed of being caught at his office of an early afternoon, since it would appear that he had to work for a living.

A charming description of one of the last representatives of this ideal appears in a short story by Isak Dinesen (1942). It is worth quoting a passage here, as it provides a lucid delineation of what we mean by the loose term "passive-receptive-dependent":

He was an observer; it had amused him to find that the pretty girl had not lived a day, and probably was incapable of living a day, without an attendant at her heels. She had never opened a door herself, nor pulled out a chair at table or picked up her handkerchief when she dropped it, nor put on her own hat. Her absurd, childish clothes, like her own dainty person, were exquisitely arranged and kept by someone else. When one day her sash became undone she tried to fix it, blushed and stood motionless until Miss Rabe hurried up and tied the bow for her. She must be, he reflected, dressed and undressed like a doll. Her helplessness was like that of a person without hands. Her whole existence was based upon the constant, watchful, indefatigable labour of slaves. Miss Rabe was the silent omnipresent symbol of the system; therefore he dreaded her. . . .

He decided, sadly, that he could not give his wife the slaves which to her were a necessity of life. He wondered whether her own freedom would fully indemnify her for their loss, whether his personal love and care would make up for their service. Or would she, within his own house, so to say within his arms, yearn for Miss Rabe herself? This was a fatal thought. Besides, he distrusted and condemned the principle. It was sweet, both droll and pathetic, when represented in Mizzi's person, in one otherwise obviously ready to meet her destiny. But it was in itself contrary to his idea of a dignified human existence.

Social standards differ, but there is something biological and fundamental in human development (as well as in that of other mammals) in the conflict between the parasitic tendencies which grow out of childhood dependence on the parents and the independence and interest in the world and in others which reflects a mature grasp of the realities of life and the capacity for independence, responsibility, love and productivity, both sexually and socially.

ON PREVENTION

The normal emotional growth and the normal balance between the developmental and the regressive forces can be disturbed in many ways. If life is too easy, stimulus for development is lacking. But if life is too hard, a person loses pleasure in the exercise of his powers and yearns for escape. Of course, how life is depends mostly on how men make it. And how they make it depends on how mature they are. How mature they are depends on all the factors that we have mentioned, their endowment, the social scene in which they are reared and live, and, above all, the emotional influences which they have undergone especially during the earliest hours, days, weeks, months and years of childhood.

The primary task of the parent is to facilitate the child's emotional development, and to do this, just as if they were raising flowers, they must provide the soil, the warmth, the light, and let the enjoyment derive from watching the complex growth unfold. Urging or retarding, neglecting or preparing, denying or overindulging, pushing out or overprotecting, frustrating or spoiling—all kinds of interference with nature are risky. Of course, domestication and socialization are necessary, so all interference cannot by any means be avoided, but it can be applied judiciously with as little disturbance of the development as possible. In the enjoyment of the child, the relationship to the flower remains a good model—to enjoy it for itself with no thoughts for oneself except the satisfaction in its maturing. The child has the right to its own personality and cannot live as a projection of the parents' ambitions, or as an instrument for the satisfaction of their desires and demands, without warping its development. "Love them and leave them alone." From birth, the only safe rule is to treat the child as an individual, with the fullest respect for its complex, immature, flowering personality as it develops toward independence, responsibility, and productivity, which, with love, are the hallmarks of maturity. Responsibility matures, and it is doubtful if anyone matures without it (Gregg, 1957).

REFERENCES

Alexander, F. (1942): *Our Age of Unreason*. Philadelphia: Lippincott.

_____ (1961): *Scope of Psychoanalysis*. New York: Basic Books, pp. 501–510.

_____ and Healy, W. (1935): *Roots of Crime*. New York: Knopf.

_____ and Saul, L. J. (1937): Three criminal types as seen by the psychoanalyst, *Psychoanalytic Review* 24:113.

_____ and Selesnick, S. (1966): *The History of Psychiatry*. New York: Harper & Row.

Cannon, W. (1929): *Bodily Changes in Pain, Hunger, Fear and Rage*. New York: Appleton Century.

Dinesen, I. (1942): The invincible slave-owners, *Winter's Tales*. New York: Random House.

Freud, S. (1927): The future of an illusion, *S.E.* 21.

Gesell, A. (1940): *The First Five Years: A Guide to the Study of the Pre-School Child*. New York: Harper.

_____ (1972): *The Embryology of Behavior: The Beginnings of the Human Mind* (1945). Westport, Conn.: Greenwood Press.

Gregg, A. (1957): *For Future Doctors*. Chicago: University of Chicago Press.

Groddeck, G. (1928): *Book of the It*. New York: Nervous and Mental Disease Publishing Co.

Rosen, J. (1968): *Selected Papers on Direct Psychoanalysis*. New York: Grune and Stratton.

Saul, L. J. (1972): *Psychodynamically Based Psychotherapy*. New York: Science House.

_____, T. Snyder and E. Sheppard (1956): On earliest memories, *Psychoanalytic Quarterly* 25:228–237.

3 | The Need for Love

RECEPTIVITY

General Formulation

A. *Source and Intensity.* There is no more fundamental force in the human mind than the craving for love. The reason for its irresistible intensity is, as we previously surmised, that it is essentially the libidinal aspect of the child's utter dependence on the parents, primarily the mother. Receiving love, i.e., a feeling, affectionate interest in its well-being, is the helpless child's assurance that its wants will be satisfied, so that it will not die. Later this need for love forms the nucleus for friendship, and sexual love and for social acceptance. This interrelation of mother and young is powerful but delicate. Once deranged, whether in humans or animals, the whole development and adjustment of the offspring becomes disordered, and it may perish. This has been shown in humans by René Spitz (1956, 1971) and in experimental animals by Howard Liddell, Eckhardt Hess, Harry Harlow and many others. It is being observed in nature by ethologists like Jane Goodall.

The craving for love, then, originates in the child's needs toward its parents, and it survives in the adult. It comes to expression in many forms. It appears as needs to be dependent on others, as demands for praise, recognition, understanding, acceptance. It comes to expression in a hunger for superiority or fame or money. It seeks satisfaction in sexual love and infatuation. If it is turned toward those of the same sex, it is powerful enough to generate homosexual desires. In some persons it intensifies self-love. Some seek to sate it with food or drink, and its cravings can cause gross overeating and alcoholism. Unsatisfied, these yearnings apparently can disorder the stomach in some people, causing ulcers; in others, they can precipitate asthma and certain skin disorders. These "receptive" love needs are closely related to the dependent desires, and both are manifestations of the same basic biological needs of the organism. The term "receptive" is far from satisfactory but if used broadly it is convenient because it includes active demands as well as passive desires for the many forms of what one person wants from another.

These cravings may be intense enough to prevent the child from leaving its parents or otherwise hinder its adult development. Though partly overcome, under life's pressures, these longings for good parents and for all the gratifications desired of them can be reawakened. They are one of the most important sources of frustration and hurt pride and so of hostility, which is also generated as a defense against them. And hostility plays a vital role in life, in neuroses and in many physical disorders, such as headache and probably, high blood pressure. The indiscriminate demand for any kind of help or advice from almost anyone who offers anything, the slavish attachments to the most obvious charlatans, belief in all sorts of purportedly medicinal preparations—as in fortune tellers, astrologers, and others who cater to human superstition—these and many other observations bear testimony to the power and the ubiquity of this craving for parental attention. As Voltaire said, "if God did not exist, it would be necessary to invent him."

Such elemental dependent love needs are never fully outgrown. But for a satisfactory life, they must be of such form and intensity as to be workable and satisfiable and not impair the enjoyment of mature functioning. Assuredly, the adult has less need for them than the child, whose very life, let alone its pleasures, depends on its parents. Enjoyment of adult life, social, sexual and occupational, depends on fusing the infantile and the adult pleasures in workable proportions. It is largely because of these infantile demands that so many persons, instead of enjoying the realities they have, chase but never find the potentialities they dream of.

The need to be loved being the libidinal aspect of the child's dependence, it is natural that the cases discussed in the previous chapter should grade into those of another type in which the main issue is not so much passive dependence as, rather, the gratification or the frustration of receptive desires to be affectionately valued.

B. Receiving and Giving. In adult life one learns to give love as well as to demand it, just as one learns to do constructive work and to take nonlibidinal responsibility. The giving of love often takes as much energy as doing constructive work. Some persons can more easily exert themselves to provide the physical necessities for another, for the spouse or children, than they can give them real emotional interest, affection or love. The father may work indefatigably at his occupation but be worn out by a weekend of taking care of his children. In other persons the opposite is true—they can give the libidinal interest but cannot take adequate responsibility for the mechanical, nonlibidinal care. Some mothers are inexhaustible founts of love, understanding and care for the children but cannot tolerate practical responsibility of a business kind.

Love and sex are important in the giving and the receiving between persons, for both giving and receiving impulses find expression in these forms. Receiving is more fundamental for the individual even than sex because it is closer to self-preservation. In childhood, what is of first importance is the receiving, the sex of the giver being secondary. The essential is to be taken care of, whether by male or by female.

With maturity the capacity for giving comes to the acme of biological expression in reproduction, the rearing of children and the responsibilities of family. Reproduction is relatively easy; but the care and rearing of the young upon which the survival of the species depends requires enormous and endless efforts for all of one's life. A poor job foredooms the children to criminality or other forms of emotional disorders. This often causes protests in the parents against all the giving necessitated by these needs of the young, and becomes a source of much family discord. But probably no one can go counter to the course of biological and psychological development without paying a price. The person who uses sex only for pleasure and receiving and shuns its connection with mating and reproduction, in the end generally feels a lack of fulfillment in his life.

Often both husband and wife see marriage in terms of what one will get from the other. The husband finds that the wife expects all sorts of attentions, has her own needs and is not satisfied with running a home for him in which he can be free of all responsibility while accompanying him when he wants to go out. The wife finds that, instead of providing everything and satisfying all her wishes, the husband expects much, and the home and the children turn out to be full-time jobs to which she must give her energies interminably. In the past it has perhaps been easier for women than for men to fuse their receptive demands into their sexual attitudes and seek to satisfy them through love and the sexual life. However, the result of receiving such love is reproduction and all the responsibility and giving entailed in the rearing of the children and the care of a family. The maternal functions and attitudes probably entail the highest degree of direct, physical, biological giving with the least immediate direct return—a point noted by the women's movement. As we have said, these demands can cause difficulties if the woman is overly dependent and receptive and resents these claims on her. This is often one factor in the postpartum neuroses and psychoses which are precipitated by the birth of a child. This holds for men as well as for women. Often the man is very emotionally dependent on his wife, with strong needs to receive attention, interest and emotional support from her, and when her time and energies must go in so large a part to the new arrival and when additional demands are made upon himself, he feels frustrated. Often alcoholism as well as many other neurotic manifestations begin or are exacerbated at the time a child is born.

C. Protest and Frustration. A common masculine problem seen by the analytic psychiatrist centers around passive dependence and competition. On the other hand, the most common problem seen in women is frustration of receptive desires. "Men must work and women must weep." This is probably due, in large part, to the fact that in our culture men tend to fight their dependent, submissive, receptive wishes, which are in conflict with their masculine trends and ideals, while women more easily accept these wishes and incorporate them into their feminine attitudes and seek to satisfy them in this form. Our cultural standard has been for the wife and children to be supported financially and emotionally by the strong, independent, responsible husband. With the women's movement this is now changing, and for the good or misfortune of the world is not yet clear.

In women, the frustration arises in some cases chiefly from the external situation of lack of satisfaction from the man, whose energies are absorbed in his own competitiveness and flight from passivity, or in unavoidable struggles with life (Alexander, 1961, pp.

384–411). In other cases, it arises from something in the woman's own make-up, which is usually a result of traumatic childhood emotional influences. Very often these experiences * are in the nature of rejection or deprivation at the hands of the parents, although spoiling and various other experiences can produce somewhat similar results. A common way in which they result in internally caused frustration in both men and women is the following: These depriving or spoiling experiences in childhood increase the desires for love, attention and the like and cause them to persist overstrongly in adult life. Because of their intensity, the person defends himself against them, so as not to be too demanding, too easily hurt, and the like; and, also because of their intensity, the desires are inevitably frustrated, causing anger. The receptive demands on others and also this anger estrange people, causing further frustration and also causing guilt feelings, feelings of depression and an unwillingness to let oneself enjoy (i.e., internal inhibition and consequent frustration). This increased frustration, in turn, causes more demands and anger. This neurotic vicious cycle can be schematically simplified as follows: Frustration—anger, defenses and demands—guilt—frustration. The individual is in the tragic situation of longing to be loved and at the same time feeling that this is impossible. The girl who has been rejected as a child would fall madly in love with a man, but in a week or two would demand emotionally more than he could give, would become enraged at him, lose him, and, being beautiful, would soon repeat this pattern.

The frustration in this type of case is primarily occasioned by the internal emotional reaction patterns of the individual, and relatively little influenced by the real external circumstances. Two women, severely frustrated for purely internal neurotic reasons, had quite opposite histories and life situations. One of them had a childhood of poverty, rejection and exploitation and in adult life

---

* Throughout, in using the word "experiences," long-term emotional influences are meant, e.g., a depriving mother, an overindulgent father, a hated uncle, a weak brother, and so on. It is such chronic forces which shape a personality and only rarely any single, isolated, traumatic event. Where such an event is intended, this will be stated explicitly. The relations of these traumatic influences to emotional disorders and to treatment will be discussed later. For a review of the major studies on this subject over the last 30 years, see Saul, L. J., 1972a.

remained poor, overworked and deprived. The other was spoiled by a wealthy father and in adult life was married to a well-to-do man and had two children. Yet the second was also in a state of frustration because her demands were not satisfied.

D. Forms and Ways of Handling. The demands are usually for "love," either in the unsublimated form, culminating in heterosexual satisfaction, or with equal intensity in the forms of being wanted and valued, of receiving attention, time, money, help, support, praise and the like. The emphasis falls on different demands in different individuals. In the extreme cases the demands are frank, overt and insistent. In the more repressed cases they are still discernible in life and usually are expressed frankly in the dreams. Some individuals with this kind of problem can and do make their demands insistently and with full intensity on behalf of others but cannot even passively accept what is given to themselves, let alone make any demands or even requests for themselves. Usually it is found that these persons have been frustrated in childhood by unfortunate external reality. Now in adult life they themselves neurotically maintain the same feelings of frustration.

One such girl, personally attractive, could never believe that a man was interested in her and could never accept a man's love. She could not even let herself be treated to lunch or dinner, and if she were invited to a meal in a private home, always had to bring a gift, which was for her not simply a friendly gesture but meant emotionally "paying" for the meal. However, she could freely demand help and favors for her friends.

Some persons look upon their more passive wishes to receive as something childish which hurts their self-regard, and they react to these wishes by retaining their quality and direction but making them active and aggressive. This makes them more acceptable, particularly to the masculine self-esteem. It is even the main mechanism in certain criminals. Their egoism is satisfied by the emotional logic: "I ask nothing of anyone. I take what I want" (Alexander and Healy, 1935). Although the aim may be parasitic, this active, aggressive component is more consonant with the masculine ideal. This is like the widespread and fateful mistaking of unproductive, hostile aggressiveness for mature masculinity. Apart from this prestige reaction, mounting frustration generally increases the urges actively to go after what one so strongly craves and does not receive.

Receptivity, especially in passive form, being so close to the small child's feelings toward parents, seems usually to hurt the self-esteem. The relatively normal man does not feel his pride hurt by his active, masculine, sexual interest in a woman and his advances toward her. On the contrary, it is apt to hurt his pride if he feels inhibited. But the woman, receptively dependent on the man's activity for her sexual, financial and other satisfaction, may feel that it is a blow to her pride to admit that she longs for the man's attentions, and she feels that she should wait for him to show his interest and that he should make the advances and want her.

Illustrations with Some Dynamic Connections

A. Animals. As with other fundamental biological needs, the effects of the frustration of receptive demands can be observed in animals as well as in human beings. As a homely example, a family with little or no interest in dogs endeavored to raise a cocker spaniel from the age of two weeks for the sake of their five-year-old boy. Gradually, it became apparent that the child too had very little interest in the puppy. The little boy had a one-year-old baby brother and took out on the puppy his resentment of this baby rival. It was winter, and the facilities of the house were not adapted to housebreaking a puppy. The vicious circle began. The more of a nuisance the puppy was to the household, the more the family reacted against him; and the more the family reacted against him as a nuisance, the more the puppy misbehaved, the more difficult he was to train, and the more of a nuisance he became. He was never subjected to any actual abuse or mistreatment but he was not loved. At the age of six months, just when the family had finally decided to be rid of him by giving him away, he ran away from the house, like a human being who avoids a direct rejection by leaving. He was picked up by a friend the following day but showed no joy in returning to his home, which provided bed and board but no love. Two days later he ran away again and never returned. Such interpretations of animal behavior are, of course, open to criticism. Puppies cannot talk, but actions often speak louder than words and the circumstances in this instance were so transparent as to leave little doubt as to the pup's reactions. He reacted just as a child might have, and as children in similar circumstances are known to do. Moreover, the rejection of the puppy had influenced his attitudes toward people and had impaired his normal development, at least as far as a friendly, easy, well-trained canine relationship to human beings was concerned. Whether these alterations in attitude and behavior were still only reactive to the rejection by this particular family and were correctible by a different, very accepting home environment, or whether they were already internalized and destined the puppy to permanent changes in personality, is not known, but such observations indicate a rich field for animal experimentation with emotional dynamics and the development of personality. This field, pioneered by Masserman, Liddell, Gantt and others, is being further explored by Harlow, Hess and ethologists such as Goodall, as we have noted.*

The operation of frustrated demands for love in the situation of rivalry between children is well known, and no emotional reactions are seen in children which cannot be observed operating with full force in adults, even though the grown-ups may not themselves be conscious of them. *For within every grown-up lives the little child he once was.* Wherever there is a group—in a factory, office, business, state or nation—and a head of the group—one sees the members unconsciously repeating emotionally, in some degree, the relationships they had in their own families to the head as a father or mother and to the members as brothers and sisters. The receptive competition for the chief's favor is often overt and usually unmistakable and creates the same undercurrents and even open interplay of rivalry and hostility that one sees among children. This need for love is so deep-going and biological that, as we have pointed out, it is easily seen in animals. Probably one reason why

---

* Masserman, Jules H.: Principles of Dynamic Psychiatry, Philadelphia, Saunders, 1946; Liddell, Howard S.: Emotional Hazards in Animals and Man, Springfield, Ill., Thomas, 1956; Gantt, W. Horsley: Experimental Basis for Neurotic Behavior, New York, Hobart, 1944; Seitz, Philip F. D.: Infantile Experience and Adult Behavior in Animal Subjects, Psychosom. Med. 21 (No. 5): 353 ff., 1959; Goodall, Jane, In the Shadow of Man, Boston, Houghton-Mifflin, 1971; Carrighar, Sally, Wild Heritage, Boston, Houghton-Mifflin, 1965; Saul, L. J., The Childhood Emotional Pattern in Marriage, New York, Van Nostrand Reinhold, 1979. A convenient resumé of modern studies on interrelations between the human and animal emotional life will be found in: Masserman, J. (ed.): Science and Psychoanalysis, Vol. 12, 1968.

various animals, including skunks and prairie dogs, have the capacity to become pets is that they develop this powerful receptive attachment, which depends not on food alone, but is a true attachment, thriving on attention, which, in the broad sense, spells love. This supposition has received support from the work of the animal ethologists. Konrad Lorenz, for example, attributes the one-man devotion of the dogs descended from wolves to transference to the master of the attachment to the leader of the pack. He contrasts this with the readiness to promiscuous attachments of breeds descended from jackals (1952). Sally Carrighar's *Wild Heritage* summarizes the extensive pertinent literature and must interest every student of "human nature."

This is a correct use of the term. Children want pets as something alive to love, and there is no doubt that the pets love them back. How intense the need for love is in pets is shown by the fact that such animals as dogs and monkeys, and probably others also, become depressed, exactly as humans beings do, refusing food, showing no interest, slowing up in their actions and being obviously low in spirits, if love is withdrawn. And just like human beings, they may even die in such circumstances. At the beginning of World War II, the newspapers all over the country carried a day-to-day story of a collie, dying because of his young master's departure for the army; the dog was saved when they were reunited. Probably one reason children and their animals feel so close and understand each other so well, is that they both have these intense receptive needs so strongly, the child's attaching primarily toward its parents. Not only do the pets have the same needs but also all the other reactions that go with them—the joy at receiving love, the loyalty to the giver, the pain at losing it, the violent jealousy at any threat to it. The jealousy of pets is well known. Just try bringing in a second pet. But even if one does, then, as with children, the initial rivalry often gives way to a predominating companionship and identification with each other, with some potential or open rivalry and jealousy in the background. People, and animals too, like the central receptive position, to have the attentions of those to whom they are attached assured to them solely, to be the only or favored child. No one likes to be pushed out of the baby position, and few tolerate this without a powerful, usually hostile, aggressive reaction—that is, a fight to maintain or regain it. Many a fight for a girl or a man in adult life, ostensibly sexual jealousy, lacks mature "object interest" and is really, beneath the veneer, a childish rivalry for mother's or father's love. In children it is easy to observe the undisguised original edition, which, if it is not outgrown, may become a pattern of excessive neediness for love which persists for life.

B. Children. The younger of two children was an unusually sweet, demure, golden-curled, blue-eyed little lady of three. When I saw her after an interval of about eight months, she greeted me with a kick in the shins and a blow in the abdomen, and I soon learned that during my absence she had earned for herself the nickname of "Battleship Mary." Her parents were distressed and puzzled and did not associate this access of hostile aggression with the birth of an unusually cute little brother, who was the new cynosure of the family and the neighbors.

A little boy of five suffered from night terrors, which were reactions to his hostility to his baby brother, who was just learning to walk. Although he made a great ostentatious show of loving the baby, the parents had reason to fear that his hugging might seriously injure the child, and he liked to play wildly with sticks, which somehow would accidentally hit the baby. During the nights following such displays of aggression he would have anxieties and nightmares, so intense was his anger and hostility because of being displaced from the baby position in the family.

C. Adults (Neurotic). A pretty girl of 25 suffered from occasional hysterical tremors, from terrifying nightmares, from a severe, vague anxiety without specific content and from a fear of people which cut her off from almost all social contacts and precluded her going with men, although she craved love and romance.

She had lost her parents in childhood and was not really accepted by the relatives who had reared her. A male cousin, some years older, was her only real friend in the family, and later, because of her neurosis (i.e., her excessive distorted childish reactions), her only friend in the world. Her symptoms, which had previously been mild, broke out in full force when this cousin married. Now she felt entirely deserted and alone, and besides her other symptoms, she feared that she would lose her mind. As is so often the case, the symptoms develop, the breakdown occurs, and *the danger point is reached when the last emotional ties are threatened or severed.* With few exceptions, no one can live without some close human relationship and some love. This final desertion and the frustration of her receptive attachment to her cousin intensified her rage, which was directed chiefly against the cousin's wife as jealousy. This sudden exacerbation of rage and hostility threatened to overwhelm her forces of control and the orderly operation of her thinking, and this is what she felt as the threat of losing her mind. Patients often tell that before the development of neurotic symptoms or of psychotic episodes they had the feeling that something would have to give way because the emotional tension was becoming too great to be borne. This tension can disturb or partially disrupt the forces of control, judgment and reason (ego forces); it can find some form of distorted or substitute expression in symptoms; it can place such a strain on the physiology that psychosomatic reactions occur, such as heart or stomach disorders; and, because it is usually largely hostility, it can break out in violence. Sometimes a patient says that when his acute psychosis began he could feel something in his head snap.

This girl had four main reactions to the emotional rejection from which she was suffering: (1) hurt self-regard and loss of self-confidence; (2) an abnormal intensification of her receptive desires for love and esteem, and of an overt, aggressive, demanding attitude; (3) rage and hostility because of frustration and jealousy; and (4) guilt and anxiety because of this rage and hostility, which inhibited her receptivity, sexual and otherwise, and so perpetuated the frustration.

Her hurt self-regard was of a kind typical of the rejected child. She felt that because her family did not want her she was not valued by them and she took over this low regard and valuation of herself. This was graphically represented in a *dream* in which her family discussed selling her for a very low price. Since her own relatives did not really love her, she could not believe that any other person could or would. Because of this, she withdrew from people and alienated herself and them. Thus she carried over into adult life the childhood pattern of being rejected and also her habitual responses to it.

Another reaction was the intensification of her desires to be loved and of her demandingness. These appeared in both sexual and non-sexual forms. She looked to a man's love to give her all that she had missed in childhood. The fact that her receptive desires were so largely in the form of cravings for sexual love is characteristic of hysteria. These desires intensified her sexual longings but gave them a too strongly childish, receptive, "getting" component. This attracted men but also made them wary. In this case, as in many others, one got the impression that his mechanism of attempting to satisfy all her heightened receptive needs by sexual love was an important element in her obviously strong "sex appeal." Another fact or element in this seemed to be her *masochism*—her desires to be attacked, caused by her guilt and her self-punishing tendencies. These she felt chiefly in sexual form. But the hostile component in this wish to be attacked sexually was too strong and caused so much fear that although it may have heightened her "sex appeal," she dared not even have a date in reality.

People who have been overindulged and spoiled in childhood are also apt to be abnormally receptive and demanding in later life, but their demands and expectations of love are usually quite different from those who had been deprived—warmer and less hard—for their feeling is, "I am a wonderful person whom everyone loves and takes care of and gives to. I've always had it, so I of course expect it. No one can refuse me." And because they have indeed received it, they are usually able, at least in some degree, to give it in kind, and this means warmth and helps win it.

But this girl, apart from her love life, was openly and aggressively demanding, a trend which was bound to provoke rejection by others. The emotional logic is generally to the effect: "I have never had my just due from the world and I have therefore suffered—now it is my right to have what was denied me or compensation for it." It is this feeling which often contributes to the hard quality of the demandingness.

This girl feared people and was therefore shy and shunned them, and her sexual life was completely inhibited. She partly covered her anxiety by a veneer of social superiority in her manner.

This veneer of snobbishness was a defense, which said, "I do not want to associate with you because I am so superior." This was more tolerable than the true feeling which it sought to spare her, namely, "I don't dare try to be friendly or expect any love because you will surely find me worthless and reject me." Snobbishness not infrequently hides such shyness, insecurity and pain. It also vents hostility and can have other motivations as well.

The third chief reaction of this girl to her family's rejection of her was direct rage and hostility. Sensitized in childhood, she continued in adult life to react with fury to the slightest frustration of her exaggerated demands for love, help and attention, and at such times she even became threatening. Her periodic hysterical tremors were primarily spells of literally "trembling with rage." When a person has neurotic fears and anxieties, an important source of these is usually her own hostility. This girl's sexual wishes, as well as her general wishes for love, acceptance and being valued, were so fused with this inverted hostility that she could think of love and sex only in terms of being attacked, and she had many terrible nightmares in which she would flee in fear from the threatening man, just as in life she fled from any sexual or even harmless social advances. This girl's dreams afford another example of how dreams reveal the ways in which a person handles his emotions, his methods and degrees of repression.

Her hostility, as well as her expectation of rejection, through the steps of guilt and anxiety, estranged her from people, made her fear them and made her unable to accept the love she craved. She was cut off from even a little acceptance and friendliness by this reaction within herself. She had a relatively normal, feminine personality organization and orientation, but her reactions caused the continuation of her rejection and frustration. *How ironic, inexorable and unfair the mental life can be!* Through no fault of her own, this girl is rejected as a baby. She reacts to this automatically, biologically, according to the laws of the emotional life. She develops into a beautiful girl, but the original feelings of rejection still live within her and, by the dynamics we have described, prolong themselves and force her to continue to be utterly frustrated and rejected all her adult life, just as she was as a child. The emotional dynamics of such persons find poignant expression in the myth of Tantalus, chained in the center of a lake which rose to his parched lips but receded every time he bent his head for a life-sustaining draught.

In another case, the deprivation was more severe, occurred at a much earlier age and left demands for love which were of a more primitive, dependent nature.

An attractive young woman of 30 had lost her mother when she was one and one-half years old. This great deprivation was followed by her father's giving her over to some relatives of his to rear. At first, the child showed two main reactions: (1) an intensification of her infantile, dependent, receptive longings for her father, all her desires for her mother now being transferred to him; and (2) rage, chiefly directed toward him, because of his rejection of her. She never, even as an adult, established any other close attachment and never succeeded in weaning herself from her father. She maintained that in spite of his rejection he had also tried to hold her affection and to keep her dependent on him. Only very late in life did he remarry.

Her rage from deprivation and rejection was not directed exclusively against her father but was manifest in a general extreme irritability, hostility and readiness to become angry at everyone. This is especially apt to occur when an individual does not know who or what is making him angry—and usually the child does not know. Apparently, she was driven by this anger reaction, which she did not understand and could struggle with only blindly, and this aggressiveness and hostility antagonized people so that she was driven back into her dependent attachment to her father. This was, in turn, so full of conflict that more rage was generated—a common vicious circle—and another person alienated.

When she was preadolescent her father one day took her to some distant elderly relatives and left her there. This strained her only close emotional bond nearly to the breaking point. But instead of an outbreak or exacerbation of her symptoms, as in the previous case, something different occurred, which affected her whole personality. She turned in an open rage against her father, but with only vague and incomplete insight into her reaction, and from then on she harbored a resentment against all men.* Although pretty enough and sought after for dates by the boys, henceforth she never would go out with them, for she would become very agitated

* This "spread" is well recognized in conditioning and painful experience may turn a person against a whole city; a child may turn against the town or whole area in which he was reared.

whenever she was in the company of a young man, because of her own anger, her consequent guilt and anxiety and her resistance against her too infantile, dependent, receptive attachment and demands, which underlay all her human relationships. She feared relationships with other persons, in part because she became too childishly dependent on them. This continued in adult life, and she could only tolerate being with men who were very dependent on her. For example, one man she knew was often in financial and personal troubles. She would help him out both with loans and with advice. She could be friendly with him because she was always in the giving role and hence in less danger of becoming intolerably dependent, receptive and demanding toward him. Also, she was attracted to him through partial *identification*—because, like her own, his unsatisfied needs were so great.

As an adult, there was another motive for her shunning men. She would not allow herself to develop her powerful receptive desires toward any man, becoming emotionally dependent on him, and so lay herself open to the possibility of having to endure a rejection at his hands. Only with a man toward whom she did not look in this way, but who was dependent and receptive toward her, could she feel sympathy and identification and relax her defenses a little. She was too vulnerable to rejection to risk developing expectations, the frustration of which she could not endure. Her early experiences, while yet a helpless baby, had sensitized her to rejection, so that she overreacted violently even to the slightest signs of it—just as in allergic sensitization if a man—or a mouse—is given an injection of serum and rendered sensitive, then for years the tiniest drop causes a reaction so extreme that even death may result.

Sometimes she craved a person's interest and solicitude and would weep violently at the least hint of frustration. But this reaction was not conscious. She could not bear to face the fact that she cared in the slightest. Although her feelings and reactions were so much on the surface as to be obvious to anyone, she herself was blind to them—so painful and intolerable were they for her to admit. It is not uncommon for patients (and, as A. A. Brill, 1946, said, we are all patients) to dread insight, not only because it hurts, but also because of the feeling that admitting tendencies or emotions will mean releasing them in dangerous and overwhelming force and being swamped by them. This is thought to derive from early childhood, when the impulses are strong and the forces of control and judgment weak, and so to *feel* strongly means to lose control and to *act*. But in adult life, when the understanding, judgment and control are not grossly disturbed or undeveloped and infantile, the opposite is generally true—to recognize an unconscious reaction in oneself is regularly the first step in learning to handle it better. Of course, preparing the patient for the insight and imparting it in digestible doses are fundamental to good psychotherapy. Denial of it and failure to recognize it, that is, repression of it, generally has an effect similar to compressing a gas—it increases the emotional pressure. Insight properly reached is the first step in relieving the pressure and decreasing the force of the disturbing trend.

Returning to our patient's life with her elderly relatives, the rage at her father, the spreading of this against all men and her isolation left her dangerously alone and without any close emotional relationship. As we have noted, few persons, if any, can live without such a relationship and without love. So it is not surprising that she turned to an older girl who was kindly disposed toward her and temporarily took her father's place as her only close human contact. This relationship had two main roots. This girl was sympathetic and satisfied in considerable degree her receptive needs for acceptance and love, these having been attached originally to her mother, a woman. The second, and probably an important reason for picking this particular girl, was that she represented the epitome of gratification to the patient, for she was the indulged daughter of wealthy and doting parents. She represented all the satisfactions for which the patient yearned. This bond was through identification and vicarious gratification. Beneath it was the inevitable envy.

As time went on, the patient became increasingly tense with other women because of her envy of their ability to go with men, marry and have children. So she turned to a career as a means of maintaining loose human contacts and a source of interest. This step succeeded only in part. Isolated as she was, her fantasy life became unduly emphasized. Just as the attachment to her girl friend, if intense enough, could have taken on a sexual coloring, so this exaggerated fantasying represented a tendency which, if it had gone far enough, would have been schizoid. But it did not represent so deep a regression and dependence nor such complete withdrawal of feelings from others. This is mentioned to show again that *psychological differences between the normal, the neurotic and the psychotic are primarily quantitative. We all have such tendencies or potentialities in some degree. (Of course, we are studying only disorders of function in intact bodies and not problems arising from brain damage, infections, biochemical disorders and other physical impairments.)*

Her attitude toward babies was significant. She always sought to avoid the subject. It was painful to her because she had not achieved marriage and children, but also for a deeper reason, namely, her underlying wish to *be* a baby and to have the love and the care of which she had been deprived in her own early childhood. This was expressed in her dreams and in her life by her infantile attachment to her father, which she was never able to break despite her hostility to him. Her deepest yearning was for a mother, to return to the time when she was a baby and had a mother's love.

The impairment of her development and the consequent disturbance of her personality and of her emotional life were caused by the severity of the traumatic situation (loss of her mother and rejection by her father) and by the time in her life in which it had begun (at one and one-half years). These are probably important factors in determining the severity of disturbance in all cases.

Defenses

Sometimes the defenses against risking the repetition of painful rejection and frustration play a major role in shaping the personality. In the case of a certain man, the central traumatic childhood situation was neglect. While the children were still small, his mother went to work, as well as his father, leaving the patient and his little brother to such makeshift care as could be found. The patient developed an attitude of *denial:* "I do not want or expect anything from anyone, for then I will not be disappointed." He grew up as a very independent child and man, but one who was lonely and unhappy, for although he denied to himself his craving for love and interest and indulgence, these cravings continued powerfully though silently within him. Yet he could not permit himself to risk any close friendship or attachment. But, if someone he knew did not greet him warmly enough he would go into a rage; and if he heard of someone unsolicitedly doing something for another person, the tears would come to his eyes, although he would still deny any feelings about it.

His defenses were not even relaxed toward his wife. They were a fixed part of his personality. He could not ask, he could not demand, but he also could not give, for he too deeply resented not having received. "I do not receive, therefore I will not give" is a common emotional syllogism (Alexander, 1961, pp. 129–136).

Neurotic Parentalism

The maternal functions are often disturbed as a result of early emotional deprivation and probably especially when there is a deep underlying longing to be a baby and have a mother. In some cases they are inhibited and impaired but in others they are exaggerated. One woman had lost her father when she was only a year old. As so often happens, her mother, left without adequate support, found the child a burden and a handicap in her efforts to remarry. The child's reactions were feelings of being unwanted, an extreme hypersensitivity to the slightest rejection, a rage and hostility largely turned against herself and felt mostly as depression and an intensification of her maternal impulses. We wish only to illustrate this last and therefore will not go into details of her personality structure, which was determined almost entirely by her rejection. On reaching adulthood, she married and soon had a baby. She then reacted to every frustration and to every situation which she took as a rejection with an irresistible urge to have another baby. Since she was a beautiful girl and a most conscientious mother, this was not too disadvantageous—except in one way. For it led her into so much giving out of love, interest and energy that it kept her emotional balance sheet in the red and caused an undercurrent of dissatisfaction and fatigue.

Her maternal and giving urges had many motivations (were "overdetermined"). There was the element of making up to others for her own deprivation, with the attitude: "I know what it is to suffer with frustrated longings for a mother's love and care and I will do all I can to prevent other creatures from having to endure this." Then there was the vicarious satisfaction, through identifying with the recipients of her giving, especially, of course, with her own babies. By identifying with them she could enjoy being a baby herself and having all the love and the care that she had missed and still craved. Also, giving serves as a defense against the painful desires to receive love with the inherent risk of anguish should they be frustrated. In this relationship she was the giver and so ran little risk of expecting love from another and again suffering that rejection to which she was so poignantly sensitized. This position eased her self-regard, which, as is usual, was hurt by having the underlying attitude of wanting to receive from others, like a child for parents. As the giver, she was in a position much more satisfying to her self-esteem. In the well-known French play *Le Voyage de M. Perrichon,* the man whose life was saved has difficulty in being grateful to his rescuer because he was the recipient of this supreme favor while his rescuer is acclaimed a hero. Giving also serves as a means of winning love, and failing to get it from parents does not preclude trying to win it from those who, like children, are not in the parent category. (But too strong dependency in love needs of parent to child is a reversal of nature and can have dire consequences for the child. It is a common cause of neurotic symptoms, mental breakdowns and emotional acting out—as with drugs, protests, militancy and even violence-proneness—during adolescence, symptomatic of the rage and efforts at the emancipation from parents.) Another element in overly strong maternalism and giving is often competition with the mother and a reproach to her, which takes this constructive form. Its intent is: "You were a bad mother—I am a better one and I will show you how you should have been."

A further motivation very frequently is guilt. A child is rejected and regularly reacts with anger at the parent. But *one cannot be hostile to one's parent with impunity.* The child's anger reaction is not its fault. It is an automatic response. *It cannot occur without good and sufficient provocation. Yet it probably always interferes with development and produces baleful results* of some kind. It generally causes guilt, and this often takes the form: "You do not deserve to receive, to get what you want, but only to give it to others."

The receptive desires themselves often, because of being frustrated, become actively aggressive and cause guilt as well as shame. This can lead to a great hunger to grasp, grab, have everything and an intense envy of everything others have. As a defense against this the reaction develops: "Because you want to grab everything and hate everyone who has what you want, whether love or material things, you deserve to get nothing but only to give." Thus from the guilt and the shame comes the denial: "I am no grabber—I am a superior person, a giver." In many cases the hurt to the pride then causes competition, and in these cases this often takes the overt form of the maternal functions—having babies, mothering, housekeeping, giving. In such ways, then, some women react to internally frustrated needs by intensification of their child-bearing and maternal functions and so recreate the longed-for child-mother relationship—only in reverse.

In Marriage

Frustration in childhood often disturbs marriage in later life. A young woman in her thirties had been a rejected child, the youngest of many children of rather irresponsible, childish parents. She sustained an unremitting rage against them. This estranged them still further and generated the usual vicious circle. This accelerated her determination to be free of them and to marry as soon as she was old enough. She married a gentle and devoted man, but, as usually happens when the childhood feelings toward the parents are not resolved, these feelings developed toward the husband. This is really the process of "transference" described by Freud.* Always pressing for expression, always hoping for satisfaction, these patterns of feelings inevitably enter in some degree into every relationship—not only in the analytic situation but also toward every doctor and every person.

In marriage there is ample time for every such emotional pattern to generate toward the ever-present partner. This woman unconsciously looked to her husband for the gratification of her unsatisfied childhood longings and for compensation for the rejection by her parents. But no man can satisfy fully in an adult woman

* Apparently, Freud's modesty and sense of proportion played a significant part in his discovery of this phenomenon which is of such vital import in life as well as in causal treatment of these problems. When his early patients idealized him and "fell in love" with him, he judged that this was not to be accepted as a natural reaction to his charms, but rather a transference to himself of needs which originated elsewhere—which he succeeded in tracing to childhood. "One must be humble, one must keep personal preferences and antipathies in the background if one wishes to discover the realities of the world" (1912).

these imperious demands of a bitter child. So she was doomed to disappointment, and then reacted as in childhood with anger and revenge. She developed feelings of depression, severe headaches, suicidal impulses and withdrawal from her responsibilities and former interests. She was a charming person, intelligent, able, with refined feelings. But her early experience of rejection had impaired her development out of excessive love needs into mature feminine attitudes to husband and family and resulted in misery despite a very satisfactory position in life.

A simple way in which early spoiling, in contrast to rejection and deprivation, can cause neurotic difficulties later in life is illustrated by a married woman of 35. She had been the indulged favorite of her father, who was a successful businessman, and as a result of this she had formed an extremely strong attachment to him. In this woman's overly strong attachment to her father was the lively desire to continue to receive from him, both emotionally and materially, as she had all her life. Her receptive desires toward him had a considerable sexual coloring and were fused with her sexual wishes. As a result, it was hard for her to separate herself sufficiently from him, and from the gratifications of childhood which he represented, to marry. She finally did marry, though, and had one child. But her development to independence and to a mature, responsible, giving attitude and interest in her family was impaired by the alluring expectations toward her father. Her husband was a steady worker and devoted to his wife and his child. But she was destined to be disappointed, for he was not the figure to her that her father was. It has been said that a man's greatest rival for a woman's affections is the unconscious image of her father which she carries in her heart. Compared with how the doting father looked to the small child, no mere man of her own generation, however superior, could look like such a promise of fulfillment, nor could any man satisfy these needs of the child persisting in the adult woman.

As her feelings of frustration mounted, her anger did also. Marital friction resulted, and also neurotic symptoms and behavior. These, too, were in typical small-child form. She would get in a pet and then withdraw from it all by going to bed. She began to neglect her house and child. She developed insomnia. Soon she was threatening suicide.

Since her receptive demands formed a component for her sexual desires and she tended to try to satisfy them through this channel, she developed sexual interests in other men, but here, too, she was frustrated because she could not permit herself to take any active steps in this direction. In this case, there was no evidence of any tendency to handle her frustrated childhood receptive demands by any maternal or child-bearing reaction. There was too much of the "accept no substitutes" in her receptive attachment to her father. In *Deux Femmes* (Balzac, 1889), two women exchange letters, one praising the joys of sexual love, the other the joys of maternity. These attitudes and components are seen in various degrees and proportions in different women, as exemplified by those described in this chapter.

A college student was brought up to think of himself and his own happiness and career as the center of the universe. He did not really know what it meant even to be interested in, let alone love and take the responsibility for, someone else. He wanted a wife and married, but he did not want children; and his parents, like other parents who are too much attached to an only child, resented the wife and tried to convince him that she was a millstone about his neck, interfering with his career. So many parents do not know that *the way to keep the child's love is to be interested in the child for the facilitation of its own growth and development toward independence. Trying to hold their children, they so often drive them away*—that is, if the child, for its own salvation, succeeds in escaping. Meanwhile, the wife, a girl with considerable musical talent, accustomed for over 20 years to being the center of the universe herself, became terribly frustrated by the attitudes of her husband and his family. She still did not know that adult life involved enjoyment of one's interests in people and things outside oneself and the enjoyment of the exercise of one's powers, whether feminine or masculine. Instead, her aim was to get from marriage all the indulgences she had had from her parents, with sexual satisfaction in addition. Her husband had been overindulged in childhood like herself. That is no doubt why they had appealed to each other—like called to like. They identified with each other because their dynamics were so similar. Her continuing disappointments caused a mounting anger, which led to temper tantrums, headaches, nightmares and hysterical spells in which she wept and threatened suicide. Interestingly enough, these two "babes in the wood" had considerable capacity for development, because a good psychotherapeutic result was achieved. They had not known what adult attitudes were and what part they played in marriage, nor, in all their education, were they ever taught anything about this. But like other persons who are not too strongly *fixated* to infantile attitudes and have reasonably normal developmental drives, when these young people began to understand, after a few interviews, what was holding them back and what development was, the pathway was reopened and they made excellent progress. Gently disengaging themselves from their parents, they are apparently laying the foundations for a satisfactory marriage; let us hope that with insight they will grow into the enjoyment of its responsibilities.

Suicide

Frustration severe enough to lead to a serious attempt at suicide is illustrated by a woman in whom the demands took primarily a heterosexual form. She was an attractive young woman in her middle thirties who had achieved a good business position. She was apparently well adjusted, although a second glance revealed considerable underlying emotional tension. This tension was a manifestation of acute frustration and rage because she had always been unable to achieve a satisfactory sexual life in marriage or otherwise. As her twenties passed, she felt her chances for marriage waning and her sexual tension mounting, and she began to become desperate for some sort of sexual life. Not that she had lacked proposals of marriage—but, significantly, she had always found something wrong with the man and had refused. Now she saw that other women had accepted these men and had apparently happy homes with them, and her bitter regret and jealousy heightened her frustration. She began having repeated *dreams* of missing trains, boats and buses—and these conveyances were always bound for the towns in which the men she had refused now had their wives and families. In her, the receptive cravings took the form of marriage and sexual life. The frustration of these wishes to which she looked almost solely for gratification made life seem not worthwhile and engendered a rage reaction against herself. She began to feel irresistibly impelled to suicide. She kept these impulses to herself, and no one suspected their sinister power beneath her cheerful surface manner.

Her work and her few friends were the only things which kept her going. Her work occupied her time and attention, took her mind off her distress and provided a certain stability. It was some satisfaction, although not enough, for she felt that to work was to be a man, and in that she found no gratification of her feminine needs. She established a liaison with a relatively undesirable man. She was frigid, the relationship went badly, and the man finally broke it off. Then she found that she was unable to have children. She felt that this cruel blow, along with the passing of her youth, sealed her fate. She felt that this fact made it utterly impossible to hope for a marriage of any sort. Never to have a man, never to have children, she felt robbed of the means for love. But the more she felt love denied her, the stronger were her cravings, for she had no other way of satisfying her needs. And these needs were not only libidinal, but also were egoistic and aggressive in competition in this field with other women.

Her dreams reflected her frustration. She *dreamed* of sitting down to a meal but then finding the food meager and inedible, thus representing her desires orally, in terms of food.

Then came two more blows from life, which often can be not only more strange but also more cruel than fiction. She had two last slender bonds to other persons. One was to the woman who was her superior at her place of business and the other was to a woman somewhat younger than herself. She had had a mother and a younger sister, so that these women, including the man who had abandoned her, exactly reproduced her family constellation, and with uncanny precision she repeated her childhood emotional pattern in her relations with them. At this point, the older woman, the mother figure, was transferred to another department. Now the patient felt everything in life toppling, represented in a dream as a great tree falling, and only through the bravest struggle did she manage to resist her urge to commit suicide. But then came the crowning blow—the younger woman married after a brief engagement. Now jealousy was added to direct frustration and complete emotional loneliness. This raised her underlying tension to such a pitch that it became obvious in an agitation which disturbed her usual cheerful surface manner. The impulses to fight and flight—to anger and to escape—were becoming more than she could control.

Each person has his own particular emotional patterns and ways of seeking to satisfy or relieve his feelings. Just as this woman had no means of satisfaction in life except receiving the love of a man, so she had practically no outlet for her anger except against herself. By suicide she could foresee relief from her frustrations and from the hurt to her pride, caused by her failure to achieve a feminine adjustment. Also she could foresee a sort of indirect revenge on life and the gratification of her rage, even though on herself, and an escape from the whole struggle and pain to the peace of infancy— flight as well as introverted fight. She dreamed of death as a return to being an infant with her mother's full love and without all the frustration and struggle of later life. In her dreams she often repre- sented her mother as the sea and dreamed of sleeping on her bosom, even though this peace could be found only through the sleep of death. So her choice of the mode of suicide was through sleep—in the sea or by hypnotic drugs.

Again we look to the childhood history for clues as to why an intelligent and attractive girl should lead so frustrated a life that she should seek surcease in suicide. And again we find in childhood the original of the pattern which we found repeating itself in adult life. Here the traumatic situation was a very close, dependent attach- ment to her mother coupled with her father's open preference for her mother and younger sister, combined with an excessive amount of physical demonstrativeness, with much fondling and kissing. The parents had wanted a girl, but had had two boys, with a gap of many years before the patient was born. But her favored position in the family was soon disturbed by the arrival of the younger sister. The father's rejection of the patient, after her initial spoiling, led to her deep resentment against him and, as is usual, to her transferring this hostility against her father to all men in later life. Rarely if ever does a person have good relationships in adult life, especially close ones, as in marriage, when the relationships with the parents have been bad.

Even more hidden than this hostility toward her father was that felt toward her sister and her mother. This hostility arose from feminine envy and jealousy because the father so openly rejected the patient and adored them. Her mother was a very superior woman, a model wife and mother and socially popular. In addition, she had spent some time in a good business position. She was good to the patient but with so little love that all the patient's normal resentment and envy were turned into guilt feelings.

Another source of guilt in the patient was her envy and jealousy of her younger sister. Normal sibling rivalry is intensified by disorders in feelings toward the parents—in this case by the excessive closeness to her mother plus her father's rejection despite exaggerated petting. The patient's envy became more open later in life when her sister married, had four children and became, like the mother, a symbol of the full feminine love life. The patient's competition with this sister was one reason why she insisted on having all her satisfactions out of life in this form and could not tolerate failure in the feminine sphere. After all, many women do not marry and do not have children. They may not be as happy as some who do—and some who do are not as happy as some of the unmarried women. But they do not all feel driven to suicide by their failures and frustrations, which, after all, everyone must bear in high degree.

Guilt was probably the chief single cause of her masochistic self-frustration. The patient was unconsciously envious and jealous of her mother and sister because of their love lives, and her punishment was the inhibition of her own love life. "Because you hate her for having it, you shall not have it yourself"—this is the precise and logical reaction of the conscience, and it determines the specific nature of the inhibition. The punishment fits the crime, even when this is only an impulse. *More accurately, the punishment fits the source. The punishment is directed to the source of the hostility. What makes the patient angry because he does not get it becomes ironically what he deprives himself of unconsciously* (Saul, 1950).

This woman was saved from suicide because there was one other human tie which she did not lose: the transference, the attachment to the psychiatrist. This tided her over until new ones were formed in her life.*

---

* Apropos suicide, if a person is consciously determined upon this act, little can be done to prevent it except continual hospitalization; and even hospitals as well as companions and private nurses at home are not complete safeguards. The physician is sworn to relieve suffering and prolong life, but the broad question cannot be avoided of the morality of invading a person's privacy and liberty by blocking his determination on suicide. In many cases, the suffering occasioned the patient and those connected with him is so intense and prolonged that in retrospect we must agree that he was correct in his judgment and should not have been forced to live.

Of the many severe cases in the practice of the author, over four decades, only one was lost. It is mostly sympathetic understanding of the dynamics and confidence in the patient and his wishes not to hurt others, including his psychiatrist, which see them through. Where psychosis, alcohol, drugs or sudden uncontrollable life situations are involved, the problem is different.

D. Adults (Psychotic). Early frustration can result in psychotic as well as neurotic reactions. The following case shows this and shows a passive, dependent trend in a very pathological but also an unusually pure and naive form. This patient was a young giant of 22. But this powerful creature had been a severely deprived and rejected child. He did heavy manual work and lunched in a small lunchroom. Here he became attached to one of the waitresses. "Orally" deprived people are apt to be particularly susceptible to waitresses. The term "oral" is used because in these cases desires for love and attention are expressed largely in the form of getting, particularly food or drink, just as in infancy, nursing and being fed are expressions of the mother's love. In the lives, fantasies and dreams of these persons, receptive desires appear repeatedly in this form. They seem to be especially prone to react emotionally with disturbances of stomach or gut. This dynamic is also often a factor in addiction to cigarettes (Saul, 1972b). Especially in such persons is the way to the heart through the stomach. Many men melt at the ministrations of waitresses (and also of nurses). In so doing, they repeat the childhood relation to the mother, in which being fed by her plays such an important role all during infancy and childhood. Be this as it may, our patient developed an irresistible longing for this girl, and he soon dated her. She was nine years older than he, which again is often a sign of particularly strong dependent, receptive tendencies in the man. The patient, infatuated, insisted on marrying her, but she refused. When she refused to see him, he proposed by mail. He gave her gifts and got her a ring, which she refused. It became impossible for her to keep him away and eventually, and reluctantly, she notified the police. He was arrested but was soon released and went directly to her home. After a little time she felt forced to notify the police again. This time the patient was given a month in jail. On his release he again made a beeline for the girl's home. He was arrested for a third time and sentenced to a year in jail. This time when the police asked him what he would do when released he said, with complete obliviousness to the desires and welfare of the person he thinks he "loves," that he could do no other than persist in trying to marry her. True to his word, on his release he went to live with his sister but told her that no matter how much he was jailed he could not but pursue his "love" and again tried to see the girl. Because of his irresistible devotion he was sent to the psychopathic hospital. Here his attitude was the same, namely, that he was driven by a force stronger than himself, that he could not help his behavior, and that what would be done with him was not his responsibility!

Whence comes so strong but so infantile a longing and attachment? As always, the individual's personal history gives the clue. Although hereditary factors may vary considerably from person to person, nevertheless in every case seen clinically, except those in which there is some definite organic disturbance (for example, as reflected in the electroencephalogram), one sees that "there are no problem children but only problem parents," or, at any rate, problem environments. The behavior of the most "ornery" child invariably becomes intelligible as a natural reaction of the child to the treatment to which it is being subjected, and the personality make-up and emotional reactions of the adult to his life situation generally become intelligible in terms of these childhood reactions to the emotional forces to which he has been subjected.

In the present case the development of the pathological longing of this boy of 22 for a woman of 31 was not difficult to trace. Briefly outlined, his story was as follows: His mother died when he was three months old, leaving him and a sister nine years older. The father married almost immediately a woman with three children. The patient, deprived of his mother at three months, was entirely pushed out by the new family, and the stepmother showed no interest in him whatsoever. His only friend in the world during his childhood was his sister, and it may be no mere coincidence that, like her, the girl with whom he became infatuated was nine years older. Probably, as in similar cases, other characteristics of appearance or personality also enabled him to identify her with his sister. When the patient became adolescent, he began to support himself, went out with other boys but was not much interested in girls before the eruption of this infatuation. This powerful fellow, with strong cravings, had but one point of emotional attachment—his sister. When he grew up and his sister married, even this attachment became attenuated; and all his longings for the love, which is the right of every infant and child but which he never had, became fastened on the waitress. His own statement was undoubtedly correct. He "could do no other," for he was driven by a force stronger than himself. Groddeck (1928) was always impressed by this—the fact that "our lives are lived for us" by the emotional forces within us, which are sensed but dimly if at all and in the end are mostly beyond our control. This patient was seen in consultation in the hospital where his emotional life could not be explored further, and it is not known why the outcome was just this, nor what else was going on within him. His behavior led him to a mental hospital where he could satisfy some of his infantile, passive, receptive needs in the form of being given care and freedom from responsibility, but at what a price!

E. Displacements, to Animals, to Things; Addictions. Some children are raised not predominantly with deprivation, rejection and frustration on the one hand, or spoiling on the other, but with a combination of the two, alternately or more or less simultaneously. The effect of such treatment is usually not only to increase the childhood receptive demands but to inject elements of uncertainty or confusion as well. In some cases, it is not so much emotional deprivation by the parents as actual physical deprivation in the form of poverty and fears of not having adequate food or protection that play an important role in the personality development.

In still other cases, parents who reject their children emotionally feel guilty about this and endeavor to compensate for it by providing *things* instead of *love*. It is not uncommon to see parents substitute money for love when the financial situation makes this possible—the "poor little rich child." Sometimes the children themselves substitute animals or inanimate things for people. This is apt to occur when getting love becomes fraught with intolerable uncertainty or when there is a special frustration.

For example, in one such case, the child, a boy, was idolized by his parents. But there had been serious friction between the parents since the very beginning of the marriage, and there were repeated episodes in which the parents separated. They were constantly on the verge of divorce, and there was no family stability or security. The patient transferred his attachment in part from the parents to the house in which the family lived. If he were away with the parents, he felt unhappy, insecure and anxious and insisted on returning home; but if the parents went away, he did not feel insecure or anxious so long as he could be in the house. The impersonal thing, the house itself, represented to him greater security and faithfulness than he could hope for from people, who, after all, are but delicately balanced colloidal suspensions, unpredictable in mood and behavior, without the solidity, steadfastness and permanency of a brick house or a neighborhood.

Such turning for love and security to impersonal substitutes takes other forms also, as we have seen. For example, one man, following the death of his mother, turned to drink as an impersonal substitute to which he clung until he married and could cling to his wife. Other people turn to food and still others to money as impersonal substitutes for the love that they crave. Thus regressive receptive craving can form an important component of addictions, two others being guilt and anger.

F. Alienation, Therapy and Other Groups. The less the love needs are attached to people, animals or things, the more blocked the capacity to give and receive love, the more the person tends to be withdrawn, alienated. So frequent is such blocking in some degree that most people are painfully lonely; and many of the attempts to assuage this emotional isolation are sad, even pitiful, and often bizarre. There is the bar fly, the girl who feels that she is only tolerated as a person if she gives her body sexually, the man who buys companionship with money, and so on. Kurt Lewin and his co-workers were among the first to study the interactions in groups, which with trained professional leadership were called Therapy Groups or T Groups (Lewin, 1951).

But the alienation, especially of the young, half of our population since its explosion being 25 years of age or under, has caused a mushrooming of groups of all sorts—Sensitivity, Confrontation, Scream and dozens of others. "Communication," really emotional rapport, is sought by all devices the imagination can conjure up. In some groups, members tell their life stories and feelings to the group, who comment freely, the purpose being to become more sensitive, more aware of their own make-up and those of others. In other groups, members verbally attack each other. In still other groups, perhaps a dozen nude members of different ages and sexes embrace each other, all intertwined together. Then there is being tossed in a blanket, one member in a circle of others, falling over until caught, the idea being to build trust in others. Then there are the larger assemblages where the sense of belonging is sought through public sexual promiscuity, being paradoxically physical sensation without personal feeling.

Of course, the natural route to closeness is *identification* mentioned above, the normal attraction of those with similar emotional dynamics, the similar emotional forces which underlie community of interest. Certain of the alienated, including those so ill as to be schizophrenic, find identity, acceptance, and some exchange of love in being part of what was called in the 1960's a hippie group or subculture. Their immediate "friends" may be very ill mentally, severe drug addicts, almost completely withdrawn, unable to work or to take responsibility sexually, for self-support, or in any other way, and may have criminal tendencies—but if the child is so alienated, so devoid of ability to love and be loved, but finds here people who accept him or her because of being in some degree like themselves, then to get this love, he drifts into this circle in preference to being totally alone or even being hospitalized. Sometimes good therapeutic results are obtained if the balance of forces in the personality is propitious. Thus a 15-year-old daughter of a relatively affluent family, pushed too hard to climb socially and in other ways, went into reverse. She was totally abandoned sexually, in respect for others and for herself, in all ways. She existed in poverty in a foul, dirty backwash, in a drugged haze, and was in trouble with the police. But there was enough parental love in her dynamics for her to accept treatment eventually, and for her today, now 21, to be married to a reasonably stable boy and to enjoy some security, friends and amenities of life in our country.

G. Violence Proneness: Vandalism, Militancy, Crime, Murder. The receptive dependent love needs can be pathologically intensified by all sorts of mistreatment of the child through omission or commission; in general, the younger the child, the more dire the effects. We have already noted that sudden deprivation of affection, with excellent physical care and no abuse, can cause refusal to eat and death (Spitz and Wolf, 1946; Bowlby, 1956; Mahler, 1965). And these exaggerated needs hurt the pride and are inevitably frustrated in our world of immature adults, where everyone craves love and affection, support, care and direction, and few there are who can give it. Few have the surplus energy let alone the capacity for natural, unselfish giving "object interest" after taking care of themselves and their families. From the hurt pride and thwarted needs for dependence and love come rage, and rage produces a whole range of effects, from internal psychosomatic symptoms or neuroses, through addictions to all sorts of *pathological acting out*, against self as masochism or against others as crimes against property and against persons. If many persons with like dynamics of violence-prone acting out get together, as a mob or organized group, then we see all the forms of force, coercion, and violence with which we are so distressingly familiar. We are speaking only of neurotic violence, symptomatic of personal emotional disorder, however rationalized as political or otherwise. Our point here is the central role that exaggerated receptive dependent love needs can play in this; we will illustrate it in the next chapter after discussing some of the other motivations and reactions that are involved in this outcome.

IN TREATMENT

Dependent love needs are of central importance in treatment. They can help a patient's progress toward cure, i.e., maturity, through his wish for the approval of the therapist, although ultimately he must improve for his own sake and for those who need him. The power of the dependent love needs is great and can also cause difficulties if not fully recognized and dealt with. A young matron with three children goes to a therapist because certain external pressures (death of one close relative, illness of another and other problems) have been causing enough tension to disturb her sleep for some weeks. Several sessions with a young therapist for two months result in adequate improvement. However, the therapist then says that what has been done is superficial and advises full-scale orthodox psychoanalysis five times per week, with the patient lying on the couch. All has gone so well that the young woman reviews the family budget with her husband and concludes that since the doctor advises it, somehow they can manage to swing it.

With her history of early, severe emotional deprivation (including loss of father, then of mother and rearing by a cold grand-mother), the analyst, if he took a careful history, may have suspected that beneath the healthy ego, formed during the excellent first three years with both parents, slumbered intense dependent love needs; and he may have hesitated to advise a procedure which would mobilize them in a person whose life was going so well. But he may have thought they were a threat for the future and that preventive treatment was indicated at this time. I do not know if he began dealing with them immediately as a central issue. Freud never wrote a paper on dependent love needs; hence, although recognized, they are not emphasized in training, and their fateful power in life and in treatment is only beginning to be realized.* Indeed, a recent book by an eminent psychoanalytic authority states that a regression occurs regularly in the process of treatment, and that the reasons for it are unknown. Nor did our highly intelligent, well-read and psychologically sophisticated young woman suspect, in agreeing to full-scale analysis, lying on the couch five times a week, that her conscious reason was largely directed by her underlying dependent love needs themselves. These attracted her like iron to a magnet, like the small child to the mothering which it craves, from the inner and the outer tensions and struggles of adult living to surcease and sympathy, to understanding and support from the analyst.

After three years, during which she learned many interesting things and during which dependence was mentioned, she was utterly "in love with" the analyst and dependent on him, feeling depressed, anxious and trapped. She proposed stopping, but the analyst could only see going on. Two more years passed; her turmoil increased, and she decided to tear herself away despite the analyst's insistence that she continue. She did so—but after two months was so upset that she returned. Two more years went by. Now she was under almost unbearable emotional pressure, keyed up, tense, barely able to control herself or to function, holding herself together by the will power of her good ego, but unable to sleep without increasing dosages of hypnotics or to get through the day without more and more tranquilizers, unlivable with at home, fearing to face other persons. So she finally came for help in breaking out of the transference attachment into which her dependent love needs (DLN) had trapped her securely.

* For an exhaustive though somewhat technical summary of the psychiatric literature on this subject, see Parens, H., and Saul, L. J.: Dependence in Man, New York, International Universities Press, 1971.

As she bitterly poured forth her story, the dynamics emerged clearly. She had transferred to the analyst those biological longings for parental love and care which are so intense in all young mammals. These needs shape the relationships of the young for life and are being studied as "imprinting" by animal ethologists and psychologists (Parens and Saul, 1971).

These needs were intensified in this young woman and less diminished in force through maturing because of the early loss of the parents and the repression of the longings for them by the puritanical grandmother. As these longings were mobilized toward the analyst with mounting power, the young matron, happy with her devoted husband and three children, can think of nothing and no one but her therapist. The frustration of these longings in childhood now recurs, and also, following the childhood pattern, the unrelieved rage which it generates is again controlled, repressed, just as in childhood when she feared that any expression of hostility would bring only coldness and punishment from the grandmother, threatening to diminish what love she had.

Not only the frustration of the hopeless longings caused rage, but also the realization of being trapped, and with this, the blow to her pride, in fact to the most elementary self-respect, of being thus enslaved by her feelings. She could not break away, not only because of the dependence and the love needs but also because the hostility that they engendered created such fear of loss of love and of punishment, that is guilt, just as it did toward her grandmother in childhood.

Another aspect of this is that the analyst too thoroughly became the patient's superego (see Chap. 5), meaning that the patient felt toward the analyst as if she were a small child and he were her parents and grandmother together. If he said, "Stay," she stayed. She dared not go, could not go. If he said she was a poor patient because she did not free associate well, she was cast down in depression. She saw him as punitive and rejecting toward her, partly because of her own guilt for being hostile to him, but partly because, conscientious and ethical though he was, these major motivations had not been sharply focused upon. Much of interest and truth had been discussed, and these motivations had been talked about, but the fundamentals had lost out to the peripheral. Many leaves and twigs were described, but the trunk and the main limbs were not clearly seen. The central core of the transference was not analyzed effectively. Hence, this young woman was dependent for her own opinion of herself on the therapist and not on her own conscience and standards. Her integrity as a person was in abeyance and with it what is intrinsic to it, her self-respect and her self-confidence. Even as she forced out her story through hysterical sobs, she could hardly talk for guilt, because only a few days before she had terminated treatment with her analyst and now felt that she was being critical of him, disloyal to him in her plea to me for help in regaining her independence.

If this sounds critical, it is not meant to be so, except insofar as training in this field is too much directed to "orthodoxy" and has not yet achieved full freedom of observation and thought. This book is an attempt to present the major motivations. Every analyst should discern the interplay of these (main psychodynamics) in most patients in the first interview, but to evaluate *quantitatively* the force of each of these in a given person, including the strength and the adaptability of the ego in controlling these wild horses, is a difficult task. More than the analyst at first suspects may lurk latently beneath a wholesome area of ego—a tendency to severe depression, to paranoid projection and to other severe psychopathology. In this case the dependent love needs became almost overwhelming, but the ego was so strong that no one (apart from her husband, who remained a pillar of strength) suspected what fury threatened it beneath its surface. This is written to demonstrate the power of the dependent love needs. It also shows how little we really know a person, even wife, husband or child, seeing, as we do, only a few facets of the ego out of the whole interplay of emotional forces and the 20 or 30 reactions to them. This note also shows the power of analysis and the importance of proper training in its use, training which rests upon open, critical discussion, upon the use of all related knowledge and upon freedom from authoritarianism and indoctrination. As in all of medicine, *primum non nocere,* the first duty of the physician is to do no harm.

It must be needless to point out that psychotherapy does not create dependent love needs. It can mobilize them in full force, however, as can other situations and other persons, like milk to a kitten. Everyone craves love and care with an intensity ten times greater than he knows—which is why the first two chapters of this book are devoted to these elemental dependent love needs.

The author has dealt elsewhere with the technique of treatment, including legitimate and illegitimate failures (Saul, 1972a), but a few words are in order about this. I saw this young woman for a two-hour session. She spoke with difficulty for over an hour. Beaten as she was, I was sincerely sympathetic and sincerely reassuring, expressing that respect and confidence which she so needed but could not give herself. Everything related above was then freely discussed with her. She followed it all but denied any sense of guilt toward her former analyst, saying that this had no meaning to her. A few minutes later she said: "I can hardly go on because I feel so guilty for breaking off with him and for talking about him to you." I called this to her attention, and she was able to laugh. I explained that analytic treatment moves best when the transference of the childhood feelings toward the analyst is of optimal intensity. If it is too weak, little progress is made. If it is too strong—that she knew all too well. When the intensity is so great as to obstruct treatment and remain unresolved for years, then it is often an effective procedure for the patient to see a second analyst in order to reduce the too-intense feelings toward the first one by accurate analysis of them. I told her that she could have at least two therapists to substitute for the one she had left; that I would put her in touch with one who well understood this emotional constellation and that I would be in touch with him, with her original analyst, and with her as long as need be. I told her directly that I had confidence in her and that she, who had lost it, should have it also. Then her husband, the only other person who knew everything and had been a rock of support, was invited in, and the three of us discussed everything freely. The next days were continuing agony for the patient. She saw the specially selected analyst twice in the week, and I phoned her two other times. At the end of ten days she felt much easier, was off tranquilizers and, except for occasional small doses of hypnotics, was sleeping naturally again. Spurred by suffering, she continued to move up on the way out. After two months the biweekly visits were reduced to once a week and then discontinued after eight months. She maintained her progress on her own for the next year and, happily, has gained much of value for the rest of her life. It is doubtful whether her dependent love needs will ever so embroil her again in real life or in transference, for she is now well acquainted with them and their power. She is psychologically vaccinated against them.

SOCIOLOGICAL IMPLICATIONS

The sociological implications of these human tendencies are far-reaching. The give-get balance (between PRD, Passive-Receptive-Dependent, and RPI, Responsible-Productive-Independent) plays a major role in the degree of social responsibility and productivity that can be expected from any individual. To the degree that he is giving and can accept interests outside himself, he will be able to contribute to wife, family, business or profession and to the community. If, on the other hand, his orientation is too much toward getting or taking, our country appears only as a rich land to be exploited in which men compete only to get the most. This is reflected in certain of our ideologies.

As President John F. Kennedy expressed it in his inaugural address: "Ask not what your country can do for you, but what you can do for your country."

Much of the turmoil, strife and man-made suffering in our nation and in the world results from pathological dependent receptive love needs in so many individuals. That is why history records changes in the *form* of hostile aggression but little or no basic amelioration of it or increase in good will and cooperation. A first step toward our goal should be the slogan of Planned Parenthood: "Every child a wanted child." This would at least insure every newborn a proper start.

REFERENCES

Alexander, F. (1961): *The Scope of Psychoanalysis,* edited by T. French. New York: Basic Books.
_____ and Healy, W. (1935): *Roots of Crime.* New York: Knopf.
Balzac, H. (1889): *Deux Femmes.* Paris: Calmann-Lévy.
Bowlby, J. (1956): *Mother-Child Separation, Mental Health and Infant Development,* ed. by K. Soddy. New York: Basic Books.
Brill, A. (1946): *Lectures on Psychoanalytic Psychiatry.* New York: Knopf.
Freud, S. (1912): The dynamics of transference, *S.E.* 12.
Groddeck, G. (1928): *Book of the It.* New York: Nervous and Mental Disease Publishing Co.
Lewin, K. (1951): *Field Theory in Social Science,* ed. by D. Cartwright. New York: Harper.
Lorenz, K. (1952): *King Solomon's Ring.* New York: Crowell.
Mahler, M. (1965): On the significance of the normal separation-individuation phase, in: *Drives, Affects, Behavior,* Vol. 2, ed. by M. Schur. New York: International Universities Press, pp. 161–169.
Parens, H. and Saul, L. J. (1971): *Dependence in Man.* New York: International Universities Press.

Saul, L. J. (1950): The punishment fits the source, *Psychoanalytic Quarterly* 19:164.

—— (1972a): *Psychodynamically Based Psychotherapy*. New York: Science House.

—— (1972b): Dynamics of cigarette addiction, *International Journal of Psychoanalytic Psychotherapy* 1(2):24–30.

Spitz, R. (1956): Chapter in *Mental Health and Infant Development*, ed. by K. Soddy. New York: Basic Books, pp. 103–108.

—— (1971): The adaptive viewpoint: its role in autism and child psychiatry, *Journal of Autism and Childhood Schizophrenia* 1(3):239–245.

—— and Wolf, K. (1946): Anaclitic depression, in: *Psychoanalytic Study of the Child*, Vol. 2. New York: International Universities Press.

4 | Egoism, Competitiveness, Inferiority and Power

GENERAL FORMULATION

An old friend and wise physician once said to me, "We all have more ego that we wot of." (He used the term to mean egoism.) Freud remarked that one's ego is the yardstick by which one measures the world. Freud introduced the term "narcissism" to signify the libidinal form of egoism, after the myth of Narcissus, who fell in love with his own image in the pool.

1. Source

Why this enormous self-interest? Its nucleus is intelligible enough as an expression of the tendency to self-preservation ("primary narcissism"). As such we might expect it to be especially strong in childhood when the energies of the organism are normally directed so largely to its own growth and development and when the emotional interests of the family are so centered upon it. If the child has some weakness or defect, the parents may tend to compensate for it by lavishing still more attention and affection upon it. And, just as the cat licks a wound, the child tends to compensate with self-love for weaknesses or feelings of inferiority of all sorts. Such self-interest and self-love represent a tendency to heal the defect or compensate for it ("reactive or secondary narcissism"). Demosthenes had to become an orator to cure his speech defect, to overcome it, hide it, compensate for it. Many a daredevil is "counter phobic," i.e., feels compelled to prove his fearlessness—because he must deny the deeper feeling, his fear. Most persons have certain attitudes, needs, desires, inhibitions; or the like, which hurt their self-esteem, and they react with anger and efforts at compensation.

The child is, in reality, weak, helpless, dependent. He tries to overcome these feelings by making himself stronger; but this is a slow process, so he also tends to hide them, deny them, compensate for them, by insisting on his superiority in all sorts of ways and by fantasying it himself and through such characters of the comics, radio and television as Tarzan, Superman and other all-powerful, invincible figures.

But why the tremendous egoism of the adult, who is full-grown and holds a place in the world? In the adult it strikes one as childish—and this is what it comes down to. We have seen that the childish reactions persist in every adult and remain powerful, if more or less unconscious, motivations in his life. Among these tendencies we have discussed the needs for love, care, attention and dependence, and we have seen that they run counter to the trends toward independence, productivity, responsibility for, and giving to, others. When they are too strong and not in normal balance, the adult feels that this part of him is still the weak, receptive, help-seeking, affection-craving, dependent little child—quite different, usually, from the strong, capable, mature, self-reliant, interested, giving adult which he and the rest of the world expect him to be. So he must try to heal, hide or compensate for this weakness or defect which causes the feeling of inferiority, the threat to his security, the wound to his self-regard and the threat to his esteem by others. And so adults continue to escape into exaggerated self-love and they tend, as in childhood, constantly to compare themselves with others, to measure themselves against others and to strive in one form or another to believe in their power and superiority or actually to achieve these in reality.

2. Early Model

The model for the comparison and the competition is the child's relations with the members of its own family. Competition between brothers and sisters is usually intense and obvious. When it is not evident, nevertheless it may be even more intense because the parents have suppressed it. The competition with the parents, although usually much more hidden, is apt to be even deeper-going, particularly with the parent of the same sex. The father and his emotional attitudes are of great importance in the forming of the son's goals and ideals. We see in adults a re-edition of the childhood emotional constellation of passive-receptive-dependent needs, which cause continuing feelings of weakness and inferiority and then a compensatory heightening of the self-interest, self-love and vanity, with all sorts of efforts, in fantasy and reality, to overcome these feelings and a constant comparison with others and intensified competition with them. Many people—very many, for this is a common emotional constellation or complex, in our culture—live their whole lives trapped in this vortex, reacting in a way which, on our scale of development, is normal for about middle childhood when a person first feels his oats, tests his strength and tries himself out against others and the world. (This period was called by Freud the "phallic phase," power and masculinity being symbolized by largeness of the phallus, unconsciously and in conscious wish.) Could they but disengage themselves from this automatic, unconsciously operating pattern and free their energies for devotion to their families, friends, interests and productive accomplishments, they would be stronger, more effective and more free of their inner dissatisfactions. Of course, this competitive drive carries many to worldly success but hardly to true satisfaction in life. Sometimes it leads only to futile attempts to overcome the feelings of inferiority by all sorts of fads, pretense and artificiality.

3. Feelings of Inferiority

The passive-receptive-dependent desires are not the sole source of feelings of weakness and inferiority. These can arise from all sorts of disturbances of development, from physical defects and from such impairments as intellectual retardation. Shakespeare's *King Richard III* justifies his brutality and lust for power by saying that it is only a second choice, forced on him because he is deformed and cannot be loved by women like other men. (1916) Guilt can cause feelings of inferiority; and fear is felt by many as a terrible affront to the pride. One man killed another whom he thought cast some aspersion on his bravery.

Another source of inferiority feelings is the emotional, regressive force in one's own nature. If the individual is emotionally mature, his various defects do not throw him into the vainglorious competitive struggle. Such people find it much easier to live with their defects if they *live and let live,* follow their own interests, their own loves, their own accomplishments. They minimize the handicap—while others exaggerate it, let it alter their whole lives, i.e., overreact to it emotionally. Many people do so even with minor defects—this one wants to be taller, this one shorter, this one cannot tolerate thinning hair or advancing age. If a person keeps *busy and useful and lives for his loves and interests* and not for his vanities, he is freed from this whole strain, which is otherwise inevitable, for, after all, no one is perfect, no one can be superior in everything. If he lives for vanity and always compares himself with others, he is sure to be constantly hurt. So his defects diminish in importance the greater the emotional maturity and object interest of the individual. But when the defect itself consists of emotional immaturity, the problem is more difficult. Hence, in all cases, regardless of what defects are obvious or are advanced by the person as a reason for his feelings of inferiority, we must look for a deeper reason in the emotional development.

4. Relation to Hostility

The emotional constellation which we have been discussing has a deeper, more sinister side. Probably any threat to the organism, whether from the outer world or from within, causes physiological mobilization for fight or flight, manifested psychologically as hostility and anxiety. Weakness and inferiority are wounds to the self-regard and are also sources of insecurity socially, sexually, occupationally. Small wonder if they are sensed as dangers and felt as constant irritants against which the individual is powerless. All these mechanisms may be predominantly unconscious, the person not realizing the source nor the complex chain of emotional reactions that is set in operation. He can but rage impotently because he feels something to be wrong about himself but cannot define or overcome it. Hence, anger, resentment, rage, however hidden, are the usual accompaniments of this reaction. The feelings of weakness and inferiority cause such hostility, in some cases, that not only neuroses and psychoses result, but also criminality (Saul, 1976, pp. 52–58); the individual tries to overcome a sense of weakness through violence, mistaking hostile aggression for masculinity, and striving with it for power as a denial of weakness. The importance in human affairs of this neurotic overcompensatory will to power cannot be exaggerated. It is amply evident in many current movements, especially the disruptive ones.

An incident was once told me of a man who did not object to appearing in court but begged that it not be made known that he was caught with only a .38-caliber revolver and not a .45. At least part of the appeal of some criminal careers probably lies in the fact that they offer the egoistic satisfaction of feeling independent, adventurous, tough and masculine without the usual cost in social accomplishment and productivity. It also offers outlets for hostilities from many sources, including those from feelings of weakness, and can serve as a denial of anxiety and a protest of fearlessness.

5. Envy

The hostility and anxiety have another closely related source. They spring not only from the person's feelings about himself but also from his envy of others. He feels inadequate, compares himself with others, competes with them, envies them. It has been stated that nothing is so hard to look upon as someone else's good fortune. "Anyone," said Oscar Wilde, "can sympathize with a friend's misfortune, but it takes an exceptionally fine character to sympathize with his success." This envy and competitiveness generate a hostility which is usually deep-going and can be of murderous intensity. Misery loves company. The hostility causes guilt and fear of retaliation and so augments the anxiety caused by the weakness. This anxiety increases the desire to escape it all and to regress to the protected, dependent situation of the child, thus forming a vicious circle. Omitting various interrelationships, and with no pretensions to a well-rounded formulation of the organic reality, we can represent this now well-known emotional constellation in schematic form in Figure 2.

The commandments of the great religions and the basic principles of law preserve society against these neurotically heightened motivations in people. If all were reared with good feelings toward parents and therefore matured into adults of good will, there would be little need for law. As it is, the fundamental commands and prohibitions reveal clearly the tendencies in exaggerated infantile,

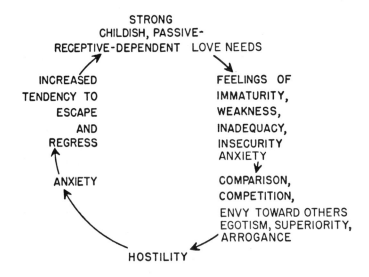

Figure 2

emotionally sick people to do the opposite. "Love thy neighbor" would not be so great a commandment if people did not tend to do the opposite. It is not necessary to tell people to breathe. "Honor thy parents" is a commandment because so many parents raise their children in ways which, by fiat and example, do not inspire honor. Adultery and murder are forbidden because there are enough emotionally ill people to commit these. And among the primary prohibitions is envy—"thou shalt not covet"—things, nor animals, nor people, including wife. Thus, envy ranks with the fundamental tendencies and when neurotically heightened, threatens individuals and society. And jealousy is largely envy when affection, love and sex are involved. Envy has at least two components—the wish to take for one's self what the other person has, and anger and hate against him for having it.

Pride precedes a fall often because of the envy it excites. Envy, like so much in the disordered unconscious, irrationally knows no age difference. A child of 14 feels murderous hate against a man of 60 because the latter, after a lifetime of arduous work, has won income and position and drives a fine car. Envy has played a central note in student and racial disorders and is a very important part of the irrational, emotional motivations and methods. This envy is intensified, of course, by inner feelings of weakness and inferiority. It may be that even relatively mature youth of good-will, inexperienced as yet in responsible work and breadwinning of the kind that makes a nation hold together, harbors some envy of those who have already made their way, achieved money, position and power. It is well known that poverty alone does not cause great unhappiness or revolution, but that it is the relative position, the comparison with those who have more. An example is the Caribbean Islands, long quiet havens, but now, seeing the affluent vacationing in luxurious hotels, resorts, and homes, seething with envy and hate which, of course, takes form as crime and revolution. Of course, the Communists are specialists in recognizing and organizing this envy and drive of the weak for power, and our defense has been the prevention of too wide gulfs between haves and have-nots; but these gulfs are not made *entirely* by the system, or any system, but in part by the emotional disorders of individuals—more by the irrational, emotional, than by what could be if mature, realistic motives and behavior ruled in everyone. And one dire effect of this is the population explosion which multiplies all of our problems manifold. (Do any parents have the energy and patience to rear *properly* more than four children?) Envy is a basic force in cruelty and violence in all their forms. Therefore, it is perhaps appropriate that a much needed comprehensive study of envy has now been written by a sociologist, who deals with it as "a fundamental problem of man" (Schoeck, 1970).

6. Typical Pattern

We have said that the dynamics diagrammed in Fig. 2 with all sorts of individual variations, are extremely common. The competition can take innumerable forms; so can the escapes; the hostility comes out in many different ways, and the anxiety is variously handled, but the basic pattern remains. With almost monotonous frequency, one finds such a state of affairs as this: The patient was, as a child, spoiled, overprotected, forced out too early, dominated, deprived or otherwise so treated; he still craves love and protection. He finishes his education, reaches adult life, faces his career. But his whole being rebels against standing alone, taking responsibility, fending for himself and for a family. He wants too strongly love, care, admiration, support, protection. Of course, he may not know this consciously, or if he is aware of it, he does not appreciate its power in his personality. He only feels that something is wrong, that he does not have the same interest, outlook, attitude and independence in his relations to people and to his work that so many other men seem to have or that his father had. He keeps measuring himself against them, consciously or unconsciously. He envies them their positions, poise, assurance, independence, grasp of reality and other qualities of maturity—and, consciously or unconsciously, he hates them for those attributes. The greater he feels the discrepancy to be, the more enraged is he apt to become. But he dare not express this, for he feels that they are strong and he is weak, still like a child in relation to his parents. So it only increases his anxiety and may cause many other symptoms—insomnia, nightmares, headaches, phobias and so on. He feels that he cannot hold his own with them, so he shunts his ambitions into a different field. His father was successful in a profession, so he goes into business, or vice versa. Or he may feel that he cannot compete in these ways and so seeks to be superior in other ways. At any rate, he finds some field in which he competes directly or indirectly. But his insecurity and inferiority are still with him, because of his immature emotional orientation, and they drive him to excessive work and competition. He feels driven, and this is unpleasant and a strain. He works not simply out of interest and enjoyment, to produce, to give and to win what he needs; his energies are not free to love his family and to enjoy his hobbies and amusements. He works because he feels driven and he works in an atmosphere of competition and hate and so of guilt, retaliation and fear. He never achieves security, for his insecurity is within, and his outlook makes of life a race and a struggle, with his hand against others as rivals and their hands against him. The anxiety mounts and his rage mounts, and with it perhaps his blood pressure and his drinking. The strain begins to tell, and by middle life he shows all sorts of effects of the strain, physically and mentally. He wants to escape, to find a refuge, to be cared for, but this he dare not do—it increases his insecurity—he is caught in the merry-go-round. He may fail or he may become a model of success and achievement. But on our scale he is a struggling, suffering child.

Such a person is apt to envy and compete in two directions—

toward those who are stronger and more mature and also toward those who satisfy their receptive and dependent desires.

Another vicious circle can result, in a rather paradoxical fashion, from needs for admiration. It is readily exemplified by a young woman who felt that she must be attractive to and admired by every person she met. This need to create such a very favorable impression soon operated as a strong resistance in treatment. It was a continuation of her childish needs for parental approval. In life it put her at the mercy of everyone she met. Unconsciously, she felt that she must be subservient to every person and never could be herself independently because of being so dependent on others for admiration. This made her feel inadequate, childish, inferior, but now she sought to assuage these feelings of inferiority by show- ing that she was attractive and admirable. Hence, the more she sought admiration, the more childish, dependent and inferior she felt; and the more inferior she felt, the more she sought admiration. The resolution of her resistance and the reopening of her emotional development followed the resolution of this vicious circle.

In the emotional life all is quantitative. "Infantile" and "quan- titative" are two of the most important keys to the life of the mind. Within limits, all the motivations and the reactions which we have been describing are perfectly normal. They become "neurotic" only as they exceed these limits and interfere with development to mature attitudes and the operation and the enjoyment of these. Self-interest is natural and normal, insofar as it works, for the individual and society. But pride goeth before a fall. Exaggerated egoism and competitiveness so often arise as reactions to underly- ing dependence and inferiority that when they appear some such underlying weakness must be expected. Further experience has confirmed this. For example, one would expect a snobbishly reared child to become a snobbish adult because of this simple condition- ing. However, in the author's clinical experience, where one goes beneath the surface, it is not at all unusual to find a very liberal person who comes from a very snobbish background (which may be obvious to an observer), but never yet have I seen real snobbery which did not stem from some underlying disorder of emotional development, often somewhat as described above. Probably it is always a sign of hidden difficulties.

ILLUSTRATIONS WITH SOME DYNAMIC CONNECTIONS

1. Narcissism

Despite an occasional brief, schematic, metapsychological definition of narcissism in the psychoanalytic literature such as
"cathexis of the self" (Kohut, 1971) the concept of *narcissism,* if
not as Freud originally advanced it as self-love (1914) then as it has
come to be generally used by analysts today, and as this author has
read it and heard it used, remains broad and imprecisely defined.
This breadth impairs its sharpness of definition but gains the convenience of covering many components. Freud of course took the
term from mythology but there is no reason why, more than half a
century later, scientific study should continue to be restricted by
the picture of Narcissus who, after heartlessly rejecting lovely
Echo, falls in love with his own image in the silvery pool. One of
our tasks as analysts is to dissect this conveniently broad term into
its components.

Taking a random clinical example, John feels superior to all of his
classmates in engineering school and at the same time inferior to
them. These two complexes of feelings seem clearly interrelated:
the sense of inferiority derives from the fact that his classmates
have outwardly happy or at least workable marriages and they are
moving toward recognizable goals in life. John feels desperately
alone because he is not married but goes home each day to an
empty apartment where he has begun to try to relieve his loneliness
by drinking. Without a wife, John can formulate no goals for himself. He is attractive and had once nearly married, but the girl with
whom he was intimately involved emotionally had broken off the
relationship and left him. They were still infatuated with each other
in a mutually destructive way. Without her, John all but gave up
completely on life and went through a suicidal period lasting several months. This near-psychotic episode revealed the depth of his
dependence upon the girl, Marge, and also the intensity of his
needs to be accepted, valued, esteemed, and otherwise highly regarded. These needs were violently wounded by Marge's rejection
of him.

Since that rejection he has felt inferior rather than superior to all
his peers; he says he is like a dependent, crawling baby, dependent

for companionship, without which he cannot exist but would commit suicide, dependent on those very peers he once felt were beneath him intellectually, esthetically, academically, physically, creatively, professionally and in sophistication. John had always been popular with many of his own generation but had never maintained an individual close friendship with boy or girl until Marge broke down his defenses by her persistent pursuit of him over a period of four years. Then when he yielded to her attractions, she immediately perceived the emergence of his extreme emotional dependence upon her, complained about it bitterly and fought it off as best she could. Her efforts were unsuccessful, and in failing generated a hostility between them that was destroying them both until she separated from him.

John's dependence threatened and impaired his independent functioning in life, and wounded his needs for self-esteem and feelings of ability and worth; this caused his feelings of inferiority, to which he reacted with over-compensatory needs to prove his superiority. But then these needs for superiority caused exaggerated competition with his peers, with extremely hostile envy of them and subsequent guilt and anxiety, which in turn reinforced inferiority feelings, forming a vicious circle with intensified feelings of both inferiority and superiority and fight-flight reactions of rage, anxiety, depression, masochism, alcoholism and suicidal tendencies.

As John struggled with all this he was, of course, much occupied with his own feelings, needs, emotional struggles and survival. Overall, these comprised the human needs to receive attention, status, prestige, to be well regarded, to be valued, esteemed, admired, approved of by himself and by others, both as an individual and in comparison with others. These seem to be the elements of what we generally call "narcissism," or at least some important components of it.

One incident clarified the point and revealed how similar Marge's dynamics of extreme dependence and narcissistic love needs were to John's: during John's relationship with her they were attending a small, purely casual early-evening social gathering of a half dozen couples. He happened to be standing while his friends and acquaintances were mostly seated, and at one point most of the group was attentively listening to John. Marge could not stand to see him receiving all this approving attention instead of receiving it herself. Her facial expression, attitude and subsequent actions and remarks unmistakably conveyed her envy, anger and rage from her own hurt narcissism. She wanted for herself everything in the attention being paid to John. Just as pure sunlight is in reality composed of a mixture of violet, indigo, blue, green, yellow, orange and red, so too normal narcissism is composed of a mixture of components. Clinically we often see any one of these components or any combination of them in exaggerated form.

Narcissism, then, seems to have many components, and through quantitative factors these can be healthy or pathologically exaggerated, inhibited or distorted, overall or in part. We can see reasons for the variations by examining the childhood emotional pattern in each case. The universal factor in childhood is the smallness, weakness and helplessness of the child and its utter dependence upon its parents or other adults and upon how much attention, adulation and feelings of value it receives from them. The child grows up feeling this combination of inferiority and superiority. The degree to which it outgrows these feelings or is fixated in them, in general or in particular aspects, depends upon the specific emotional and physical influences (such as acceptance, rejection, etc.) upon the child during his earliest, most formative years from conception to age about six. John, for example, was a first child, fervently wanted, loved and adored. He grew up feeling loved in spite of other interactions which made problems. He enjoyed his parents' adulation and continued to desire it from others; also, this attitude of his parents he took over toward himself. It made him continue to feel he was "the best," superior to others. But insofar as he was fixated in this residue of childhood and had failed to outgrow it, he felt like a small child in a world of adults. Compared to them, he felt inferior and reacted with exaggeration of his feelings of superiority. In fact, narcissism can be defined very roughly and in the popular but perhaps not most accurate sense as an exaggerated need to be "the best," in a word, as "bestism."

Another clinical example is Leonard, who at age three lost his father in an accident. Leonard and his baby brother were burdens to their mother who was seeking a job to support them and also seeking another husband. Leonard grew up in the universal inferiority of child compared to parent, affected by the very specific interaction of loss of father and the subsequent partial neglect and deprivation by mother. The form of his narcissism, therefore, and its conflicts were different from the previous example of John.

We have remarked the two additional regular contributors to the intensity and form of each individual's inferiority and superiority feelings and their interactions: the oedipus complex and the sibling relations. A boy child is in reality weak and helpless compared with his father. And depending upon his position in the age line of children and also upon the personalities of the parents and the sex and personalities of his siblings, he lives through his 0–6 in certain situations of inferiority and superiority to each and all members of the family.

We can conclude that the components of the inferiority-superiority feelings, i.e., of the narcissism and its conflicts in the individual, consist of and are specifically determined (1) by the *general* inferiority of the baby and small child he once was in relation to the adults upon whom he depended; (2) by the specific factors of the individual's oedipal and sibling situations; and (3) by the particular personalities of his parents and others close to him and responsible for him, especially from 0 to 6. And we can see why narcissism in all its forms and conflicts is so universal an element of human nature, in health and in psychopathology, and why it is so difficult to outgrow, overcome or diminish.

Not infrequently, the term "narcissism" is used in a pejorative sense and equated with vanity, pride or egotism. In light of the previous discussion, however, it seems that narcissism is not all pathological or deplorable. Rather, it is like any other "instinct," such as sex or the dependence or love needs that vary in their form, intensity and objects, from healthy to deviant. Pride, vanity and egotism appear as special forms of narcissism in which an individual praises himself excessively. As in all of the emotional life, it is mostly quantitative, a matter of degree, as we have emphasized throughout.

2. Pre-natal Fixation

The therapeutic struggles were considerable to keep John realistic enough and motivated sufficiently to get through engineering school and then to hold his job against his almost irresistible dependence upon Marge and his mother, and his passive desires to give up all effort and live on his parents' money so long as it was being provided. During these struggles I often wondered if his extreme dependence and hostility were entirely reactive to the pressures upon him in babyhood or if there might be some genetic impairment of the drives to independence, interest and accomplishment.

I often would think of Bill and Karen, as emotionally healthy a couple as I had ever met; my wife and I saw them when they were proud parents, a few weeks after the birth of their first child. My wife, as soon as she held the baby, remarked, ''You are a tense little thing.'' He was indeed—not only with us but with Karen, his mother, and so he remained. Little Billy was never as warm, cuddly or responsive as his two brothers who arrived after him at two-year intervals. This emotional distance, alienation even, that was so evident from birth continued as part of Billy's personality. He was never close to his parents or brothers, and showed little warmth to anyone. He made no close friends and was not popular in school and with the neighborhood children. This was partly because he was so self-centered, so inconsiderate of others and so readily hostile to them, whether boys or girls. Billy antagonized people and then complained that people did not like him. His parents were truly loving and sought advice on how to help him, for they feared for his future if these patterns continued, patterns that were easily traceable to birth and certainly not reactive to any lack of true love and tender care.

And often I would think of Julie, a young woman of 30 who complained violently about her inability to marry or achieve any rapport with others, or to have any interest in anything, much less hold a job of any kind. In this case also the absence of rapport with others, including her parents, her dependence on them and her hostility to them and her passivity were extreme, and from what I could learn from many interviews with her parents, traced back to the first days after her birth.

The overall impression (and there seems to be no way to establish or disprove it at present) is that there is a fixation of a part of the personality at a pre-natal stage. Something failed to develop adequately in the transition from the placental, unborn condition to the neonatal stage of interpersonal relations between child and mother. And it is this inability to relate emotionally to the mother which so distresses the child and the parents as time goes by. The child grows physically but fails to socialize fully or form truly close, gratifying relations. One controversial theory is that minimal brain damage (MBD) exists, too slight to be detectable, and therefore unprovable.

It is a difficult and lengthy process to ascertain that this partial pre-natal fixation is present in the psychodynamics. It usually carries a guarded prognosis and means that analytic therapy will be even longer and more difficult than what is required to correct interpersonal traumata that occurred in the first year after birth.

It is likely that partial pre-natal fixation is present in the borderline or psychotic characters, and may well turn out to be the key to understanding them.

3. Literature

Narcissism, egotism, is so strong a force in people that it is almost impossible to overestimate it. Object interest signifies the enjoyment of interest in people and things outside the self. This is illustrated in Shakespeare's *Julius Caesar*. The speech of Brutus portrays Caesar as ambitious for himself and advances this alone as sufficient reason to have slain him. But Mark Antony claims that Caesar was not motivated by self-love, by the prestige and power of being emperor, but by a genuine unselfish interest in the people of Rome. The physician who is interested primarily in his patients, or the businessman in his clients, has "object interest." When the emotion attaches only to personal advancement, this is "narcissistic." Accomplishment and success, with inner satisfaction instead of neurotic suffering, are better achieved with object interest, which is an expression of emotional maturity. When the self-interest fuses with object interest, the result is apt to be maximum accomplishment and maximum satisfaction. Working for self-love alone, without object interest, is apt to be the wrong way to achieve real satisfaction. As Ibsen expressed it in *Peer Gynt*, his beautiful, semimystical study of egoistic compensation for boyish immaturity: "To be yourself, lose yourself"—forget yourself in outside interests and you find and realize your full capacities and adult nature. (In Matthew 7:7: "Who shall lose himself for my sake shall find himself.'') Without this, something is always lacking despite all outer success.*

4. Animals

How fundamental egoistic competition is, becomes evident from a glance at a few of its manifestations in animals. Perhaps it is one reason why certain horses insist on being in the lead and why some cows fight for priority in going through the gate. An owner of dog kennels told me that a bitch will be frightfully upset if her pups are taken from her while the other bitches still have theirs. But the same dog will object hardly at all to the removal of her pups if the other bitches do not have any. This does not mean that the only motivation in these cases is self-esteem; but these examples show that this self-regard or narcissism is not an exclusively human psychological refinement but is a biological reaction seen in varying degree in members of other species.

5. Children

Its manifestations begin at a very early age. Before the age of two, a child may show a tremendous drive to be the equal of the grown-ups and may bitterly resent being treated as a baby. It may insist on opening the door by itself or on carrying its own plate from the table if the parents do (this may, of course, have other motivations). It may refuse to obey commands because its pride is hurt, but very soon may carry out the order with a show of doing whatever it is, not on the command, but of its own volition.

When self-love becomes exaggerated through wounds to it and

---

* GOSPEL OF ART

Who works for glory
Misses oft the goal.
Who works for money
Coins his very soul.
Work for the work's sake
Then, and it might be
That these things shall
Be added unto thee.
    Author unknown. From
    Dr. and Mrs. Hallowell Davis.

through reactions against inferiority feelings, one common mechanism is the reaction: "If others do not give me the praise, interest, admiration and love that I crave, then I will give it to myself." But self-love can also be cultivated directly. One young man was so much the center of his family circle that he grew up impervious to any realistic judgment of himself or others, feeling about himself as his adoring parents had felt about him throughout his childhood—that he was a most superior person whose slightest wishes should be the first concern of those about him.

Let us consider a little boy who showed clearly the sort of regressive reaction described in the preceding chapters, but also an egoistic rebound and defense against them. This little boy's regressive tendencies were stimulated by his baby brother. When away from home he was his usual self-reliant little self. But as soon as he entered his house and saw his baby brother being fed and cared for and the center of attention, he fell back to his own baby attitudes. He demanded to be dressed and bathed and fed, although he had taken pride in being able to do these things for himself and often had refused help even when his parents wanted to assist him. When the baby crawled, he often crawled, and sometimes he demanded his milk from a bottle. He became generally sloppy, careless and dirty when in the house and in this way forced from his mother the kind of care and attention he had had as an infant, which his baby brother now enjoyed. If the baby were given praise or attention, he would become demanding and aggressive and often ended up by dashing out of the house, frequently hurting himself by falling down or in some other way, thereby taking out his hostile feelings on himself. These regressive manifestations in young children have long been known to mothers and to other observers of children. The new child and the care and the attention it receives stimulate the older child's regressive envy and jealousy, arousing in him strong wishes for the same attentions. Outgrown so far as overt behavior went, these wishes can remain latent, and seeing them gratified for the baby by the child's own parents brings them again into the open. Also, there is usually resentment on the part of the older child because of being forced out of the baby position by the new child.

The child, even the small child, usually has another reaction also, a prestige reaction. The little boy we have mentioned had been proud of his achievements and his independence and had a great urge to be grown up. Now that in reality, in reaction to the new baby, he behaved in infantile fashion again, he placed exaggerated emphasis on being grown up. He made a great issue of his age and became very angry when he was told that a friend of his was a few months older than he and not younger. His boasts about his knowledge and his prowess became extravagant. He began to speak of other children as "dumb" and "silly." He crossed the street without permission, like the big children. In short, the more the babyish desires came to the surface in his thoughts and behavior, the greater became his egoism. The more he competed with his baby brother for infantile goals, the greater the prestige issue and the more he competed for adult goals and the more he depreciated anyone over whom he could find any superiority, chiefly, of course, the baby brother. He was no longer his sweet self but quite aggressive and hostile in his behavior. Also, he began to pick at his skin, to suffer from nightmares, to want a night light and to show subtler signs of fear and anxiety. That is, he developed symptoms which signified unrelieved anger turned against himself. He showed the same conflict which we have described in adults, regressive trends → inferiority feelings → compensatory egoism and egoistic competitiveness → hostility → anxiety.

The fact that when the little boy was away from home or even alone with his parents his infantile and aggressive behavior vanished was a favorable sign, for it showed that the process was reversible and that he would go on with his development, without having it greatly hindered by the infantile, regressive forces. This conflict represents a psychological manifestation of the biological forces of development and regression.

The reactions of the first child to the second are strong, but if both are loved wisely no serious problems result.

6. Adults

A. Marriage, deplorably, is often a place to observe narcissism in operation in all its meanings. Most common is male chauvinism, seen in the husband who wants a divorce because he sees himself as so superior to his wife intellectually that he is "bored" by her. To him the wife's love, devotion, warmth, loyalty, hearth, home and fine children mean little. He is so narcissistic in the sense of his own egocentric, selfish desires that he rationalizes his actions in seeking everything *he* wants, even believing that if his wife loves him she should be happy to allow his comings and goings with no regard to her meal schedules, having other women and bringing these women to the home. In addition, such a husband takes it for granted that he is superior to his wife in all ways and should therefore pursue *his* own career and desires because only *his* life is important, not hers. Such feelings are often straight oedipal, a repetition of his relations as a baby or small child with his mother. He expects his wife now, as his mother once did, to serve him and adore him, giving, giving, giving, without his seeing her as a human being with her own needs. Often this failure in mature "object interest" toward his wife and "identification" with her go so far as to reveal an emotional withdrawal that is definitely schizoid. Of course women who are subjected to mistreatment as small children also grow up with narcissistic problems although usually in slightly different form.

B. Neurosis. A brilliantly successful young man of 30, with an income in the higher brackets, had a lovely wife and children, was immensely popular, a pillar of the community, a church supporter, a member of the best clubs and a fine athlete. Let us call him Mr. Q. He was entirely self-made. But one flaw spoiled everything. He suffered from attacks of palpitations (essentially rapid and over-forceful heartbeat) and when these occurred he became acutely anxious and feared that he would die. Then he would see his physician, who kept him going by reassuring him. But after a few years the attacks became more frequent, he grew more and more tense, he no longer slept well, and the anxiety attacks became so severe that they handicapped his work. So the physician referred him to a psychiatrist as a neurotic problem.

An inquiry into the circumstances in which the extrasystoles and anxieties occurred yielded an immediate clue to the causes. He had had such an attack on the preceding day, although he had felt fine all that morning. He had met Bill by chance at lunch. When he said, "How are you?" Bill replied, "Wonderful—just closed a $50,000 deal." At this the patient felt a trifle dizzy; he ordered lunch but felt his heart pounding. The patient knew that his doctor insisted that his heart was perfect but wondered what this could be. During the afternoon the over-action continued. He became more anxious and began to fear that he would die young. He did not relish his dinner and retired, feeling tired and tense. He could not fall asleep for a long time, and when he did he had a nightmare about climbing up a hill with men attacking him.

Bill turned out to be one of a half dozen men in the patient's group who were "friendly" competitors in the same business field. Bill and he watched each other's incomes, dress, cars, houses and social standing. In a word, it soon came out that the patient was intensely competitive. But why, when he had everything? For neurotic and irrational reasons—that is, from motivations left over from childhood—natural, inevitable reactions, intelligible then but no longer appropriate in adult life. That is the meaning of *"neurotic"* in the broad sense: *inappropriate ways of thinking, attitudes, moods or behavior which arise from infantile motivations or their derivatives or reactions against them.* This young man's behavior was certainly inappropriate insofar as he vitiated his enjoyment of excellent health and a most enviable life situation. It was infantile in terms of his failure to develop sufficiently from the envy and competitiveness of childhood. Why did he not mature beyond this childhood phase of development? As usual, his history will give a clue.

This patient was the youngest of four brothers. His family was desperately poor. The three older brothers at a very early age began to work and to contribute to its support. They were all strong and energetic. The patient was the exception; he was often ill and was the special object of his mother's solicitude, care and indulgence. He did not work and contribute to the family but went to school. He felt keenly his father's and brother's lack of respect for him, and the compelling purpose of his life became the drive to prove to them not only that he deserved their respect but also that he was superior to them and was not a mother's baby. At the same time he strove to continue to be her favorite. After college, where he distinguished himself in studies, athletics and personality, he continued this intense competition, chiefly in the field of money-making. This form of competition was largely determined by his reaction against his lowly and poverty-stricken origin, which hurt his pride cruelly. He rose rapidly and was a model of popularity and success, but he paid for his competitive hostility to his colleagues with severe anxiety, attacks of palpitations and fears of financial failure and of death. This man was brought up with high ideals, and his conscience and training would not permit him to accept this hostility to his own colleagues and, basically and unconsciously, to his own brothers and to his father, whom he revered. He was driven to compete mercilessly but also to be a morally superior person. Therefore, his strong conscience reacted something like this: "You want to climb to success over father and brothers and colleagues—so you deserve to slip back and have them climb above you."

Mr. Q. had a mild fear of heights, which is worth passing interest since it casts light on the nature of neurotic symptoms in general. Personal ambition often takes the form of "going up," "rising in the world," "social climbing," and so on. This patient's dreams expressed this repeatedly. The majority of them were of climbing up a mountain, going up in an elevator, driving his car up a steep hill and so on, always to have something go wrong, so that he fell back down to the bottom and then began to struggle up again. These dreams expressed the essence of the patient's outlook and revealed what an emotional struggle life was to him—even though he had achieved more money than he could spend, a secure business and a fine home and family. With every external success, yet he lived like the mythical Sisyphus, who was forced forever to push a huge rock up the mountain, only to have it hurtle down just as he reached the top. He experienced his whole life as striving upward above others and struggling against slipping back down. This was reflected in his interest in heights and also in his fear of heights. In this case we see an early physical weakness, overcome fully by adolescence, and also poverty as wounds to the self-esteem. The deepest wound however was neither of these but, as usual, an emotional impairment, namely, the exaggerated dependence, in this case on his mother. It was the most important direct cause of his inferiority feelings and his intense competitiveness with father and brothers. This hostile envy and competition cause the conscience reaction and the tendency to fail and slip back, as a punishment. In addition, this making of life only an arena of vicious competition, this struggling to rise over the competitors externally against the force of his own conscience internally, made living so anxious, such an effort, that it generated the longing to give up, withdraw from the struggle and regress to the early days of childhood when he was cared for by a solicitous mother and all was provided. The slipping downhill in the dreams, and the conscious fear that in reality he would lose his position and fail, thus represented not only the guilt reaction of his conscience but also the regressive tendency to relinquish the battle. This is typical in that the tendency to regress depends not only on the *pull* back, the attraction of the childhood position and the protest against adult giving and responsibilities, but also on the *push* back caused by the difficulties and the anxieties of adult functioning. In this case these difficulties were in no part external—the patient had everything in real life that anyone could desire, including as much real security as life affords—the difficulties were entirely in his own emotional attitudes, the persistence in a big, capable, successful adult of childish, competitive patterns, encouraged and abetted by the ideology in which he was reared and the milieu in which he lived. Here again we see clearly the old pattern: dependence—inferiority—competition—hostility—guilt, anxiety and strain—increased tendency to give up and regress, causing further inferiority and anxiety and closing the vicious circle.

Exaggerated intellectual competition all but paralyzed I. G., a young instructor. This young man was physically frail and was excessively dependent emotionally on his overprotective mother. His brother escaped some of this overprotection and restrictiveness by running wild and compensated for much of the feeling of inferiority which it caused by being an outstanding athlete in school. The patient could not compete with him in this but resolved to follow the well-known mechanism of "retiring in favor of" his brother in these fields and shifting to another. Let the brother rebel and be physically strong—the patient would be a giant intellectually. Learning became for him not a subject of interest but a means to an end—the means of proving his intellectual superiority to his brother and, following this pattern, to his colleagues and competitors. He thus sought to compensate for the feelings of inferiority and weakness which arose from his extreme dependence on his mother. He would do brilliantly until the examination. Then he would get "examination fever," becoming so anxious that he would be unable to write. His anxiety was a reaction to his hostility. He was not interested in the subject but only in the defeat of his competitors, his hostility aimed eventually at his envied brother. His conscience would not permit this but turned the hostility against himself, as though he felt, "You want your own brother, your own colleagues, your own friends to fail and you hope to triumph over them—therefore you deserve to fail yourself." In dreams such hostile competitive feelings very often appear in the form of killing the competitors or being killed by them—revealing thereby their power and their true primitive nature. *What is consciously only competition to the unconscious may be a death wish.* Against this the conscience may react strongly, as it did in this case, and might have been expected to do, in this gentle-mannered, well-brought-up, academic person. The reason for his own failure was his own masochism. His intellectual activity was sterile without the saving grace of productivity. He did not compete through trying to do something or contribute something better than his brother or his associates, but only through cultivating his mind and passing courses. Alexander Dumas once said, in reference to taking a certain amount of poetic license with history in his novels, that one may violate history if one has a child by her. And Tannhäuser was promised forgiveness if his staff flowered.

C. Psychosis. How this same type of conflict can result in psychosis is illustrated by a patient committed to a state hospital. A well-built young man of 25, Y. T., lumbers in, obviously acting the tough, bad man. His dress would be appropriate on a ranch. (This was 30 years before the hippies, but there he was: hair long in back, dungarees, high shoes, broad studded belt, even the old army jacket.) He assumes an air of exaggerated poise and deliberateness. Our method is to comprehend the present emotional situation and to try to understand from the history its genesis in relation to the present life situation ("genetic-dynamic"). We learn that in reality he is inadequate and dependent. He tries to overcompensate for these tendencies by a show of roughness. He does not realize these tendencies in himself but only feels them as a sense of weakness, which makes him feel inferior to others and enrages him. We find further that he is unable to support himself fully, and although he does simple manual work, he is largely financially dependent on his brother, who is five years younger. This young brother is not only a steady worker but is married and has his own home, in which the patient lives. The patient suffers from paranoid ideas of being persecuted, chiefly by his brother.

The essence of paranoia is "projection," that is, attributing to others impulses which, whether they are really in the others or not, are certainly in oneself. In paranoia these impulses are typically hostile in nature. When our patient accuses his brother, and occasionally the brother's wife, of hating him and even of making attempts on his life by poisoning, we must suspect, since there is ample evidence that the patient is mentally ill and misinterprets reality (the hallmark of psychosis), that this is a delusion and that it arises as a defense against his own hostile, even murderous impulses against the brother and his wife. Why does he hate them? For the answer we look to his history.

The patient is of good stock. His father had a difficult time because of the Depression and died when the patient was six and his brother two. The mother was kind but not very strong or practical, and she found it difficult to make her way during the Depression with two children. Here was a situation to test the balance of regressive versus developmental forces in her. She managed to stand her ground but sought all the help she could get, and the person to whom she looked chiefly was the patient. He was to care for the younger brother, help with the house, sell newspapers after school. She forced him into responsibilities far beyond his years or capacities. Soon he was in the position of the father himself. But through all this he got great emotional support from his mother, and whatever the demands on him, his position in the family fed his self-esteem. When he was 24, his mother died. This was a tremendous loss. He had never freed himself from his emotional dependence on her and had not reduced the intensity of his needs or transferred them to other men and women. His brother had always looked up to him and was used to accepting a dependent attitude toward him. The patient's pride would not let him accept a dependent attitude toward his brother. However, no person can live without some such receptive satisfaction. He worked along, unhappy and relatively alone, for, as we have said, he never had learned to develop other emotional attachments to satisfy his dependent, receptive needs. In spite of his pride, these needs attached more and more to his brother. Meanwhile, the brother, with less traumatic childhood experience, was getting on more normally. He was in no such conflict over his dependent needs, which he was accustomed to accepting more freely, never having felt that he must act the part of the head of the family. Also, they were not intensified by the frustrations of being forced out of satisfying them and into premature effort and responsibility. He pleased his employers, worked steadily and even became physically larger and stronger than the patient. Then he married.

The patient felt more and more inferior and inadequate in comparison with his brother, and his envy and rage mounted proportionately. Finally, he felt compelled to accept dependence on the brother and his wife, both emotionally and financially, and took up his abode with them, but this was intolerable to his pride, envy and jealousy—to feel like a weak, lonely, dependent child in the home of a now married and successful younger brother, toward whom he had once been in the role of father and family head. As his hostility mounted, something had to give. In this case, what gave was reality, and to the extent to which it gave, he became psychotic, believing the brother to be plotting against his life, whereas it was really he who was plotting against his brother, at least in his unconscious wishes. As a result of this reaction, he was committed to a state hospital, and so, finally, he could escape the struggle which was too much for him and thereby satisfy his passive, dependent needs in spite of his pride. There he could have the shelter, food, attention, leisure, dependence and passive indulgence from which he was so rudely ejected in childhood and therefore craved too intensely. Moreover, he could feel that he was not there because of his own wishes but was forced to stay there by the machinations of his brother against him. The intermediate stage and the central factor in the paranoia was the hostile competition with the brother, pathologically intensified by the history and the life situation that we have described. The paranoia developed in this case as a defense against his hostility, in part because his love for his brother made the hostility intolerable. Because of loving him, he could not believe that he hated his brother and he denied it by "projecting" his hate upon the brother—"I do not hate him—he hates me" (Freud, 1911; Saul, 1976, p. 60). Moreover, this belief then justified his hostility in the name of self-defense. But the question why he developed only paranoid projection as his main method of handling his hostility, rather than some other psychological mechanism, would require more detailed investigation.

Competition takes innumerable forms and has many goals—one envies others and tries to outdo them in strength, beauty, talent, money, power, fame and other areas. We have mentioned but a few, since we are more interested in the basic constellation than in the form taken by the competition. We have briefly sketched the operation of this particular emotional constellation in a child in the course of normal development, in two adult neuroses—a work inhibition and an anxiety-cardiac neurosis—and in a committable paranoid. The wide differences in outcome seem to depend on differences in the balance of the emotional forces, determined by various factors such as age, past emotional conditioning experiences especially in childhood prior to age about six, and current pressures. The particular neurotic symptoms—fear of examinations, anxiety attacks, palpitations, even paranoid delusions—are special forms of expression of the emotional forces which shape the whole personality and dictate the course of the whole life.

However conflicting, inconsistent and chaotic emotions and motivations may be, they can become more or less organized into constellations, complexes or patterns. Each is not an isolated force, living its own life, as it were. Rather, there is an inner logic which dictates complicated interrelationships (Alexander, 1961). Vicious circles are easily established, but, fortunately, the situation works both ways; often judicious therapy hits at one point only but breaks the whole circle. A little reduction in the dependence, inferiority, competitiveness, hostility or anxiety may cause reductions all along the line because of the ways in which these forces are related to one another.

In order to broaden our grasp of these forces and to show how much remains unsolved, let us approach these reactions from a different angle—that of the conditioned reflex (French, 1933). If a certain tone is sounded each time a hungry dog is fed meat, he soon salivates to the sounding of the tone, even when no meat is offered. If another tone is sounded in connection with which no food is ever offered, this tone serves to inhibit salivation. Now, what if the two tones are made so close, say a quarter step or less, that the dog cannot discriminate? Then he is conditioned both to salivate and not to salivate. The result can be a "nervous breakdown, which is cured or improved by a rest in the country, far from the whole experimental situation, or by being brought repeatedly into the experimental situation where good treatment is consistently given instead of experiments'' (Liddell, 1956).

Now if we recall Mr. Q., the successful man with the anxieties and the palpitations, we see a similar state of affairs. He was conditioned by his mother to be the dependent one, to make no responsible productive effort but to receive freely love, care, support, adulation. But he is also conditioned by his independent father and brothers to be self-reliant, contributing, giving. Small wonder that he finds life such a struggle with these two opposite drives in his breast. Thus, spoiling is like a short circuiting. The child is conditioned by its rearing to the necessity for ''success''—but the means of achieving it are not given him. These means consist in maturity and the enjoyment of self-reliance, effort and accomplishments. Instead of this, all is provided, so that he is conditioned to expect and to receive from others and not to make his way himself. He is oriented to get the fruits of success without the effort—a short circuit in which the current sparks across instead of turning the motor and so doing productive work. The result is a burning need for success plus a sense of helplessness in achieving it, which results from the passive-dependent-receptive attitude and the lack of a mature, independent approach. And the ''success'' is often a false goal—basically a childhood need for prestige.

Another man rose from rags to one of the top positions in industry in the United States. Yet he never could relax or enjoy anything but was a poor husband and a worse father, being driven mercilessly from within, still competing as bitterly as ever with the tiny handful of men who had any more money or power than he.

D. Criminality; Murder. Y. X. was the unwanted child of an unmarried mother. His father disappeared on hearing of the pregnancy, and his mother did not want to risk an illegal abortion. Two months after his birth, his mother left him with relatives; but they soon passed him on to other relatives, who, after a year, persuaded still others to take him. The vicious circle was inevitably established. The child reacted to being unwanted with the automatic reflex response of fight and flight. He became angry, irritable, uncooperative, withdrawn, not a healthy, happy, warmly responsive baby. He was unpleasant and difficult because he did not get the affectionate, accepting love that babies require for normal growth as a tree needs sunshine; but because he reacted with this universal response and was therefore resentful and unattractive, he was further rejected and deprived. So the cycle spiraled downwards, and he became a juvenile delinquent.

Barely into his teens, his personality had given up hope of satisfying his deepest craving—satisfaction of the baby's original needs for maternal dependence and love. Of course these needs continued, undiminished and even heightened by the rejection, but repressed, defended against, denied, unconscious. Not only did he ask nothing, he could accept nothing; no one could reach him. In appearance, he was attractive, and people now responded to him because of his intensity and his youth. At first, they always believed the best, and not until his hate-filled delinquent acting-out forced the realization upon them did they reluctantly see some of the dynamics that operated not far beneath the surface.

There was enough love and care in his past to save him from a complete psychotic breakdown in adolescence, but not from a warping of his personality into a semipsychotic, schizoid, criminal machine. Could treatment in adolescence have saved him, for himself and for society and his innocent victims? Most unlikely. The unsophisticated talk glibly of treatment and rehabilitation as though these were easy. But most even relatively mild neuroses can be influenced only with difficulty, through many hours of individual treatment, in persons who suffer and make sacrifices to get help. Here the trauma, the long-term injurious influences began almost at birth and operated for years with so little relief or compensation that it is questionable whether their effects could be corrected appreciably. Nature's forces of cure are powerful, especially when facilitated by modern professional understanding and methods, but they cannot straighten the tree that was too badly bent as a twig. There are hopeful cases with good prognoses, but this was not one (Slovenko, 1966). For in his mind was formed, from birth, a composite image of other persons as rejecting, depriving, ungiving, hostile, and not as benign parents using their power to love, understand, and help him; and this composite image with these feelings toward those who were in authority over him as a child, he now projects onto the authorities of society. He feels toward society as he did toward his long series of rejecting substitute parents and sees it in their image.

The craving to be loved and valued continues although denied by his front of defiant independence, and keeps him constantly and deeply frustrated and angered. The craving is now unsatisfiable and it is felt to be so. To acknowledge it would be to experience again the suffering and humiliation of rejection. And now, in adolescence and young adulthood, it is also felt as too childish and therefore intolerable to his pride as a grown-up. This normal pride is further offended by taking over toward himself the rejecting attitudes of his parents and their substitutes—if his own father and mother abandon him and those responsible for him pass him on to others, of what worth or value as a person can he be? In reaction to this he becomes overly vain and proud, in fact grandiose. And the infantile longings for love and dependence defeat all attempts at adult responsibilities. All during childhood in the power of others, now grown, he cannot take sustained mature responsibility, he remains weak and all but helpless and, hence, frightened. For these reasons his "primary narcissism," his basic needs to be valued, to have the respect of others and of himself, are badly wounded, are, in fact, all but shattered. Trying to be strong, effective, mature, he feels himself to be weak, in the power of others, childish. These hurts to his self-esteem combine with the frustrated dependent love needs to generate mounting rage. And this is further fed by envy, by his sense that others have what he lacks and that he can never succeed in competition with them. They have self-respect, are valued, they know how to make their way in life, to make friends, marriages, families, money, position, names and power. These are all impossible for him because of his dynamics, which he does not understand. Hence, he burns with defeated competition, humiliated pride, unassuageable envy, and impotent rage—that he cannot have all this and he revenges himself on them for what they have and he envies. He becomes an *irrational, pathological, hostile acting-outer.* He vandalizes, he steals, he rapes, he is a potential murderer; it is only a matter of time and opportunity. He is in and out of jails, repeatedly breaking parole. His pattern throughout childhood of hating his parents and their substitutes is transferred to society and its authorities—to the police, the wardens, the courts, to all who are stable and secure, to the Establishment. He burns to smash them all—that is the big thing. Understandably, he has some sympathy with underdogs (but not really), and his egotism, expanded beyond all reality by the depth of his sense of inferiority, makes him see himself as a great liberator. Not weak and in the control of others, he will be the leader who smashes the Establishment, revenges himself on those he envies, taking what they have, liberating the poor, with himself wielding absolute power. Thus, the child's fantasy of destroying the bad parents and taking their place and power, in a desperate bid to achieve a modicum of maturity, the nature of which he does not comprehend.

He is, however, sexually potent. Now nearing 30, he can, in sexual relations, feel for the moment in full command, with the girl completely in his power. There is little or no love. There is no mating, psychologically. There is little or no parental urge to have children. It is almost completely the urge of the weak for power. This he can act out with those emotionally frail, immature teenage girls whose own dynamics resemble his, but who are attracted to this kind of masochistic sexual relationship. With the incoming era of the late 1960's, Vietnam, the assassination of Bobby Kennedy and Martin Luther King, and the riots at the convention in Chicago, a time of so much immature sexuality and violence, of hatred and defiance of authority of church and state (derived so largely from defiance of parents), of egotism and irresponsibility, and of masochistic regression through drugs, small wonder that Y. X. should attract to himself others like himself, but not so old and not so extreme in feelings and behavior. Thus, he becomes a little leader of a little gang of like feather. The rest is quickly told. Time and opportunity arrive and several murders are eventually traced to him. These were all irrational, purely emotional, *pathological, hostile acting out.* There was no monetary or other gain, only the infantile emotional gratification of exercising absolute power and venting absolute rage and hate in the murder of completely innocent and helpless victims. Unwelcome and fearsome as the conclusion is, we must fact it: Until every child is not only wanted, but reared with love, understanding and respect as a person, we shall continue to manufacture psychotics, neurotics and private, organized and political criminals and murderers, who threaten to destroy our country.

SOCIOLOGICAL IMPLICATIONS

When one sees a person like our successful man with the anxieties, Mr. Q., he has food for thought as to the nature of man, his standards and his civilization and our concepts of mental health. What poignant irony is this man's whole life! He has achieved everything—a fine scholastic, athletic and social record, a meteoric rise in business, financial security, a charming wife and children, a beautiful home and great popularity in a wide circle of friends and acquaintances. Moreover, he is a leader in his community, respected by young and old. He is in perfect physical health. A happy man and, indeed, one to be envied. So he seems to all except those very few who know his suffering, who know that he is a frightened child, driven and harassed, fearing that any moment he will crack under the strain or die of heart failure. Were it not for his few symptoms, no one would know, and he might deny the truth even to himself. Is he perhaps symbolic of Western man's plight?

Our patient's neurosis fitted his competitive social milieu. Because of his neurosis he gravitated to this milieu, fitted it and was a success in it, at least outwardly. It is not easy to develop or even to hold mature attitudes and "object interest" in such thoroughly competitive circles pervaded by such an ideology. Many a young man has begun his career, including the practice of medicine, with a mature orientation of accomplishment and service but has been caught in the whirl and has succumbed to it, changing the basis of his life from a primary interest in his patients, while still taking adequate care of his family and himself, to almost complete absorption in personal climbing, competition, and self-promotion. Much in the world is accomplished through competition, but it often defeats itself. Its saving grace is productivity—if the results are of some constructive social value and not purely sterile self-interest.

Perhaps competitiveness is even more prominent in our American life than in other cultures. But it is always present in some degree as a biological force and is not confined to human beings. Obvious examples are almost any two neighboring individuals or groups. "A prophet is not without honor, save in his own country and in his own house"—largely, we surmise, because of the local envy of him and because those near to him know his weaknesses, which makes it is easy for them to express the hostility that arises from their envy. As between families, competitiveness is seen in "keeping up with the Joneses." Usually neighboring schools are the bitterest rivals, and the hostile reactions of most neighboring countries are notorious.

Sterile, hostile, trouble-making competitiveness riddles our society and does much to mold it. Such clinical examples as we have given are all about us. In his autobiographical *Of Human Bondage,* Maugham (who stuttered) describes Phillip's suffering, not so much from his clubfoot itself but from the cruelty of people directed so unerringly to this defect. Thus do people seek to raise themselves by depreciating others. They search out defects—social, financial, religious, racial—or inconsequential mannerisms—and if no defect is obvious, then it is invented. But who has none, for who, as Dr. Kenneth Appel says, is better than 70 percent? The Catholic Church, with its long experience, makes malicious gossip a sin, for gossip is always ready to believe the worst. And this, as we have seen, is largely because people feel inferior if they have real inferiorities, namely, childhood attitudes and patterns, which they have not outgrown. Almost everyone feels himself to be a child and wants to be adult. Perhaps all the striving *upward,* the climbing, is a symbolic representation of the small child's wish to be as big and tall as its parents, with all the status and the power that the parents have in relation to the children. I think there is only one true aristocracy, and that is an aristocracy of maturity—without pride (for almost all pride is false pride).

The undue prominence of any part of the dynamics described in these three chapters—dependent love needs—inferiority—competitiveness and envy—egotism, vanity and pride—hostility—regression from responsible productivity—is a symptom of some form and degree of emotional disorder. It requires considerable experience of one's own in life, out from financial and emotional dependence on parents and making one's own way by responsible, productive and giving work (a value for a value), before one reaches the tolerance, grasp of reality and constructive motivations of maturity. The student who is still dependent on his parents, who has never made his own way by constructive work, who has not yet undertaken the decisions and responsibilities of career and marriage, is not apt to have wisdom about people in their local, national, and international relationships no matter how high his I.Q., for the intellect is only a servant of the emotions. Most people have disturbed emotions; if most were mature, we would have few problems. If he has not solved the problems of his own personal life, he is not likely to be capable of solving the complicated problems of universities let alone of national welfare to which great minds have devoted a lifetime of conscientious effort. Those who are so sure they know all the answers advertise an egotism that makes one suspect the vicious circle mentioned above. Of course, strong dependence upon parents is felt as a carryover from childhood, does make a sense of inferiority, does hurt the pride and exaggerate it and cause resentment, dogmatism, and even a proneness to force and violence. Disruptive behavior usually signals something very wrong in the relationship with the parents, something which has generated excessive hostility, conscious or unconscious, the emotional pattern to the parents being transferred wholly or in part to society and its authorities, thus making extremism of the left or of the right.

This is why so many young people, so passionate, so prone to certainty, dependence, egotism, power and hostility, are so readily and uncritically mobilized politically.

It must be obvious that our purpose is not exemplifying nor evaluating social, political, racial or other situations, but exclusively reporting what we have observed clinically about the *inner, personal* motivations as these shape each individual's views and opinions, behavior and actions.

REFERENCES

Alexander, F. (1961): *The Scope of Psychoanalysis,* ed. by T. French. New York: Basic Books, pp. 116–128.
French, T. (1933): Interrelations between psychoanalysis and the experimental work of Pavlov, *American Journal of Psychiatry* 89:1165.
Freud, S. (1911): Psychoanalytic notes on an autobiographical account of a case of paranoia, *S.E.* 12, p. 59.
———— (1914): On narcissism, *S.E.* 14.
———— (1916): Introductory lectures on psychoanalysis, *S.E.* 16.
Kohut, H. (1971): *Analysis of the Self.* New York: International Universities Press.
Liddell, H. (1956): *Emotional Hazards in Animals and Man.* Springfield, Ill.: Thomas.
Saul, L. J. (1976): *Psychodynamics of Hostility.* New York: Jason Aronson.
Schoeck, H. (1970): *Envy: A Theory of Social Behavior.* New York: Harcourt, Brace & World.
Slovenko, R. (1966): *Crime, Law and Corrections.* Springfield, Ill.: Thomas.

5 | Training and Conscience

GENERAL INFORMATION

1. Grouping of Mental Activities

When we speak of the "mind" or the "personality," we refer to the way in which the brain operates and mediates the various motivations of the organism insofar as we are able to sense, perceive, be aware of these motivations, reactions, processes. Those we readily and customarily perceive are conscious; those which we grasp with difficulty are "preconscious"; others, like the interplay which creates dreams, are "unconscious" but because they can potentially become conscious they are still "psychological"; but such elemental physiological processes as secreting bile from the liver or increasing white cells in the blood to combat infection are "subpsychological," not susceptible of entering the mental awareness.*

The way the mind works suggests a certain arrangement of its activities in a psychological "structure." This "structure" is only a way of *grouping* the activities of the mind and is not fully established scientifically, but it is a great convenience, for it brings order and organization to a complex interplay of emotional forces. (See Chap. 20, Determinants of Personality.)

A. Id. Each person is a biological organism filled with manifold, powerful biological impulses, some of which have already been discussed in this book—forces of development, dependence, self-love, envy, competitiveness, power drives, receptive demands, hostility, love, sexuality, giving and the like. Because the sources of these impulses lie in the impersonal physiology of the animal organism, Freud called this source the "Id."

* For a more detailed discussion of these "levels" see Saul, L. J.: Bases of Human Behavior, Greenwood Press, Westport, Connecticut, 1972.

131

B. Superego. But people do not give in freely to all their crude physiological and biological impulses. Each child goes through a long period of training by rewards and punishments, by lessons and examples, by modeling himself on parents and others important to him. His immediate family stimulates all kinds of reactions, as we have seen in previous chapters, by their treatment of the child, making it dependent or demanding or angry, facilitating or retarding its development. They also teach it to control its reactions so that it can function as a member of a social group. Its eating, excretions, sexual urges, anger, demands and other impulses all must be restrained. The long years of training and of establishing codes and ideals produce controls which are largely automatic. This means a great saving of energy. One need not at each impulse consciously decide and make the conscious effort to inhibit. A dog, after having a light flashed every time he eats, salivates when the light is flashed alone; after having his toes stepped on often enough, he learns to walk properly beside his master. So the conditioning experiences of human beings operate to a large extent without requiring conscious effort. "Superego" is a convenient term for all the forces of restraint and inhibition, domestication and socialization (Freud, 1923, Part III). It includes the results of training, conditioning and identifications, the ideals, standards and conscience. (It has been referred to as the part of the personality which is soluble in alcohol.)

Almost all animals (Allee, 1951; Carrighar, 1965) and certainly men cooperate with each other socially. The training, domestication and socialization are probably built upon this innate biological nucleus of *social cooperation,* which in turn must stem largely not only from identification but also from needs for love, and develops with maturity.

C. Ego. Between these agencies and forces in the personality—the animal urges (Id), selfish, egotistical, and the inhibitions and ideals (Superego), basic to social living—is the "Ego" (Freud, 1923, Part II). This term is used in this technical restricted sense to designate the conscious, rational part of the personality—the consciousness, judgment, memory, reason, intellect, will power and the like, the capacity for perception, integration and executive decisions. (It has nothing to do with egotism.) The ego can be "strong" or "weak."

A person who is extremely upset emotionally, or perhaps tends to be emotionally confused, dependent or infantile, may carry on well through sheer force of his ego, that is, his will power, conscious controls, intellect, judgment and so on. Some persons suppress severe neuroses or even actual psychoses through sheer ego control. (Conscious deliberate control is called "suppression"; relatively automatic, unconscious restraint is called "repression.") Other persons with weak ego functions have little control or "character" and give in to their impulses of all kinds and may show lack of restraint in both their animal impulses and their guilt and shame reactions. A weak ego is characteristic of infantile and also of impulse-ridden personalities.

The ego mediates between (1) the primitive urges of the id and (2) the standards, ideals and restraints of the superego, and (3) the outside world. That is, each person tries to satisfy his powerful, manifold and often conflicting needs and urges in the outside world—and this is a hard enough task. But in addition he can do this only in accordance with inner training, standards, ideals, inhibitions and conscience. No one fully realizes and appreciates the nature and the power of his animal urges, or of his conscience. Both are partially unconscious. Thus, as Freud observed, man is both more moral and more immoral than he thinks. Although this formulation of a basic "structure" of the personality is not fully established, and its terms not yet fully accepted, if we use them descriptively to include those tendencies and functions outlined above, we shall we dealing with a useful organization of observable facts.

2. Forces of Conditioning

A. Inanimate. The forces of conditioning and of inhibition are various and complex. There is, for example, the impersonal conditioning of experience with the inanimate environment. By touching the hot stove the child learns not to do so again. Once burned, twice shy. Similar reactions occur against other kinds of hurt, for example, early poverty, which the individual dreads ever after. There is the example of the self-made man who always kept an excessive supply of the finest shirts, for in his childhood his family had been so poor that he generally had to do without any shirts at all.

B. Fear. Conditioning also results from fear. For example, to attack another person, especially a stronger one, brings the fear of being attacked. This fear may be important in forming the fundamental mechanism of turning impulses against the self. Then there is the whole experience of training and inculcation of models and standards, begun by the parents.

C. Formation of Conscience. The conscience represents all the effects of training and identification in establishing standards, ideals and ethics and is the internal moral arbiter of right and wrong. Psychologically, the conscience is in essence the internalization of the once external training and experiences. (It may, however, as we have suggested, have a biological nucleus in the id, in the instinctual impulses to social cooperation and love.) If anger is controlled only through primitive fear of retaliation, this is not conscience. But if it is "learned" (Hilgard, 1948) that anger must always be controlled or some form of retaliation or suffering will always ensue, then conditioning takes place, and an internal control develops. In the next stage, the moral and ethical concept of right and wrong enters the reaction. One accepts control of the anger not only because of fear or because of inhibition, but because it is "right" and "proper" to control it, because it is necessary to social living (Erikson, 1964), and social living is our most effective security in the face of the inexorable universe. The term "conscience" is commonly used in this restricted sense.*

The conscience reaction, whether caused by past misdeeds or by current hostility or by any other deed or impulse for which "one reproaches oneself," results in a tendency to self-punishment. The feeling ("affect") of being reproached and attacked by one's conscience is chiefly guilt † or shame. The action of the conscience, the tendency to self-punishment and the sense of guilt may be conscious or may be hardly realized or quite unconscious. Often a person knows that he "feels like kicking himself." Sometimes he may know that he hates himself. Often he does not know the extent to which one part of his personality militates against him.

* Throughout this book the conscience is dealt with only insofar as it can be studied as a natural phenomenon, and apart from the question of divine origin.

† The relation of guilt to night terrors has been delicately delineated by Eugene Field in his poem "Seein' Things." Reprinted by permission of Charles Scribner's Sons, New York.

Generally *shame* reflects a feeling of weakness, one is ashamed of being childish; whereas *guilt* results from injuring someone and results in the sense that one should be harmed in return. Training, conditioning and the inculcation of standards take place in various ways (Freud, 1930).

D. Methods: Love, Dependence, Identification. If one loves a person toward whom one is angry, then the love serves as a check. The child who is hostile to a younger brother or sister learns to control this hostility not only through training, rewards and punishments, promises and threats, but also because, to a degree, he can identify with and love the younger child. The dependence on the parents and the need for their love are also powerful forces in teaching the child control and standards of behavior. Loss of parental approval and love is a devastating experience for the small child who needs his parents for very survival. The emotionally dependent person tends to be readily submissive to those whose love he needs and to model himself on them. This is seen in the ''hero-worshipping'' stage of boys who tend to obey and imitate their heroes.

I ain't afeard uv snakes, or toads, or bugs, or worms, or mice,
An' things 'at girls are skeered uv I think are awful nice!
I'm pretty brave, I guess; an' yet I hate to go to bed,
For, when I'm tucked up warm an' snug an' when my prayers are said,
Mother tells me ''Happy Dreams!'' an' takes away the light,
An' leaves me lyin' all alone an' seein' things at night!

Once, when I licked a feller 'at had just moved on our street,
An' father sent me up to bed without a bite to eat,
I woke up in the dark an' saw things standin' in a row,
A-lookin' at me cross-eyed an' p'intin' at me—so!
Oh, my! I wuz so skeered that time I never slep' a mite—
It's almost alluz when I'm bad I see things at night!

An' I am, oh, *so* sorry I'm a naughty boy, an' then
I promise to be better an' I say my prayers again!
Gran'ma tells me that's the only way to make it right
When a feller had been wicked an' sees things at night!
An' so, when other naughty boys would coax me into sin,
I try to skwush the Tempter's voice 'at urges me within;
An' when they's pie for supper, or cakes 'at's big an' nice,
I want to—but I do not pass my plate f'r them things twice!
No, ruther let Starvation wipe me slowly out o'sight
Then I should keep a-livin' on an' seein' things at night!

Identification means that the child takes as models persons close to it and tries in part to imitate them. They exemplify the satisfaction of certain needs, and the child tries to do likewise and be like them, to take them into his own personality as part of himself (introjection). For example, a football hero at a certain boys' summer camp as counselor refrained from smoking cigarettes while there because he was an idol to the boys, and they tended to take him as a model for what to do and what not to do. The conscience is not only a restricting force; it tells one not only what *not* to do, but also what *to do*. How the training is accomplished and what persons the child is in close contact with, to imitate, to model itself on and to identify with, are essential factors in the child's emotional environment, and as such are of first importance for *the facilitation or the impairment* of its development. Good training is usually accomplished not by authoritarian commands but by winning over the child to social behavior. This takes much time and patience, and depends upon "the inevitability of gradualness," while avoiding hostility, rebellion against authority and conflict with his own conscience.

E. Assimilation. In the course of normal development the forces of restraint become well integrated with the rest of the personality. Ordinarily, the stronger the infantile impulses and patterns are, the greater is the need for the forces of inhibition and control; hence, the higher the tension between them. The more infantile and hostile a person is, the more he fails to live up to his standards and training, the more ashamed, guilty and inferior he usually feels. The failure to assimilate training and to achieve a relatively harmonious relationship among the primitive urges of the id, the conscious judgment of the ego and the results of training, the superego, marks an impairment in the normal development. Of course, no one is fully mature, fully satisfied in his desires, in his relations with the outer world and other persons, or fully at peace with his conscience. Again it is a matter of degree.

It may be possible that a small core of conscience is inherited in addition to the biological nucleus of social cooperation and that gradually, over the centuries, man is becoming more domesticated. Perhaps internal restraints on father-murder, mother-incest and cannibalism are already so far established that the incidence of these crimes would not increase appreciably even if all external prohibitions were removed. On the other hand, it is not easy to accept inheritance of this kind of presumably acquired characteristic, and nothing can be accepted without hard evidence. Inhibitions of this kind can come about in a totally different way. For example, adolescent monkeys will not mate sexually with their mothers or with any mother figure; i.e., female monkeys who are older and of the type who had authority over them (Masserman, 1968).

F. Timing. Since the child's main emotional contacts during its formative years are with its parents, or substitutes for them, these emotional contacts are the most central and powerful in the development of its standards and conscience—of its character. Often persons whom he meets later or books that he reads exert profound influences only because the ground was already prepared by the early training provided by the parents and the other emotionally important persons of early childhood and by the child's identifications with them.

3. Development versus Restrictiveness

The conscience or, to use the broader, more inclusive term, the superego, is formed in part through the child's wish to grow up, to *be like* the adult. The developmental forces and the pride in them stimulate the child to take the father and the mother as models and to accept and try to achieve their standards and ideals, to identify with them. These standards and ideals, if the parents are relatively normal, mature and well developed emotionally, represent not only checks and restraints but also positive expressions of mature, adult attitudes. They exert a pressure not only to *control* the more infantile, childish, regressive reactions but also to *outgrow* them in favor of the more mature, developmental ones. *This is the key to human living, to happiness or to misery: the socialization of the child by the parents must favor, not oppose, good human relations with them and healthy maturing.*

The sense of restriction, whether from without or within, often results in a feeling that to do wrong is really heroic, for in this way a person shows that he is independent and fearless, not bowing to restraints, and risking the consequences. So it is said of the United

States that we pass laws about everything but have little respect for the law and expect to break it because individualism is a higher law. But duty and right are not merely something pious which the strong scorn, but represent responsibility, effort, object-interest, productive accomplishment. For they have developed out of man's age-long struggles to live together and are in principle basic conditions of social life. Often it is seen that right or duty demand a certain line of action, but it is not always clearly realized that maturity also does. Thus law and true morality do not always coincide, although no doubt they should.

4. Operation of Conscience

A. Hostility. The conscience operates in different ways. A person gets very angry at someone and out of good sense controls it, yet feels distressed and that night dreams of men or of wild animals that threaten *him—projected* representations of his own rage. This is seen in more extreme form in those cases in which acute anxiety is the direct effect of an intense rage which threatens to break through. On the other hand, a different picture is seen in such a case as that of a man who killed the girl he "loved" out of jealousy and then was impatient to be executed—or in those figures of literature, such as Lady Macbeth, in which the personality is dominated by guilt after the commission of a crime. Here the hostility arises not only from feelings of anger reflected back by the conscience but from the reproaches of the conscience itself. If the conscience is thought to include the agency which turns the primitive hostility against the self, then the distinction is only a matter of the original source of the hostility, for both in the turning of primitive hostility against the self, and in the conscience reaction itself, hostility is directed by the conscience against the self.

Conscience reactions are important in anxiety, guilt and shame. In a previous chapter a girl was described who reacted to being unwanted with a rage so strong that often she literally trembled with it. She suffered anxiety lest she "lose her mind," that is, lose control of it and have its accustomed orderly functioning disrupted by her rage. She also projected the rage and felt it as directed against herself, which caused constant anxiety. Here guilt was present but not prominent—for she felt that the mistreatment to which she had been subjected justified her demands and her anger.

In contrast with this girl is one to be described later in this chapter, a girl who had very little anxiety but whose well-organized guilt reaction dominated her life. In many such cases guilt causes a tendency to self-punishment and anxiety.

B. Shame. Let us look a little more closely at shame and guilt, mentioned above. Both are major reactions of the conscience (Alexander, 1938). Guilt arises from transgression and is an attack by the conscience on the individual, the punishment that the parent or external authority would have inflicted for such forbidden behavior. By identifying with their authority, their role is internalized. It may be that the deeper source of all guilt is hostility to other persons (Freud, 1930). Certainly hostility must be looked for wherever guilt is encountered. Shame arises from a wound to the self-esteem, caused by a feeling of inadequacy in living up to one's accepted ideals or standards. Guilt tends to depress one, but shame more often acts as a spur. We have mentioned delinquent types who show little guilt and even boast of their crimes, because they think these prove their toughness and they cannot tolerate any hint of weakness in themselves. Here shame is far stronger than guilt. It can be very powerful, as seen in the chapter on Egoism, Competitiveness, Inferiority and Power, in which feelings of weakness were seen to be reacted against in ways which affected people's whole lives and could even result in criminality and murder. Some boys confess that their great thrill in perpetrating hold-ups is the sense of power—that after years of feeling weak, now, with a gun, they can feel strong. Hitler's power drive seems to have consisted in large part of a reaction against weakness threatened by submissiveness to his father (Saul, 1976, pp. 166–174).

Sometimes hostility produces more shame than guilt. In the analysis of an egoistic man, only at the very end could he force himself to confess something. This was not some terrible deed but a childish thing. It was the fact that for several years during childhood, following the birth of a younger brother, he used to indulge in cruel fantasies before falling asleep. He was not guilty about this but terribly ashamed. Another man boasted of various misdeeds, but only at the end of his analysis and with the greatest difficulty was he able to confess shamefacedly that as a boy sometimes he would urinate on the floor next to the toilet.

C. Guilt. One of the most important aspects of the functioning of the personality consists in attempts to buy off the conscience with suffering. This has been worked out in detail by Alexander (1930), who points out that punishment is the currency with which guilt can be paid off. He tells the anecdote of the young girl who wants to read a book forbidden by her parents, so she first falsely confesses that she has read it, gets herself punished and then settles down to enjoy it with a clear conscience. (Freud's study of wit has amply confirmed the observation of G. B. Shaw that when someone laughs, look for a hidden truth—but this holds for all expressions of emotion.) Freud described a type of criminal whose behavior is motivated by an unconscious sense of guilt and need for punishment. In these cases, the delinquency has a strong element of provocation, and one of its aims is to get the individual punished. This is an observation of considerable interest in view of the fact that most criminals are never apprehended, while some are repeatedly. It means that certain acts of the criminal which lead to his arrest are parapraxes, "purposive accidents"—little slips which are apparently accidental but are motivated unconsciously in these cases largely by guilt and tendencies to self-punishment.

Probably everyone carries a great burden of guilt through life— for everyone carries far more hostility to his fellows, especially toward his parents and immediate family, than he knows. Thus everyone carries some tendency to self-punishment. This reaction underlies much of the suffering in life. Many of the ways in which people unwittingly block, defeat and injure themselves have been examined in relation to the neuroses by Alexander (1930) and reviewed by K. Menninger (1938). This subtle, unconscious tendency toward suffering is called "masochism." This word derives from Leopold von Sacher-Masoch, whose novel *Venus in Fur* portrays a man's sexual pleasure in being beaten by a woman clad in fur. But the term has come to be used in the broader sense of self-induced suffering (Eisenbud, 1968; Freud, 1924; Panken, 1967; Smirnoff, 1969). It may dominate a person's whole life. It may operate very subtly, as when little slips, or certain tastes or decisions which seem to be reasonable, lead regularly to unhappiness or even disaster. It may be manifested only in keeping a person with fine potentialities from realizing them. It may appear overtly in persons who injure themselves or get themselves injured physically, professionally or socially. It occurs in students who sacrifice fine opportunities to serve their country and themselves by ruining their careers. It is seen in women who are attracted to sadistic men who make them suffer and in men who cling to sadistic women; in men who so drive themselves in their work and lives, despite their own better judgment and the advice of their friends and physicians, that they cannot enjoy life and consequently die before their time; in people who needlessly expose themselves to all kinds of hardships; in the accident-prone; and in the sexual perversion in which a person wishes to be beaten or otherwise hurt because it affords sexual pleasure. It is also seen in persons who react to success by vitiating it, breaking down or in some way injuring themselves. The guilt and the need for punishment are far stronger than the individual realizes, and he cannot allow himself success and happiness. The conscience operates powerfully and often subtly, grinding slowly but exceeding small. It is often uncannily precise in its exaction of an eye for an eye, a tooth for a tooth. The "wrecked by success" reaction is sometimes specific: "You have envied and hated others for this particular kind of success or happiness, now you don't deserve to have it yourself" (Saul, 1950). Hence, when such a person tries to do or be what he envied others for, he is inhibited or defeats himself. Many inhibitions in work, sexuality or social life are largely on the basis of such conscience reactions.

In some cases the mechanism seems to be different. In these it seems that one part of the personality is so fixed on hating, say adequacy, or whatever the person envies in others, that it attacks this even when it is in oneself. A person may hate a man for his position, potency, possession of whatever and feel threatened by his own hate directed toward himself when he approaches this position, potency or possession. He comes to hate the adequacy, whether in himself or in others, without distinguishing. This must arise, in large part, from identification and is probably, in part, a more primitive mechanism that conscience reaction alone.

There is also a type of person who is "wrecked by failure." Some people are stimulated to blame others for their own misfortune, while some blame themselves too much. In such cases, there is usually a sense of guilt and a tendency to self-punishment and suffering, which is much stronger than the individual knows and which is held in check. Misfortune then mobilizes this tendency and breaks down the defenses against it, so that the individual castigates himself and often adds self-punishing behavior to the buffets of life. In some persons, any reproach, even for a minor matter, causes an excessive reaction because of the fact that it arouses latent guilt feelings from other sources.

We have noted previously that "the punishment fits the source" is directed to that desire, the frustration of which aroused the hostility (p. 85).

Self-injuring tendencies also are sometimes motivated by regressive *desires* to be weak, passive and dependent, desires which are better justified if one is handicapped in some way.* Often the guilt and the passive tendencies operate together to impair the development. Such a person fears to be adult and productive because of guilt from long envy and hate of those who have achieved this, and also resists this adult role from fear of leaving his old passive-dependent-receptive orientation (Alexander, 1936).

It is hard to realize the extent to which people torture themselves by the reactions of their own consciences. But just as we tend to *underestimate* the power of the conscience and its role in human life, so in other ways we are apt to *overestimate* it and hence be surprised at the frequency with which wars break out and the brutality which apparently decent people are capable of bringing to overt expression (Freud, 1915). Perhaps it is safest to say that we should not underestimate the tremendous power of the conscience, but let us also not underestimate the power of the warped infantile motivations and reactions that live on in presumably mature adults. Nor should we underestimate the role of hostile aggressiveness in these reactions. This has been portrayed dramatically by R. L. Stevenson in his *Dr. Jekyll and Mr. Hyde,* in which the crude animal impulses become less controllable each time they are unleashed. But, if humanity is to survive, we must distinguish with utter sharpness between the natural, inevitable, biological killing of, say, a zebra by a lion, or a squid by a whale, or a fly by a spider, or a steer by a man, or of any carnivore of another species for food,

---

* Freud (1924) called this tendency to be weak, childish and feminine, particularly in men, "feminine masochism." He considered it to be a part of "erotogenic masochism" or the general tendency of the organism to libidinize its innate tendency to disintegration and death. He points out that probably every impulse, if it reaches sufficient intensity, stimulates sexual excitation and tends to be libidinized and drained sexually—a phenomenon that we shall encounter in later chapters.

and the neurotic and psychotic killing by human beings of their own kind, the irrational, hostile acting out.

A harsh conscience does not always originate with harsh parents, as we have noted. It sometimes develops in children whose resentment against their parents has been aroused but who have also been treated most kindly; because of the good treatment, they are unable to "bite the hand which feeds them" and hence develop disproportionate guilt.

Freud pointed out that a great simplification of theory is achieved by assuming that guilt always arises from hostility in some form. This observation is of use practically. Beyond the simple guilt for certain misbehavior one must look for a deeper cause in some hostility. When guilt is found in connection with sexuality, for example, if one probes the matter in each case far enough, it is usually found to spring not merely from violation of training and social standards concerning sex behavior but also from hurting someone, from anger at frustration or from some kind of hostile aggressive impulses which are drained by the sexuality or otherwise connected with it directly or indirectly. Sometimes guilt for a simple disobedience is heightened because of a less apparent tendency to spite the forbidding authority. As has long been known, much anxiety is fear of the conscience, which as Shakespeare said, "Doth make cowards of us all."

5. Projection of Conscience

Conscience reactions are often projected, just as primitive impulses are. A man of fine character, who was not especially neurotic, once did something at his firm which was unnecessary and caused considerable inconvenience to several persons. This lapse caused him great pain. He, that is, his conscious ego and his conscience, judged himself very harshly. His ego was not so harsh as his conscience, for he knew that what he had done was not intentional and, indeed, amounted to little. But he could not escape the painful feeling that he had been mean and negligent. The interesting point here is that he also felt that all the others judged him as harshly as he judged himself and thought that no one who knew about it would have any use for him thereafter. He seriously believed this was the reaction of others, even of his friends, until he gradually learned that all they had felt was transient irritation and held him in the same high esteem as always. He had projected his own feeling of unworthiness into the attitudes of others.

This projection of the conscience reaction is an extremely important mechanism. Often in paranoia there are delusions of being watched and observed and having one's mind read. Into these delusions go the patient's whole judgment of himself, and this judgment is sometimes exactly like his parents' judgment of a naughty child. Here what was probably once external, the judgment of the parents, has become internalized as his own standards but is again felt to be an external judgment of others (Freud, 1911). This is seen very widely in milder manifestations, as when a person has some feeling of weakness or guilt and thinks that other persons see it and are depreciating, ridiculing or accusing him. Many belligerent, aggressive individuals are so because of this mechanism. They are really on the defensive—fighting back against the judgments against them which they feel other persons are making. There may be a kernel of truth in this, as in most projections, but it is exaggerated by attributing to others the individual's own self-censure. In *The Informer,* the man who betrayed his friend to his death for the sake of the reward feels thereafter that other persons, who in reality know nothing of it, are accusing him. In depressions, also, the patient makes the harshest judgments of himself, and he often attributes these to other persons as well. Contrariwise, the adult who was adored by his parents may always feel that people are watching him admiringly and may tend to be exhibitionistic.

6. Conscience and Internalization

The development of the conscience often can be seen graphically in early childhood. By the age of a year and a half, the child who has been taught not to touch something may be seen to touch it and then shake its own head and say, "No, No," as though it were the reproving parent.

This conditioning and the internalization of standards can be observed in the domestic animals as well as in human beings. The guilt of puppies is readily observable and has been portrayed on numerous magazine covers.

The universality of conscience reactions is seen in superstitions such as knocking wood, which are chiefly magical methods of warding off fear of projected conscience. This is felt as a sense of anxiety, lest some ill befall to balance the good. The gods who are appeased usually are the now internalized authorities. Much human behavior is motivated by attempts to appease the conscience.

How unconscious the conscience can be, how a man can underestimate its power within himself, has been the theme of innumerable stories and plays, such as Poe's *The Telltale Heart,* Stevenson's *Markheim,* Shakespeare's *Macbeth* and Dostoevsky's *Crime and Punishment.* The person who acts contrary to his conscience can subject himself to a terrible automatic retribution, which destroys him slowly and subtly from within.

7. Healthy Formation of Superego

Normally, the child's domestication and training should take place gradually and in doses which can be digested and assimilated. In the well integrated individual the conscience is a relatively harmonious part of the personality, which the individual accepts. But if the training demands too much, demands it too quickly and is too harsh or too lax and inadequate, then the normal course of learning restraint, of conscience formation and of personality development is disturbed. The upbringing should help development and not disturb good feelings toward the parents and others in the family.

Some persons have had too little training and are deficient in standards, ideals and conscience. There are others whose development is impaired by too much. In some the deficiency is due to a simple lack of training or to actually making delinquency a standard of behavior. There are also those whose training has been adequate but improperly imparted. Good behavior which is obtained too easily and quickly by violent methods, such as extreme threats or punishments, is often seen in later life to have been at the cost of lifelong intimidation, resentment of authority or some similar impairment of development.

Even adults learn best from teachers of whom they are fond, toward whom they like to be submissive, whose love they enjoy, with whom they try to identify. For in the last analysis, the chid accepts the restrictions of life and the standards imposed upon it, provided that these are within normal limits, through the fact that it loves and is loved; but if it feels that it is not loved and is trained, for example, only by domination, then its incentive to accept standards is gone; it learns only through fear of punishment and is apt to develop hatred and rebellion not only toward external authority but also toward its inner representative of these, namely, its own conscience. Moreover, hating authorities, the child cannot identify with them, and so lacks adults upon whom to model itself in its struggle toward emotional maturity. If its emotional environment provides only individuals with immature childish reactions of their own, it is difficult for the child to mature emotionally. Since in adolescence and thereafter, these patterns formed in reaction to parents are transferred in varying degrees to school and to society and their authorities, we have a central built-in source of unrest and hostility in school, the nation and the world.

ILLUSTRATIONS WITH SOME DYNAMIC CONNECTIONS

1. Insufficient Training

A. Children. How children run wild when they do not have adequate care, training and leadership was reported on a national scale in Russia following the Revolution. These were homeless children, the "wild boys of the road." In the film *The Road to Life,* these wild, preadolescent criminals were given a strong, kind young man as a leader. He did not restrain them but trusted them and expected only the best from them. His person provided a figure of authority to whom they could become attached and with whom they could identify. Underneath, like all children and adults, they craved love; and their developmental trends toward maturity led them to admire his quiet strength and to want to be like him. Thus, they gradually assimilated his social controls and standards. This type of treatment works for some children with deficient "superegos." Doubtless many a young boy has been reclaimed because it has been possible through the social agencies to provide him with a strong, kind young man who affords him the kind of person who had been missing in his life. But if the childhood pattern with its hostility is too deeply ingrained, the child cannot be reached.

Infantile, impulse-ridden, unrestrained children are an everyday type of case. They usually grow up to be infantile, impulse-ridden adults. One such sophisticated little miss of eight was a problem because of sexual play of all sorts as well as lying, stealing, begging, cruelty and similar entirely unrestrained behavior. She was, of course, intolerable in school, and because of her corrupting influence most children had to be kept away from her. There were almost no imaginable lurid types of behavior in which she had not indulged. She had also learned how to get toys from children by tales of deprivation, and tidbits from the corner grocer by plaints of being underfed. She had run the gamut of sexual experiences. In one of her cruel spells she dropped a cat down a well. At the same time she could be very affectionate and loving, and most adults could not help liking her in spite of everything she did. She knew this and boasted with glee how she managed to "work" people by holding their hands and making up to them.

The reason for her make-up was immediately apparent from her history and was a simple reflection of the early environment in which she was brought up. Her warmth with people was a direct reflection of the fact that she was apparently the family darling. She knew how to give and how to receive affection. But she had had practically no social training or discipline whatsoever. She was allowed free expression of all feelings—destructiveness, cruelty and rivalry. She would break windows freely or throw an ax at someone. Her sex play was the subject of amused recognition by the parents. Not only was she not trained, but also she felt sanctioned in her behavior by the example of the parents, who took no pains to conceal their own spontaneous instinctual reactions.

By providing suitable foster homes, it is possible in many cases to give a child some social training and examples in kind, firm parents, but it is questionable how much could be accomplished with such a child as this one, warm and affectionate though she was, except over a very long period, since her behavior afforded her such gratifications. Her development was impaired in two ways: in the formation of the structure of her personality, in that she had no chance to develop proper controls of her primitive impulses and to form a superego of automatic, unconscious standards, ideals and restraints which would be consonant with mature social functioning in our culture; and in the development of her childhood impulses to more mature forms and attitudes. Freely indulging all her childish impulses had the effect of "fixating" her to these enjoyments and blunting the tendencies to relinquish them or transform them into mature, social, constructive activities and attitudes. Such persons are not "neurotic" in the strict sense of *conflict* over their behavior and repressed impulses causing symptoms, for there is little sense of guilt or shame, and the primitive impulses are gratified directly. But it is a "neurotic" condition in the broad sense of impaired emotional development. It is a personality disorder. She is an "impulse ridden" character or personality, a behavior disorder in the category "acting out." *

In girls, delinquency often takes the form of promiscuity (which, of course, has other motivations also), and in many of these cases the absence of a stable background is found. An adolescent girl was picked up several times, after having hitchhiked around the country and having had various sordid sexual experiences. She turned out to be a pretty, intelligent girl and expressed an interest in music and secretarial work. She knew that she was unable to control her impulse-ridden behavior. The stuff of control and the encouragement, training and models for development were lacking. Her mother had been married five times and was neglectful of the daughter who from earliest childhood knew no other life than to which she had been exposed and which she was now living.

A widespread miscomprehension concerning psychoanalytic therapy is (or perhaps *was*) that its aim is to release inhibitions. Recently, someone told me that he thought the superego was a pathological part of the personality that should be removed by psychoanalysis! The aim of therapy, which operates through insight into motivations, that is, through *emotional honesty* in this regard, is to help the patient recognize and appreciate, as fully as possible, his true impulses and desires, both the childish and the mature; to bring them under the purview of conscious realization and judgment, so that rigidity and automaticity of reaction can yield to greater flexibility, conscious choice and the reopening of this hitherto blocked part of the personality to further development. To know one's impulses does not mean to act on them. In infantile, impulse-ridden personalities the aim of the treatment can

---

* Diagnostic and Statistical Manual of Mental Disorders, prepared by the Committee on Nomenclature and Statistics of the American Psychiatric Association, second edition, Washington, D.C., American Psychiatric Association, 1978 (Draft).

be only to *increase* the forces of control and by no means to reduce inhibitions. The same is true with regard to individuals who are under such severe emotional tension that there is danger of some kind of breakdown.

B. Trusting One's Conscience to an Authority. Authority, once internalized, can, to an extent, still be handed over to an external person. This is seen in hypnotism and also in groups in which the authority of the individual is given over to the leader. In military organizations and in other groups with leaders, one can see how individuals submit themselves to the orders of their leaders rather than to their own consciences. In such situations the leader replaces the conscience, and the individuals do what he permits or orders. Then one often sees how thin the veneer of civilization can be. It is in large part because of this phenomena that individuals behave in groups with an abandon they would not permit themselves as individuals. However, groups tend to attract individuals of similar dynamics. If many hostile persons join together and organize, they can dare *pathological, hostile acting out,* even violent criminal behavior, because of the personal security of the group. The group only brings out in each member what is already there.

When, as in war, the group sanctions or requires behavior which is contrary to the man's conscience, and he cannot fully transfer this conscience to the group or his leaders, then a conflict ensues. This type of conflict is one of the sources of war neuroses.

C. Releases from Restraints. The importance for the social life of release from the superego is manifold. Holidays, celebrations, orgies, demonstrations, confrontations and also some revolutions and wars, partake of the nature of releases from the conscience, in which all kinds of indulgences, otherwise in restraint, are for a while permitted.

The role of the forces of control and of repression is important to understand in every case. We have mentioned briefly two instances in which it was inadequate. In many cases these forces are not pathological in kind or extent but are important chiefly because of the nature and the intensity of the impulses which they check and turn back on the person or distort into symptoms.

2. Too Strict Training

A. Animals. Too strict training is apt to result either in too great submissiveness in the individual or else in irrational rebellion against all authority. These are primitive reactions seen in animals as well as in human beings. Horses or dogs trained improperly or too severely may become rebellious and dangerous or have their spirits broken.

B. Literature. In literature, Marquand's *The Late George Apley* affords a delightful portrayal of the effects of too strong inculcation of standards and a way of life. George Apley is subjected to the gentle but firm pressure of his family and forced to conform to their manner of living. His early school, his dancing class, his friends and associations are all selected for him. Of course, he goes to Harvard, does what is expected of him in the extracurricular activities and becomes a member of the right clubs. His position in business awaits him and, tacitly, his wife is just about selected for him. He is pressed quietly and neatly into a niche in life. His rebellion is short-lived. The family wins, and he breaks off with the girl of his own choice. But this renunciation of his own love and of all that love implies occasions a "nervous breakdown," after which he gives up his struggle for independence and accepts as his own the family's standards, attitudes and social forms. He now becomes himself a model and an exponent of them. He marries the girl he is expected to marry. He leads a cool, pleasant life, but a life which is not his own, which is not made from within but ordered by others, a life which is not quite real.

C. Adults. The life of a young woman who had been born with a silver spoon illustrates what can result when anger and rebellion are provoked but meet with the restraints of high social standards of training. A young woman of 30, from the West Coast, had been born into a social setting similar to that described for George Apley. She was subjected to insistent pressure by her family. Instead of educating her in the etymologic sense of "leading out" and facilitating the development of her personality, individuality and self-expression, with only the necessary restraints for socialization, her parents pressured her to submit to the plan of life which was given to her. She rebelled against these constraints and became very angry at her parents. Her rebellion and anger were intensified by a personal emotional factor. This was the parents' relative rejection of the girl emotionally in favor of her older brother. These two traumata produced the following state of affairs. She was angry and hostile because of rebellion against giving in to a submissive attitude and because of the rejection in favor of her brother. But in spite of her rebellion, the training took considerable effect, and she internalized it as a strict but unaccepted conscience. Her anger at her parents was a spite reaction directed at their most vulnerable spot and at one source of her anger, namely, their social standards; but because of her conscience reaction, it took the indirect form of attacking them through depreciating herself socially. In this way she both took revenge on them and satisfied her own conscience by punishing herself. She associated only with people who had no social or economic standing and with many who were on the fringe. She would have nothing to do with the wealthy, accomplished, attractive and socially prominent young man selected for her by her parents but went chiefly with inadequate, ineffectual, unstable persons on the fringe of society, and unconsciously she managed matters so that she was repeatedly in situations which shocked and distressed her parents. Here was a girl who was born to every advantage of person and background. She was beautiful, intelligent, sensitive and cultured. She had offered to her the best of education and of social contacts. She had no need for financial worry. She had her choice of the most eligible young men. Nothing in the external situation or in her personal endowment and capacities was lacking. She might have made a fine contribution to a husband and children and to society. Yet I happened to see her because she came to the clinic for help. She was dressed in the poorest clothes; her shoes were worn. She had left her home town and was tired out from struggling to make both ends meet. She lived alone in a slum area. She always became interested in men who could not decide whether or not to marry her and from whom she, in the end, after months or years of indecision, frustration and heartache, finally broke off. Except for a few girl friends, she dragged along alone, down at the heels and miserable. This young woman is a good example of the way in which both the repressed impulses and the repressing forces enter into the formation of neurotic symptoms. Here the repressed impulse was chiefly hostility, directed at the parents. The repressing force was the girl's high standards of training. She could not vent her hostility freely, like the little eight-year-old already described. She was constrained to be a lady so far as overt social usage went. Her hostility caused strong guilt feelings. Repressed from direct expression, it came out nevertheless indirectly in the symptoms, as repressed impulses always manage to do ("return of the repressed"). In this case, the chief symptom was self-depreciation. It expressed the hostility against the parents and also the punishment for it. This symptom was in the form of behavior in life. Its mechanism of formation was classically neurotic. Such a case falls into a group for which the apt term "neurotic character" has been suggested. More specifically, because her own need for suffering was the most prominent feature of her life, she was a "masochistic personality." This was masochistic "acting out." She became interested only in men with much repressed hostility who made her miserable.

Repressed hostility causes suffering, but obviously the solution is not as vulgar distortion misinterprets it, the free expression of hostility. This is usually unrealistic externally, leads to retaliation by other persons and causes even more guilt than if the hostility is controlled. The way out usually involves a recognition, reorientation and a reduction of the hostility and of the severity of the conscience. "Getting out" the hostility means getting it and its sources and connections out into conscious awareness to reduce it and the problems it creates through diminishing its sources.

A professional man was overtly aggressive but was moderately successful in spite of this. His behavior clearly expressed his poorly restrained or transformed (sublimated) hostility. But it turned out that there was also a conscience reaction in his aggressiveness, namely, the need to punish himself by making people antagonistic to him. Because of this neurotic need to get himself disliked and rejected, his behavior had a provocative motivation also. When people turned against him, he felt a sort of relief mingled with his distress, a feeling that, after all, this had to come sooner or later.

Another example of unassimilated training is a man of 40 who had been dominated in his childhood by his mother. His sister gave in completely to this domination, never left home and never married. She became a bitter, submissive, broken woman, with no life apart from her attachment to her mother, to whom she was virtually a slave. The father reacted to the mother's domination by taking to drink. The patient rebelled, but with only partial success. The mother set him very high ideals. She selected his wife for him as well as choosing his career. Everything he did bore his mother's stamp. He felt that he was not living his own life but was only carrying out her training. This filled him with a sense of restriction and restraint. He felt "caged" and unable to escape the dictates which were deep within him.

This case is an excellent example of unassimilated superego. There was nothing intrinsically wrong with his mother's standards, but he was never *won over* to accepting them as part of himself and integrating them into his personality. Instead, they felt to him like a foreign body in his personality, which he struggled to throw out but could not. He still felt impotent under his mother's tyranny and transferred this feeling to all authorities. He had his own business, for he could not tolerate any boss. His constant struggle and the terrible, continuous rage which it engendered apparently contributed to blood-pressure elevation, if indeed it did not directly cause it. He tried drinking, promiscuity and other unconventional gestures in his efforts to escape and to rebel against this unassimilated training; but when he did so, he became filled with guilt and anxiety which were even more intolerable than the submission. He was eminently successful in his profession, with a fine home and a charming wife and children, but he felt imprisoned, and indeed he was—not by stone walls but by the restrictions of his own superego.

3. Inconsistent Training

It is by no means uncommon for children to be exposed to inconsistent training, such as alternations in strictness and liberality. Sometimes one parent is strict, or simply consistent, while the other is overly repressive or else overly permissive. Confused or inconsistent and conflictful behavior is apt to result in the child. Sometimes a parent is inconsistent by laying down the law but when the time comes to enforce it encourages the child to disregard it. In still other cases, the parent tries to train the child to one standard while setting an example of the opposite.

A. Children. For example, a girl of ten stole and played truant from school, even though her father lectured her and spanked her for this. But the father had his own example to thank, for he had a history of petty thievery, and he reacted to squabbles at home by walking out and spending his time at taverns. Himself an infantile personality, he sometimes fought with his daughter over what station to listen to on the radio, until, in a pet, he would remove a radio tube so that she could not use the instrument and he would walk out with it. The girl imitated his thievery, truancy, petulance, childishness and irresponsibility. She did as he *did*—not as he lectured.

B. Adults. In some cases, both the superego and the temptation to indulge the immature animal instincts become intensified at the same time. A girl was brought up in a brothel by a racketeer father. Nevertheless, to protect her from too free instinctual indulgence, the father leaned over backward in the repressiveness with which he brought her up. He permitted her practically no pleasures, even the simplest, and absolutely forbade any friendship with boys whatsoever. The girl grew up with a striving to rise above her sordid environment. She succeeded to some extent but felt that if she did not struggle she would sink back into it. What this signified was that she felt unconsciously tempted—that if she did not strive to rise and did not continue to forbid herself all pleasure and sexuality, she was threatened with going to the other extreme, rebelling against her father's training, giving in to the examples she had seen, and losing all restraint. To avoid excessive vice she had to be excessively virtuous—like those who dare not drink at all since there is no golden mean for them, temptation is too great, and one drink means too many more. This mechanism of defense is seen in other types of cases. For example, a pampered young man later could keep himself from being a complete wastrel only by plunging himself into work and shunning even the slightest temptation to recreation or pleasure.

Inconsistent parental training shows its effects in the following example. A girl of 18 was the child of parents who divorced when she was seven, and she spent some time with each parent. The mother was extremely puritanical and repressive, looking askance even at movies. She raised the girl in a most strait-laced fashion.

The father was the opposite in outlook. When the girl returned to him at age 17 to spend a year, he and his circle were shocked to find that she did not smoke, never had had a drink, even a beer, and had never experienced sexual relations. When with the father she tried to adopt his standards—when with the mother hers. Like Pavlov's dogs, she was oppositely conditioned in the two homes. The result was a state of incapacitating confusion.

Identification with other people can be very complete and precise, be they parents or siblings or mere acquaintances, and often a person takes toward others the attitudes of his own superego toward himself. A very successful man was most strict with himself, never satisfied with his accomplishments, always striving and driving himself to do better. And this was exactly his attitude toward his subordinates—he looked down on them, treated them as inadequate, criticized their errors, rarely praising them but always driving them ruthlessly to improvement in themselves and their work. His attitudes toward them and toward himself were amazingly precise repetitions of the attitudes his own father had had toward him all during his childhood.

So, too, one commonly sees a person who has taken over toward himself the strictness his parents had toward him and then identifies with his own children and repeats this strictness (or other attitudes) toward them. Everyone has a concept of himself which is derived from the formative emotional influences of his childhood. The younger the child the more profound the effects of these external influences; the core of the personality is pretty well formed by the age of about six (Saul, 1977). The child takes over from his parents, or their substitutes, not only standards, ideals and dictates, not only their attitudes toward the world, but also their attitudes toward himself. One boy, because of the death of a previous child, is overly adored, and as he grows up he takes over this adoring attitude toward himself. Another is unwanted and senses this and goes through life thinking of himself as a poor little unacceptable outcast. In reality, the rest of his personality has matured and he is successful and popular, while secretly he eats his heart out because of this picture of himself, which, as usual, represents what was a reality of childhood but is now no longer true. Assuredly, one's feelings not only toward others but also toward himself are of prime importance for his whole emotional life.

SOCIOLOGICAL IMPLICATIONS

A person's standards, ideals and conscience are essentially the socialized part of the personality, the representation in the individual of training, customs and cultural factors. (Presumably these express the mature conclusions of his adult society. But because so many adults, perhaps most, suffer from warped patterns from their own early years, these social norms are only a sort of average of the maturity and distorted childishness of most of the individuals of the society.) It is this aspect of the personality, in technical shorthand the "superego," which has certain common factors in each culture and varies as between cultures.* It is obviously of first importance in anthropological studies (Saul, 1979). And it is essential to many problems of war and of criminology and to the whole attitude of society to crime. It is reflected in religion, which, entirely apart from other considerations, represents in essence, so far as psychology alone is concerned, a projection of man's struggle with his instincts—more precisely the struggle between the immature animal impulses and the restraining and socializing forces of a mature parental authority. This is all part of the struggle of mankind to grow up and to live together civilly (which is the essence of civilization)—an age-old struggle which is reflected in almost all human thought and endeavor from dreams to great organizations—the neurotic, that is the warped childhood, versus the mature, the responsible loving.

Prevailing ideologies reflect the status of the conscience of the group. Ideologies must be judged on a scale of biopsychological maturity as themselves infantile or mature. Their power in influencing standards and behavior is well known, but their origins have not been fully explored, nor do we, perhaps, appreciate the extent to which they affect our own outlooks (Alexander, 1942; Freud, 1912).

However, one point can be made with mathematical certainty. Any society in which most parents raise their children with pathological superegos, with unassimilated socialization to family life, with impulse ridden or self indulgent behavior or with anger

---

* The wildest dreams of Kew are the facts of Khatmandu,
  The crimes of Clapham chaste in Martabam.

and rebellion, overt or repressed, that society is bringing to adulthood a generation filled with these same characteristics in their political and social behavior, a generation rife with crime, violence and revolution, and incapable of mature, constructive solutions. The child who grows up hating his parents, hating their internalizations in his own mind as his superego, will transfer this hatred in large part to the authorities of school and state. Thus, hatred is generated internally and usually has little to do with the actual behavior of the authorities themselves. Every act or incident will be *rationalized* to justify this hostility provoked by the parents and now continuing within the adult personality. Thus parents unwittingly breed in their very young children not only neurosis but crime, revolutions, wars and the decay and destruction of nations.

REFERENCES

Alexander, F. (1930): *Psychoanalysis of the Total Personality*. New York: Nervous and Mental Disease Publishing Co.
_____ (1936): *The Medical Value of Psychoanalysis*, 2nd edition. New York: Norton.
_____ (1942): *Our Age of Unreason*. Philadelphia: Lippincott.
_____ (1961): *The Scope of Psychoanalysis*, ed. by T. French. New York: Basic Books, pp. 129–136.
Allee, W. (1951): *Cooperation Among Animals*. New York: Abelard.
Carrighar, S. (1965): *Wild Heritage*. Boston: Houghton Mifflin.
Eisenbud, R. (1968): Masochism revisited, *Psychoanalytic Quarterly* 54(4):5.
Erickson, E. (1964): *Insight and Responsibility*. New York: Norton.
Freud, S. (1911): Psychoanalytic notes upon an autobiographical account of a case of paranoia, *S.E.* 12.
_____ (1912): Totem and taboo, *S.E.* 13.
_____ (1915): Thoughts on war and death, *S.E.* 14, p. 275.
_____ (1923): The ego and the id, *S.E.* 19, Parts II & III.
_____ (1924): The economic problem in masochism, *S.E.* 19, p. 157.
_____ (1930): Civilization and its discontents, *S.E.* 21, Part VII.
Hilgard, E. (1948): *Theories of Learning*. New York: Appleton-Century-Crofts.
Masserman, J. (1968): *Science and Psychoanalysis*, Vol. 12. New York: Grune and Stratton.
Menninger, K. (1938): *Man Against Himself*. New York: Harcourt.
Panken, S. (1967): On masochism: a reevaluation, *Psychoanalytic Review* 54(3):527.
Saul, L. J. (1950): The punishment fits the source, *Psychoanalytic Quarterly* 19:164.
_____ (1976): *Psychodynamics of Hostility*. New York: Jason Aronson.
_____ (1977): *The Childhood Emotional Pattern*. New York: Van Nostrand Reinhold.
_____ (1979): *The Childhood Emotional Pattern in Marriage*. New York: Van Nostrand Reinhold, Chapter 6.
Smirnoff, V. (1969): The masochistic contract, *International Journal of Psychoanalysis* 50(4):65.

6 | Hostility and Violence

GENERAL FORMULATION

There is no more fateful motive force in man than hostility—it is essential for his survival but it also produces neurosis, criminality, war and social unrest. Resentment, anger, rage, violence, cruelty and similar aggressive, destructive impulses can be included under the term hostility. "Hostility" is more precise than "aggressiveness," which is ambiguous in that this also implies initiative and activity which are not necessarily "hostile." Moreover, hostility can be vented passively. Hostility is one of the most difficult forces in human beings to domesticate. Necessary and useful as it is in certain circumstances, such as under primitive conditions of nature in killing for food and in self-defense, it is one of the greatest sources of human suffering. We have already noted that the rational use of hostility by one form of life that feeds on another must be demarcated clearly from the neurotic hostility of human beings against each other, which jeopardizes social cooperation, man's greatest instrument for security in nature, and now threatens us not only with criminality and tyranny but also, through the atom bomb, with extinction of our species. For civilized man, neither wild beasts nor the forces of nature nor even the dread germs of disease are the greatest cause of suffering. It is the neurotic hostility within man himself which is directed against his own kind . . . man's *irrational, pathologically hostile acting out.* Can it be that, however far a civilization such as ours progresses technologically, it will not only have within its grasp the means of destroying the human race but will eventually use these means to do so?

It has been estimated that the world has known less than 300 days of peace in the past 4,000 years. In the decade from 1960 to 1970 there were wars involving 70 of the existing 140 nations. But war and criminality are only overt expressions of hostility. It comes out in innumerable forms in social life—in slavery, in racketeering, in some practices of management and of labor, in the treatment of children, in families, in gossiping and backbiting, in exploiting and misleading and all the other ways, gross and petty, which are described in the history books and in the novels and which every child and adult in some degree must see and endure every day of his life. Men find themselves upon this planet with livelihood and pleasures to be won. Cooperation has proven to be the best and obvious procedure. Yet war and cruelty have been glorified from the dawn of history. Apart from this, when people try to cooperate for the benefit of all, they succeed only to a certain degree—for they are opposed in this by their own hostilities and antagonisms to one another. These feelings are not generally recognized, for in most modern civilized men they are contrary to the social mores and are largely unconscious. Few persons, indeed, realize how hostile they are, and our ignorance does not help us in attacking the problem of this inner force which menaces humanity today, even more than it has throughout history. For men rationalize, excuse and treat moralistically, heatedly, vindictively an emotional force which they repress and do not wish to see in its full intensity within themselves—rather than facing it frankly, objectively and scientifically like a disease or any other dangerous force of nature.

Hostility causes suffering in still another way in addition to its direct and naked and its indirect and disguised expressions against others. It rebounds upon the individual himself in the form of all kinds of neurotic symptoms and as the remarkable phenomenon of "masochism."

Hostility occupies a position in dynamic psychology analogous to that of heat in physics. Thermodynamics teaches us that no physical process occurs without the generation of heat and its flow from the hotter to the cooler area. In the psychodynamics of the mental and emotional life, there is probably no impairment, frustration, conflict, anxiety or friction of any kind which does not result in hostility as a reaction, and the hostility seeks to express itself in some way. Hostility is probably the psychological correlate and perception of the body's automatic physiological response to any irritation or threat, that is, of the body's physiological mobilization for fight or flight.

This response is one of the basic biological self-preservative *"behavioral response mechanisms"* seen in all species throughout the animal kingdom. Hence, in general, exaggerated hostility can be taken as a sign of irritation or danger, external or within the personality. The internal threats almost always are the results of long-standing injurious influences (traumata) during childhood. (It is a general misconception that trauma means a single damaging event, usually in childhood. Such can occur and will be discussed in Section 3, but the everyday warpings of the personality of growing children are from long-standing abuses of commission or omission over all or most of the years of childhood and, as we repeatedly emphasize, the younger the child the more vulnerable it is.)

The causes of hostile behavior can be entirely internal, as in the compulsive or psychotic, unprovoked and senseless killers, or the cause can be predominantly external (*reactive*) as in self-defense.

The *outcomes* of hostility also can range from fully internal to fully acted out against others, and provide a simplified but accurate schema of psychiatric diagnostic categories: entirely pent up, the hostility can cause physiological disorders such as headache and elevated blood pressure; it can disturb thinking and feeling to produce neurosis, or disrupt them, causing psychosis; it can be acted out against the self masochistically as we pointed out above, the ultimate being irrational suicide; the acting out can be against others subtly and within the law (criminoid) or as every form of overt crime: at the ultimate, sadism, violence and murder.

But is not hostility more than this? Is it not also a force in the individual like sexuality or like the regressive trends? Freud came gradually to this conclusion. He saw it as essential in getting food and in self-preservation, acutely mobilized in emergencies, but like sex in the broad sense, whether latent or activated, a fundamental biological force in the personality. Just as he came to think of sex as a specialized expression of a conserving, preserving tendency of the organism to take in food, build up, reproduce, and come together in groups and societies, so he came to see hostility as a manifestation of a general destructive tendency in organisms— useful in self-defense, killing for food, sometimes sexually in dominating the female, and in these and similar situations serving Eros, the life-preserving tendency, but also operative as a sheer destructive force toward others and also toward the individual, in whom it becomes manifest eventually in senescence and death (Freud, 1930).

Sadly, it must be admitted that many people, in the ordinary course of their lives, do more harm than good to their fellows, causing them much unnecessary suffering. Society at large and many individuals would probably be spared torment and have better lives if those who do untold harm were dead or had never been born.

The extreme is the criminal who, consciously, directly and deliberately damages the lives of others, even injuring or killing them. Why should society hesitate to eliminate such violent acting-outers? The moral argument states that society must respect life, and therefore not use the death penalty for punishment. Realistically, such an argument is based on the fear that, if society claimed the right to kill even for self-protection, many hostile members of that society would feel less inhibition to kill individually and indiscriminately, and killing would increase.

The death penalty used as punishment makes little sense (as the old man said as he mounted the scaffold: "This sure will teach me a lesson!"). It might relieve the revenge feelings of society, but there is no convincing evidence that it is a deterrent to crime and acted out hostility. However, it does remove from society those members who injure innocent people, and relieves society of the expense of supporting the criminals in jails.

But punishment does not strike at the root of the central problem: criminal, hostile behavior is not entirely willful, responsible action but is mostly an expression of reactions to traumatic treatment in childhood, and as such is not really the individual's fault. The deepest moral consideration asks: can society surgically remove those emotionally disordered persons who injure others, even though their actions are the result of how they were treated as children?

It is true that in clinical experience and from psychological observations of everyday life, every single individual shows strong hostile trends, more or less overt, disguised or repressed. But in therapeutic practice it is possible substantially to alter and decrease the hostile tendencies in most cases so that they no longer cause suffering to the individual or to others. Most often childhood influences form a pattern which results in the constant generation of hostility, and this hostility and the reactions to it play their part in the symptoms, in the personality structure and its functioning, in human relationships and in the whole course of the individual's life.

It is difficult to accept man's hostility to his own kind as anything but a mental and emotional illness (i.e., a neurotic aberration), especially as it is all but unknown throughout the rest of the animal kingdom in the forms and extents seen in *homo sapiens*. Moreover, the enormous differences between the unrestrained killer and the person of good will are invariably traceable back to terrible abuse in the childhood of the former. Not all men hate and are cruel and violent to other humans—only those who were made to react this way as children.

Obviously this generation of hostility in childhood, with its far-reaching effects throughout all the rest of the individual's life, is a central problem in the bringing up of children. It probably can never be avoided entirely. Some schizophrenics were too good—in part, because their developmental drives and their instinctual demands were too weak, and they were too passive, dependent and accepting. For most, perhaps all, normal children, no matter how sweet and satisfied in their very early years, there comes a time when some situation generates deep-going feelings of resentment and hostility. It may be something in the most normal course of events, such as the birth of a new brother or sister; or even without this, it may be simply the envy which the small child feels for the adults and the resentment of being little, weak and dependent and excluded from the comings and the goings of mother and father; or a protest against growing up and relinquishing the more infantile care and attention. The only child, as well as the child in a large family, sooner or later, no matter how carefully brought up, shows some signs of repressed anger, however minimal. These signs may not be obvious but they are unmistakable if one knows what to look for—in behavior, in self-injuries, in anxiety, in bad dreams, needing a night light and so on. These are the "normal" children of normal, happy homes, with little or nothing unusual to stimulate hostility.

The first child may feel displaced from the parents' exclusive love when a second arrives. The second must always have the first a step ahead. The middle child has its own problems, inevitable in any human triangle. One or both parents may be under the strains of earning a livelihood and managing a household. Thus, even loving, understanding families with emotionally stable parents usually harbor some stresses and frustrations. But in such relatively harmonious homes the hostility is of low grade and the children handle this without appreciable disturbances to their development. But if the home is broken or the child rejected or overly restricted, or mistreated by fate or the ignorance or the malice or the neuroses of its parents or guardians—then the soil is laid for a heightened hostile reaction which can seriously warp the child's development and cause suffering to others also.

Often the individual does not realize just who or what is making him angry. This is especially true in children. There is some irritation or frustration and the automatic response is anger. In many cases this makes the person feel irritable, tense and unhappy for reasons which he comprehends but dimly, if at all. He struggles with an automatic rage response which occurs without his will or control, the extent and the source of which he does not appreciate. But there is always a reason, although it may not always be easy to find. One man's wife used to inform him when he was in a rage—it was obvious to her and others, but he did not know it himself and only felt unhappy and disgruntled. A traffic policeman once accidentally helped me in the treatment of a young woman. She was a "masochistic" girl who was not aware of her hostility and took it out subtly but devastatingly on herself, discarding every advantage of birth and endowment for a life of useless misery. She could not realize in what a rage she usually was, although this was obvious in her expression, manner and behavior as well as in her psychological outlook. One day while she was waiting to cross the street, the policeman genially remarked, "What is the matter—why are you so angry?" She looked up in surprise. "You look as though you want to murder someone," said the policeman good-naturedly. She was deeply impressed by this and began to understand what I had been trying to help her see. Morning irritability (getting up on the wrong side of the bed, "I am not worth a thing until I have my coffee," etc.) is often a result of the relaxed controls of sleep, which are not yet fully reestablished, and of anger at exchanging the pleasant self-indulgent realm of dreamland for the demands and the responsibilities of real life.

Hostility against the person (or situation) who provoked it is readily displaced to other persons. Konrad Lorenz has described this in animals (1952). The hostile individual tends to take it out wherever he can—on other persons, on the dog, by kicking something and even on himself. Conversely, some persons become enraged at themselves ("I could just kick myself") for their own weaknesses or defects or behavior then also turn this anger outward toward other persons. Often the source of the anger is unknown or forgotten and the person's main aim is *the relief of the hostility in some kind of action,* how and against whom being secondary considerations. In extreme cases, it is even a toss-up whether the individual will kill himself or someone else. The newspapers repeatedly carry accounts of persons who do both. This *displaceability,* this deflectability, is one of the features of hostility which makes it so important a problem, the source of so much cruelty, injustice and neurotic suffering. The child who grows up in a rage at a parent or other family members usually displaces this rage to others during its adult life. Hence all the problems in interpersonal relations, including those in marriage.

The extent to which hostility can become an *end in itself* is not generally appreciated. We are all great rationalizers and like to believe in good reasons to justify our emotional satisfactions. We do not like to believe that men *enjoy* hostile behavior, cruelty and fighting but like to think that there is always a sufficient, immediate external reason, that these are only means which are justified by the ends. Such reasons may exist. But sometimes they are only a precipitating factor, and sometimes they are only an excuse or rationalization for the means, which may be the *real* reason. Present or not, they do not preclude the fact that in many persons there is a secret, but often overt, satisfaction in hostile aggression. This is, in essence, "sadism." This was expressed rather neatly by a young woman patient whose anger and hostility were stimulated by rejection in childhood. She had read of a woman stabbing a man to death and gloated over this and frankly wished that she had the courage to do the same. When this was discussed—the injustice, the neuroticism, the penalty and the like—she had a single answer, "But just think of the gratification!" Under the pressure of her own hostility she wished that just once she could give in to her cruel fantasies and vent her rage. We know from the daily papers that some people do give in to these desires, sometimes even toward their own parents. Fortunately, this girl had a sufficiently well-developed personality to preclude such acting out. Instead of *pathologically hostile acting out* behavior (i.e., criminal behavior), she had neurotic symptoms. She suffered from anxieties, which cut her off from a love-life and from enjoyable human relations. She knew that the only solution to her problem was not to vent her hostility, but to reduce it by analyzing its sources, freeing herself from the childhood attitudes which prolonged it and developing adult attitudes.

Even when a person attempts flight rather than fight, there is often an important admixture of hostility—"spiteful flight."

For example, a young man meets some emotional pressure. It might result from a great variety of situations. He meets with a rebuff, the pressure of work becomes more than he can carry, his parents come to visit him—any circumstance which strikes an emotional vulnerability with force enough to throw his typical fight-flight reaction into gear. Different persons under such pressures fly into acute episodes of alcoholism, drugs, promiscuity, perversions and the like. The flight element is often obvious. Through this behavior the individual escapes from the painful situation, but, in addition, this escape is apt to contain an element of rage. It is not a quiet withdrawal but often a bitterly spiteful one directed against whoever offended him and usually turning out destructively for himself.

Such spiteful flight also can lead to extravagance, gambling and other such reactions. One woman was extremely sensitive to any rebuff and would react to it with reckless spending and also by sexual indulgences in which she was conscious of an element of revenge.

Spiteful flight is seen in extreme form in some cases of suicide. However, it is not always destructive. It may even find highly constructive outlets. Some women escape their husbands and some men escape their wives, just as some children escape their parents and relieve their anger against them, by plunging into some form of creative activity—be it study, manual work, art, poetry, science or professional activity. It is probably a matter of the mature productive drives being strong enough to dictate the direction and provide the channel.

To understand a person one must understand the status of his hostility, its intensity, its role in the nuclear constellation, its sources, its forms, its directions, the reactions of the rest of the personality to it, how it is handled, repressed and expressed. An exhaustive treatment of this vital problem of man's hostility to man would be too extensive for our main purpose. It is dealt with more extensively in the author's *Psychodynamics of Hostility* (1976). The operation of hostility is to be seen in almost all cases described in this book, although it is not always central and is not emphasized in the presentation and the discussion of cases in which our interest focuses on other tendencies. Even when simple passive dependence is the central feature, as in the cases cited in earlier chapters, this regularly causes frustration and hurt pride and results in reactions of repressed hostility. Only one case will be presented here, but it will enable us to focus on some common sources and results of hostility in the emotional life. It will also serve as a more rounded illustration of the interplay of those motivations which have been described in the preceding four chapters. Of course, all the main tendencies are present in everyone in various degrees, proportions and combinations.

Distinguished scholars cannot seem to agree whether man's hostility to man is a universal human instinct (as Freud concluded), or whether man is "born good" and becomes hostile to his fellows—in a word, is human hostility the result of nature or nurture? This "either-or" type of thinking seems to be a gross oversimplification. The reality, I believe, is that "human nature" contains many tendencies, some favoring sympathy, identification and love for others, which we properly call "pro-human" forces. Other tendencies, such as cruelty, violence and general hostility to others, may be termed "anti-human." In understanding human hostility, every one of these component tendencies must be analyzed in detail and evaluated. This subject urgently requires research, but an emotional resistance against such a study seems to exist. We hope these studies will come in time to illuminate the problem of hostility, which now threatens mankind's very existence. It does seem clear that one important component of anti-human hostility springs from the fight part of the flight-fight reactive mechanism of adaptation.

A CLINICAL EXAMPLE WITH ILLUSTRATIVE DYNAMICS

An able young lawyer of 32, A. L. was well-built, attractive in appearance and personality, sensitive, discriminating and highly intelligent. He was popular and generally considered to be a relatively normal and most eligible bachelor. It surprised all except a few discerning persons when he went to a psychiatrist. This is a frequent occurrence in practice. Many of the most ostensibly normal persons will come with problems. Sometimes these are serious but have been well hidden. Sometimes these persons have no more emotional problem than what is average, but have the interest, the courage, the intelligence and the emotional honesty to wish to deal with them. There is an old quip that psychoanalysis is a fine thing, especially if one is nearly normal.

This young man was normal by the usual standards. He had no serious neurotic symptoms; but, as it turned out, he had certain emotional trends in his make-up which were ruining his seemingly enviable life. The most central one of these was hostility.

His mother evidently had been kind, supportive and maternal but also rather passive, retiring and colorless. This is how he described her, and this is how she appeared in his fantasies and dreams, and in his real life mother figures never played any significant part. She seemed to be of minor importance in his emotional life. The central figure was his father, and next in importance his sister, who was four years his junior. In his father's mixture of attitudes toward him the leading ones were indulgence and domination, on the one hand, and ambition for him on the other.

Neurotic conflicts often have this structure (Kubie, 1943).* The patient, like many others, had been subjected to opposite conditionings—to be passive, dependent, indulged, praised, petted, supported and, simultaneously, to be ambitious, energetic, and heroically accomplishing and achieving. Both his passive-receptive-dependent desires and also his prestige needs and self-love were overly cultivated by his well-meaning father. Moreover, his expectations for gratification of both trends were prolonged by the father's comfortable financial position and the prospects of an independent income for life. He longed for his father's love and

---

* We again remind the reader that throughout this text the term "neurotic" is used not in its narrow technical sense, denoting the classical neuroses, such as anxieties, phobias, compulsions, but in its broad sense of "emotional disorder," including psychosomatic symptoms, addictions and all the behavior disorders not excluding criminality. We use it comprehensively for all symptoms, the physiological and psychological internal ones and also those with involved acting out. The term neurotic has another implication also: namely, the cause of the symptoms as a persistence of warped childhood emotional patterns.

support, but this led to anger and hostility as a defense because he contrariwise wanted to be independent on his own; but he was also angered when these desires were not gratified.

He was raised in close physical proximity with his sister, sharing a bed with her until eight years old. This appeared to stimulate and hasten, and perhaps intensify, his sexual feelings, which, however, he strongly repressed so far as she in particular was concerned. Toward her he was the superior older brother, the masculine hero—but he also envied her for her baby role in the family. He hated her for this and for any sign of weakness in herself, for this reminded him of his own weaknesses. This is a very common mechanism—to hate in another something which is present, often unconsciously, in oneself, and which one hates in oneself.

He never had gotten on normally with the other children but was always rather fearful of being attacked or hurt in rough games and constantly tried to hide his anxieties. They appeared at night after he retired, when he fantasied all sorts of dire happenings to himself and to the members of his family and often was too frightened by these to fall asleep for hours. At preadolescence he had bedtime fantasies of making all sorts of sadistic attacks. These started with little girls as the objects, but unconsciously these little girls represented his sister and he felt guilty about this and afraid of the sexual element, so, also unconsciously, the objects of his sadistic fantasies changed to little boys. These fantasies soon obtained a sexual coloring and stimulated sexual feelings in him. With the advent of adolescence and the access of sexual feelings toward girls, they changed into fantasies of sexual attacks on girls and culminated in frequent masturbation. After his first sexual experience, he became girl-crazy which, because of his hostility, meant unconsciously, in large degree, hostile attacks, with very little of love. He could not succeed in making up his mind to marriage. No single girl could satisfy all his conflicting desires. The older, more maternal types appealed to his dependence, his child to mother and father residue; those dependent and submissive to *him* were younger sister figures who appealed to his mature masculinity but did not satisfy his desires for a parent figure. Moreover, his underlying feelings contained too much hostility and not enough love. Hence, he could not sustain any longtime intimate contact with another person of either sex.

Love is much emphasized in morals, ethics and religion because it is so difficult to achieve. People try to love one another but cannot because the undercurrent of feeling between them contains too much hostility. If this is frankly recognized, then the chances of achieving the goal of brotherly love are improved, for what hinders and obstructs it then can be recognized, studied and, eventually, we hope, dealt with. This young man was a case in point. He tried to love a girl and to marry her. He tried to love his friends and colleagues. But he could not—chiefly because of the underlying hostility which pervaded his feelings toward people.

His father's funds were enough to see the patient through law school. Fulfilling the ambition cultivated in him, he did brilliantly in his studies but then his father lost his money, forcing him to face a career on his own, from scratch. After his father's death, he always found one man whom he hated and one whom he idealized and looked to for help. He thus had two men to take the place of his father ("split father image"), one for the hostility and one for the dependence, identification and idealization.

Despite his intellectual brilliance and personal gifts, he did not get on professionally or socially so well as he anticipated and never rose above a mediocre position. As time went by, he tended to withdraw from competition and gravitated toward the fringe of professional and social status. Thus his hostility was taking a masochistic form.

His sadistic fantasies now found social expression through sympathy and identification with this or that cause and hostility to its enemies. He suffered nightly from increasingly terrible nightmares so that he feared to go to sleep. In these there would regularly be a larger man who was hostile, and the patient would have to battle for his life. This man usually would have an ax or a knife and sometimes would aim to castrate the patient. This, in reverse, was part of the content of the patient's childhood sadistic fantasies—it was what he fantasied doing to others, the while experiencing pleasurable sexual sensations. Hostile impulses very often take this form. In childhood the patient *fantasied* being the *attacker,* now he *dreamed* of *being attacked.*

In another type of dream the patient expressed his passive-receptive wishes—for example, a dream of going away and marrying the large, strong daughter of a very wealthy man. Thus, dreams reflect the mind's efforts to reconcile conflicting urges. Here he represents his wish to marry, to have a sister figure, but not to relinquish the desires to lean on a big strong woman and to retain his dependence on a strong wealthy father. These are the original passive-receptive trends which were part of the core of his problem and of his hostile reactions, and also the wish to escape back to these attitudes and satisfactions from the emotional struggles which they caused. The wish to *be* big and strong in spite of this is also obvious in the desire in the dream to achieve it as a reflected glory—not by *being* independent and adult but by marrying one who was. In the dream he satisfied both wishes. This is commonly, almost universally, seen. The boy or man who is not able but strongly wishes to *act* as the potent adult, that is, to discharge the obligations of responsibility and productivity, strives for the signs of power that will make him *feel* strong and will win admiration from his fellows.

Thus this patient carried into adult life the emotional conflicts and patterns of his childhood, with his older friends and colleagues in the place of his father and mother, and with his girls in the place of his sister. Also, he remained a "little boy" in his profession. We are interested here in analyzing his reactions only so far as necessary to show the main sources and the consequences of his hostile impulses. These were studied extensively in this patient for therapeutic purposes, and the findings that follow are based on this information—not only on the meager sketch given above.

The patient's anger was not merely "reactive" to the treatment to which he was subjected as a child. It continued as a response to needs and attitudes within himself which were strengthened and prolonged by this treatment. Four main sources of the hostility could readily be discerned. They are common ones: (1) simple frustration of passive-receptive-dependent love needs; (2) a defense against such wishes; (3) hurt prestige, chiefly because of these wishes; and (4) retaliation for hostility.

1. The patient, like any other child who is used to having everything done for him, reacted with resentment and hostility against being pushed out of this position, against having to shoulder responsibilities for himself. Hostility was apparent whenever he did not get the help and the attention he desired and was used to during his early childhood. This was an especially important source of

hostility in his adult life. He longed to be dependent and take his ease but had to exert himself, after his father lost his money, and make his own way completely. This enraged him. Unlike the young man described earlier in this book who was glad to see the family fortune lost because now he could be like other men and learn to make his own living, this patient was bitterly angry and never sorgave his father for losing the inheritance.

His own ambition was also a source of hostility. It drove him from within, just as necessity drove him from without, to effort and exertion; but the more he worked the more he inwardly protested angrily against it and railed at his lot. Sometimes such protests cause "nervous breakdowns" of various sorts in part as a kind of "strike" reaction—a refusal to go on any longer. As a child, he had reacted to his younger sister with hatred for pushing him out of the position of baby in the family. And later his hostility to her, which was quite open, was fed by envy of her for being a girl, for, as such, she was not under so much pressure to live up to the standards of effort and accomplishment which were set for him as a male. This resentment of being pushed out of the baby position and his jealousy and envy of the younger child in some degree probably represent a universal reaction of children. In adult life our patient continued this pattern in the form of hostility to his girl friends and to women in general out of regressive envy. He felt that they had an easier time of it. He resented the effort and the giving—emotional, physical, temporal and financial—involved in holding on to his mistresses. He wanted to marry a girl who would support him financially and emotionally, but he also feared and resented such a dependent relationship after his experiences with his father; and his masculine and developmental drives to independence also urged him to shun dependence, and so he could not gratify this desire. Thus, any frustration of his passive, receptive desires led to anger—whether directly through not getting his wishes gratified, or indirectly through envy and jealousy of others who did or through being driven out of the passivity and the receiving that he had enjoyed as a child into the responsible productive activity and giving of the adult. As is so often the case, the course of development and external circumstances united to frustrate these desires, and anger and hostility inevitably were engendered.

2. The father's spoiling and domination cultivated in the boy an

attitude of dependence and submissiveness. The boy did not quite know what this was but sensed something in the relationship that was a threat to him. He became hostile toward his father as a defense against giving in to a passive, submissive and dependent attitude toward him. He thus mobilized hostility in self-defense against a tendency which threatened to impair his normal masculine development toward independence. In adult life he continued to react with hostility to any person, especially to stronger men, who aroused in him wishes to be submissive and dependent. This hostility to a stronger person who arouses one's regressive childhood wishes to be submissive to him and dependent on him is a reaction of first importance. It is seen most clearly in certain cases of paranoia. One is hostile and antagonistic in order to keep from being submissive and dependent. These dynamics seem to have been central in Hitler, who could not stand to be dependent and submissive (Saul, 1976). The political and sociological consequences are obvious when many people with this emotional constellation coalesce into organized groups.

3. Any hurt to the self-regard (self-esteem, self-love, egoism, pride, narcissism) causes anger. A universal hurt in childhood is the very condition of being a child in a family and a world of grownups, being little, weak and dependent for one's well-being and very life on the constant help, care and love of others. This causes anger, rebelliousness and envy of the adults, in particular of the parents and the later substitutes for them. This state of affairs, lasting throughout the years of childhood, certainly leaves its influence on every personality and must play an important role in the universal feelings of inferiority with which are associated the common "looking up" to persons in "higher" positions and the whole ubiquitous struggle for power; and also the converse of this, the common attitude of "looking down" on underlings. All this, as we have discussed above, reflects the child's efforts to escape from its littleness, weakness and dependence into the position of the big, tall, strong parent. It seems that although influencing every personality to some extent, these early years, especially before about six, can be outgrown satisfactorily and the parental orientation securely achieved, provided that nothing intensifies these reactions during childhood.

Various forces can do this. For one thing, if the mother or the father cultivates the child's opinion of and love for himself too greatly, this heightened vanity becomes all the more sensitive to wounds, and the competition with other adults is intensified.

If the vanity is not inflated by the parents, it can still be made hypersensitive by all sorts of hurts to it. A common hurt is any impairment of development or any defect—intellectual, esthetic, social, physical or emotional. We have already remarked that when the emotional development is strong and mature, the other defects can be borne without warping the personality.

A 28-year-old young woman, as a result of polio at the age of eight, lost the use of her left arm and hand, and had such minimal use of her right that she learned to write with her foot. By incessant arduous effort she became self-supporting as a teacher, developed a circle of friends and finally found a boyfriend and a chance of marriage. Then began an untreatable painful rotation of the spine and she lost all she had worked for over so many years. Yet she maintained her spirit, her pleasant mood and her determination. She considered herself one of the fortunate ones because she was handicapped for almost as long as she could remember, while those who were stricken at adolescence had a terrible adjustment. If she lost all capacity for independence she might commit suicide. If she were to become a burden to herself and others this, she believed, would be a rational decision.

Impairment of the emotional development and the presence of too strong regressive desires and attitudes are seen again and again as a source of injury to the self-esteem and of feelings of inferiority, and, as a reaction to this, anger and a hostile attitude develop, whether repressed or overt. The patient, A. L., felt this inferiority and consequent rage even as a child, although he did not realize its source in his over-strong submissiveness, receptivity and dependence toward his father. He only felt somehow less free and self-reliant than many of his playfellows. In adult life he resented his own position as a follower and reacted to it with competitiveness and hate.

4. A. L.'s father rarely showed overt hostility to him, but when he did, in the form of domination, unpleasant teasing and occasional spankings, the patient reacted with hostility as retaliation and defense. It was in large part because his father treated him well and because he expected so much from his father emotionally and

financially that he repressed his hostility and rarely let it come to any overt expression; and this led to heightened guilt feelings and the turning of the hostility against himself.

A universal source of hostility is the whole interplay of attraction, frustration, jealousy and rivalry arising from the feelings toward the parents and toward the brothers and the sisters. Included in this interplay is the oedipus complex, seen most clearly in the son's attraction to his mother and rivalry with his father. All emotional tensions seek expression in all phases of a person's life. Certain activities relieve predominantly one or another of these tensions or combinations of them. The hostility in this case was manifest in some form in all aspects of the individual's life.

Overt hostility in direct fighting or criminality was not present in this instance. The suffering was mostly internal, in his own mind. Acting-out of the hostility was chiefly masochistic against himself, as we have said, mostly in subtly ruining his life socially, domestically and professionally.

The circumstances in childhood which lead or contribute to naked hostility in people no doubt will be elucidated by further studies than have as yet been devoted to them. Of course it is always determined by the balance of forces, as in physics—the mature and warped childhood in id, superego and ego. Probably where the outcome is overtly antisocial and hostile there was always some overt antisocial behavior in the parents as models, or direct acting-out against the child, as physical violence or otherwise. One single factor in this case was that, by training and example, the patient was brought up to control such overt manifestations. Also, his dependence on his father and his emotional and financial expectations toward him were such that he dared not jeopardize these by offending his father with any open hostility or overt misbehavior. Such a situation, coupled with considerate treatment, is well designed to cause strong repression of hostility and the piling up of guilt. Physical punishment of children sometimes has the opposite effect. By relieving guilt and providing a model of direct aggression, it results in more direct hostile aggression on the part of the child. Our patient, well-treated and loved, with only models of gentleness in his family could not be openly aggressive—could not even *feel* hostile without guilt. And so his hostility in large part must turn inward against himself. He must injure himself rather than his loved ones.

A few of the ways in which hostility manifested itself in the life of A. L. were:

1. In his active, promiscuous sex life, which had, as in everyone, a complex content but served chiefly to drain his hostility. For him sex was in large part an attack on the partner.

2. In his outspoken envious bitterness against those of his colleagues who had achieved solid success and respect.

The patient was faced with the emotional problem of satisfying his dependent needs and continuing to be loved in spite of his hostility. He solved it, as we have noted, by "splitting" the object, that is, by having two objects, one for dependence and love and one for hate. Considerable hostility existed beneath the surface even to his "loved" objects, and his idealization of older colleagues was in part a defense against his hostility to these men and an overcompensation for this hostility.

Still another mechanism in the idealization was the projection of the patient's own repressed vanity. Although in reality filled with self-love and personal ambition, he hid this under cover of an exaggeratedly modest attitude, but he satisfied it to a certain extent vicariously by attributing to his friend all the wonderful qualities which he desired for himself and then identifying with the friend. This reaction can play a part in falling in love. He could boast of his friend although not of himself. He did not see the friend objectively but as a representation of all that he himself wanted to be but could not admit even to himself.

3. The patient also expressed some hostility in connection with the social scene. He was much interested in labor problems and always very heated on the subject. He vented his spleen on both capital and labor and held to no position very consistently. Labor was to him the underdog with whom he identified himself, but his pride urged him to identify also with capital, which carried more prestige. As is so common, he projected his own intense emotions onto the social scene. This made him interested in social problems but also interfered seriously with his being objective and realistic about them. The parties concerned were too much representations of his own emotional trends. This is so frequently the case that political discussions are notoriously emotional more than realistic.

And the country, the world, in fact, is kept in turmoil because so many persons attack something or someone on the outside for a problem which is really inside their own minds.

4. Much hostility was drained by his fantasy life, through his almost constant imaginings of attacking or being attacked or of war and social conflict. His dreams have already been mentioned. In these the hostility was handled chiefly by the mechanism of projection and turning against the self, that is, a large man would attack the patient. This was a guilt reaction of the superego to his wishes to attack men who seemed to him stronger than himself. Hostility often results in nightmares, as in this case.

Fears of castration are not always reactions to intimidation or restriction narrowly in relation to sexuality. They usually represent punishment for the person's own hostile impulses, especially those which are castrative or sexual in form, as in this case, in which sexuality was so largely an attack on the woman. Hostility of women to men also often takes the form of castrative impulses, and the sexual act for these women comes, in some part, to have this meaning. Castration anxiety because of masturbation seems to arise, at least in part, because of the hostile components in the sexual feelings and not only because of threats or other reasons. Hostile impulses are especially apt to take the form of wishes to castrate in those men in whom they are reactions to underlying feminine trends, with feelings of weakness and of impaired masculinity. This is seen in those passive homosexual men whose rage at being in the feminine role sometimes comes out in actual attacks on their sexual partner in the form of castration. Such details are usually omitted from newspaper accounts. Hostility tends to take the form of castration when there is envy of the other man's masculinity or whenever hostility is directed toward masculinity for any reason, or simply when it is erotized.

The ''castration complex'' was described in considerable detail by Freud in connection with the Oedipus complex. Here it expresses the little boy's hostility to his male rival, and also the punishment he fears, which is directed to the organ which most clearly yields the feelings involved, the punishment fitting the source (p. 85).

Another motive for self-castrative impulses is quite different: it is the passive, receptive wish to be helpless and cared for and rid of responsibilities. Femininity is often conceived of in this way in such cases (Freud, 1924). This component is seen in dreams in which it may be fought against violently by the rest of the personality. It is also seen in schizophrenics, some of whom actually accomplish this mutilation upon themselves. This act is often equated in dreams and in schizophrenic thinking with losing arms or legs or in other ways rendering oneself helpless so as to regress to the indulgence of the dependence, submissiveness, passivity and receptivity of infancy. These tendencies can also take a passive, homosexual, feminine form.

5. Certain neurotic symptoms, both psychological and physical, including the patient's insomnia and his nightmares, were mostly a direct result of the pressure of his hostile impulses. These caused lifelong anxiety, and projecting them generated a paranoid trend. He also had palpitations of the heart, which were apparently part of his physiological mobilization for fight or flight caused by his constant psychological hostile aggressive feelings.

Most of the results of hostility which are seen in frank neurotic symptoms can be observed in lesser degree in reactions which do not get to exceed the bounds of normality. Sometimes when a patient is intensely angered for some reason, neurotic reactions appear in *statu nascendi:* feelings of depression, paranoid projections, compulsive thinking (e.g., having to count), doubt (wrestling with decisions but unable to reach one), suicidal impulses, anxiety, psychosomatic symptoms (emotionally caused physical symptoms), fantasies of violence, and so on. Thus, a pressure of hostility can be a central cause of disturbances of thinking, of feeling, of behavior and also of physical symptoms, disorders of the heart, the stomach and the like. Unlike A. L., the murderer described at the end of the last chapter demonstrated hostility as his central feature, *directly acting out* his childhood pattern of pathological hostility against others.

6. Hostility was also an important factor in A. L.'s choice of career. He was a criminal lawyer and derived much satisfaction from his contact with open violence.

7. As so often happens, since man has more conscience than he realizes, the hostility vented itself on the patient himself. We have

noted that despite his ability and personality he was on the social and professional fringe. This was, in part, a result of his protest against the responsibilities and the efforts entailed in success, but it was equally a result of his tendency to self-punishment. The patient himself vaguely felt that he was "destined to failure," that something within him forbade him success whenever he was on the verge of achieving it.

In school he rarely entered into competition in any form. However, on several occasions, in both scholastics and athletics, at first he did well but as soon as success was in sight he went to pieces, did not function nearly up to his usual standards and lost ignobly—not wrecked by success, but by the mere prospect of it. Emotionally, he was too intensely competitive, too hostile to his opponents; to win meant to him too hostile a triumph over his adversaries and an egoistic satisfaction greater than he could permit himself. To defeat a rival meant in his unconscious to kill him, and when this follows the pattern of the original rivalry toward a father who is good to you, the guilt becomes enormous. He hated others for their success too intensely for his conscience to permit him to succeed himself. In his adult life, just as his hostility caused him to dream of bad things happening to him, so it caused him to make wrong decisions and to handle his life in such a way that he always missed out and dragged along at a level far below his capacities. He was masochistic—his own worst enemy, blocking and injuring himself in love, friendship, profession and in mental, emotional and physical health.

The pressure of hostility can play a part in causing an individual's own death, as, for instance, when a person dies because his will to live is shattered by the generation of enormous bitterness. It also appears to be central in certain psychosomatic conditions, such as essential hypertension or coronary disease, when an individual's inner drive prevents him from living a well-balanced life but keeps him in constant anger and anxiety and forces him to overdo his activities until he drives himself to an untimely death. Among the most dramatic manifestations of hostility turned against the self are persecutory paranoias, in which the patient unshakeably believes that great organizations are determined to ruin, torture or kill him; such a patient may actually carry out his hostility by suicide, or, turned outward against the delusional persecutors, as murder.

The analysis of a patient's hostility, in fact of hostility in all persons and groups, is so significant because (1) it is an indispensable element in producing the symptom or behavior and (2) because pursuing its sources leads one directly to the fears, the frustrations and the conflicts which are at the root of the matter.

Often the hostility in an individual is easily overlooked but is nevertheless the clue to an important problem of behavior. Waelder relates a remark of Freud concerning the judgment of Solomon (Waelder, 1941). Solomon discovered the real mother of the child by the fact that she would rather give up the child to the other woman than have it cut in half. It is easy to overlook the fact that the other woman was willing to have the child cut in half—probably out of envy and jealousy of the real mother. In Somerset Maugham's famous short story "*Red,*" the handsome young Red marries a beautiful native girl, and they live in idyllic happiness on a South Sea isle for a year or two. Then Red is shanghaied onto a ship which he goes to visit. The girl is heartbroken and loses all interest in life. She functions, but without feeling. Another white man, Nielson—a superior person—is convalescing on the island, and a few years later, after hope of Red's return has been given up, he finally persuades the girl to marry him. But she never gives herself emotionally, and he feels that he cannot compete with the lost lover to whom she remains true. Many years later, a fat, paunchy, red-headed ship's captain drops in, and the girl, now a large, elderly woman, with pendulous breasts, does not even recognize him. Nielson now feels cheated and leaves her. She has sacrificed him to a mere memory, not to a real rival at all. It seems to me that there was also something else in this fictional woman's motivation—a hidden clue to her hostility. From clinical experience with moods of withdrawal and with depressions, one would judge that her reaction was one of rage. In the story, surprise is expressed that this passionate young girl could be capable of so steadfast an attachment to one man. However true her love, it is likely that what was equally steadfast was her hate of Red for deserting her at the height of their bliss and for never returning. And this unremitting revenge reaction she took out on the next white man.

SOCIOLOGICAL IMPLICATIONS

1. Other Causes

We have seen that emotional influences and conditioning experiences of childhood are of great importance for the generation of hostility and the ways in which it is expressed and repressed by the individual throughout his adult life. These are not the only factors, of course. The congenital endowment is to be considered, and the social ideologies and influences, both in childhood and adulthood, and also the personal and social situations in which the adult finds himself by accident or through his own deliberate or unintentional making. For example, slum areas are of critical importance in freeing aggressive behavior, and war has various effects on a large scale. It is often easier in dealing with social problems to ignore the quantitative individual differences and to focus on certain trends of human nature which people have in common and to study the effects of social conditions in shaping, inhibiting and stimulating these trends. We here deal with the influences of *personal* emotional factors on the hostile trends in *groups* and we are brought face to face with the problem of so shaping these trends as to reduce the childhood sources of man's hostility to his fellows and so increasing the possibilities of cooperation and the reasonable settlement of differences. This is the essence of democracy. When reason and negotiation fail, force is substituted for the forum and for democratic procedure.

2. Hostility Always a Symptom of Disorder

Socioeconomic studies aim to describe the conditions under which hostility is mobilized and comes to overt expression in terrorism, wars, revolutions. Studies in criminology have just begun to explore the early environmental influences which encourage the expression of hostile aggression in the form of crime. But the actual generation of the hostility, its intensity, its objects, the ways in which the individual reacts to it, its modes of repression and expression, its full role in life, and ways to influence it at its very source—these problems have barely been touched upon. Study of the neuroses thus far strongly suggests that while there may be some irreducible level of hostile aggressiveness in everyone, as there is of sexuality and regressiveness, yet exaggerations of hostile aggressiveness, readiness to it and especially to the overt forms of it, *are always a sign of a disturbance of the emotional development and a lack of full maturity caused by traumatic emotional influences during childhood.* Therefore, we can hope that the proper raising of children will reduce materially the amount of hostility generated in them. Although some hostility unavoidably must be stimulated, children do not become enraged and destructive, do not have tantrums and anxieties, do not become malicious and permanently cruel, are not usually even unreasonable, except as a reaction to the treatment they receive. So trained an observer as Hugo Staub (1943) after a lifetime of experience as a criminal lawyer, stated that he had never seen a "normal" criminal, but that criminalism is always a reaction to traumatic emotional experiences, often the most overt mistreatment in childhood.

The last few years have shown the use of force, destruction and violence even on university campuses in degrees which seem out of proportion to the issues, which suggest their use for personal power or for forms of pathological personal gratification. We have seen failure to negotiate by reason all over the world: Northern Ireland, Vietnam, Nigeria, Biafra, the Middle East, and so on. This strongly suggests what all of history appears to demonstrate, namely, the impossibility of solving differences by reason because they are basically emotional and primarily motivated by hate, anger and hostility. Yet we have not only cold and hot killers but also men of good will. Hence the only possible solution is in the *individual*—to so rear children as to develop enough mature adults of good will in populations of warped hostile acting-outers. The basic problem is the irrational pathological hostile acting out which stems from the childhood emotional pattern. I think this should be a recognized psychiatric *diagnosis* and be included in the official nomenclature.

The turning of hostility against the self as masochism is also a problem of worldwide importance. Every good parent feels some concern lest his son or daughter damage his or her own future while still adolescent, and this is common enough. Articles have appeared in the press about college graduates, including those with master's degrees and Ph.D.'s, trained in science and engineering, fluent in several languages, talented and highly intelligent, who leave it all to become "social dropouts." Sometimes they do something requiring no special skill, but socially useful and gainful, like driving taxicabs, and spend their evenings in poolrooms. They say this is freedom—and perhaps it is—from more skilled responsibility. Asked where they are going, they reply "nowhere." They thus sacrifice a fuller, richer life for themselves, and for their families, reducing security for themselves and abandoning the possibility of making major contributions to their country, now struggling with such dire problems as overpopulation, integration, violence and war in the atomic age. Is this not hostility to country, family and selves, and a regression from productive responsibility? How many professional taxi drivers must envy their training and opportunities and deplore this masochism! One wonders if masochism, this self-directed hostility, does not play a part in the shortsightedness of so many that it influences the behavior of the nation, to see no further than their immediate benefit and immediate danger.

3. Crime Areas

Of course, slum areas breed hostility, crime and delinquency. But not *all* children reared in these areas are delinquent. Evidence suggests that the home plays a determining part in whether the child will succumb to delinquency or, like Oliver Twist, fully resist it. And the climate of the home depends on many factors. For example, it has been reported that juvenile-delinquency rates are higher in families of recent immigrants. Some juvenile delinquency may well be a normal reaction to an abnormal, insecure, frustrating environment in which the individual feels unvalued and unwanted by society. A well-organized social program can be successful through providing the youth with clubs or groups in which they can feel that they belong and have status, in which they can gain emotional support, balanced off with interest and participation in the activities (Horney, 1937). The delinquent who does *not* respond is often considered by the rest of the group to be "neurotic." Nevertheless, such correction is in part only a supplement to the home influence, since, as we have said, children from certain homes do not become delinquent in spite of the area in which they live.* In other words, the force of the conditioning within the home

---

* I am indebted to Rothe Hilger for information and discussion of these significant points.

during the earliest years far outweighs in depth and permanence of its effects any other influences short of the catastrophic.

4. The Ultimate Source: The Bent Twig—The Child from Birth to 6

Even well-meaning parents, unintentionally and usually because of their own underlying unconscious attitudes, frequently warp their children's development and unwittingly provoke hostility. So many children are so badly brought up, yet, difficult as this problem is, there is room for hope. It is in the first few years of life, while human nature is in its most formative stage, that most problems of adult life, including neurosis, criminality, social turmoil, political extremism, pathologically hostile acting out and violence and war itself, have their ultimate roots and their only possibility of lasting solution. With better developed, more fully mature adults, we can expect less readiness to hostility and cruelty, less pettiness, selfishness, greed and exploitation, less vanity and competitiveness, less hate, and proportionately increased possibilities of reasonableness, responsibility, security and cooperation for mutual interest. Perhaps hostile aggression, which still is glorified in certain parts of the world, will one day be looked upon as what it mostly is: a manifestation of childishness.

The great finding is that proper child rearing, with good feelings in the family, especially from birth to age six (0–6), from the first hours, days, weeks, months and years, deeply conditions the child to good feelings toward other persons for life, and lays the foundations for proper maturing to the capacity for responsibility, love and constructiveness, while the hostility of humans to each other is a mental disorder, the symptom of impairments and warping in the emotional development. Its consequences are very direct. Our nation is in turmoil, and even in some danger, not only because of rational reasons of unsolved inequalities, but irrationally, emotionally, because so many of our citizens hate their own country. This is not because it has treated them badly but because, in reaction to some sort of long-term traumatic treatment in childhood, they hate their own parents and transfer this hatred to their own land. Every child who grows up with hostility to his own parents is a potential threat to our country.

5. Hostility and the Nature of Man

And God saw that the wickedness of man was great in the earth, and that every imagination of the thoughts of his heart was only evil continually. And the Lord was sorry that he had made man on the earth, and it grieved him to his heart. So the Lord said, "I will blot out man whom I have created from the face of the ground . . ."

Genesis 6:5–7

The destructiveness of man to his own kind, the sadism and murder committed by individuals, by organized groups and on a mass scale as war is a phenomenon not seen to such an extent in any other animal species. Why should man—the wise one, the one with speech and knowledge—be the most destructive? A polemic continues among the ethologists. Konrad Lorenz (1966) sees man's hostility to man as an instinctual drive like hunger and the sex drive, and calls it "aggression." We have already pointed out the disadvantages of this term, by which Lorenz means only hostile, destructive aggression, but which can also mean constructive activity. Richard Leakey (1977) sees much more the ability of the human brain to be conditioned and to learn. We have previously emphasized the importance of the child's experiences from conception to about age six in developing angry, hostile, destructive trends in his permanent personality, in contrast with loving, responsible, productive trends.

That childhood experiences mold the personality seems definitely established, but this does not mean personality is strictly all nature or nurture. Rather, there seem to be a number of emotional forces which enter into making a person either more hostile and aggressive or loving and cooperative.

Favoring hostility is a too-ready fight-flight reaction combined with the frustrations, intimidations, irritations of early childhood that create sensitivities which keep the fight-flight aroused, as well as the examples of the parents' behavior that sanctions its expression. A counterforce is the tendency to good will seen in all species, to social cooperation and the cultivation of good will by the favorable emotional experiences from 0–6, especially love and respect for the child's tender, enormously conditionable developing personality as well as the model of mature, loving, tolerant parents. This brief list is only meant to illustrate the fact that a hostile or loving personality is not a sharp "either-or" but a culmination for good or ill of all the childhood experiences acting on the instincts.

Man is still a member of the animal kingdom. He survives by eating, digesting and eliminating the same way as other animals. He reproduces the same way; he works his muscles and sleeps the same way. He differs in having well-developed speech and a far greater intellect for memory and reason, but the greatest difference is that he does not live in the wilds in accordance with his animal instincts. For security he is banded together into societies, either small and simple or vast and complex. His young are born into such societies and must learn their customs and rules in order to survive for the rest of their lives. Scratch an adult and you find a child . . . scratch a child and you find an animal.

Hope lies in the 0–6. The puppy grows into an adult dog that "reflects" the home in which he was raised and his early experiences. This is true of any pet. The grown dog, cat, horse or other domestic animal will be gentle, loving, devoted and trustworthy within the capabilities of the species, or it will be suspicious, hostile and even dangerous depending upon how it was treated by humans from birth through the earliest hours, days, weeks, months and years from childhood to adulthood.

We live so much in a world of feelings and ideas that we are apt to be distressed by evil, cruel people without remembering that man is an animal with animal instincts for survival. But unlike the lion in the savannah and the porpoise in the sea, whose instincts and reflexes insure their life cycle, man must band together in societies for survival. And each society, from small primitive tribe to technologically advanced nation, has evolved its own rules and laws within which its members must live if they and the society are to continue. These involve control of the animal instinct and reflex. Even man's sex drive cannot be allowed free rein without causing chaos. Out of this control come repression and transformation of instinct into culture, expressed in literature, art, music and science.

This brings us again inevitably to 0–6, to the question of at what age a child's socialization begins. Quite simply, it begins at conception, with the way society treats pregnant women. The interpersonal relations begin at birth, with the relationship between the newborn and his mother, mother-substitute, father and remainder of the family, and even to hospital personnel if the birth takes place there. Breast or bottle feeding, demand or scheduled feedings become part of this socialization process. Interpersonal relationships and feelings are crucial for harmony or discord within the nuclear family. They affect the whole attitude and tone of the training and education of the child for life. We cannot escape the central importance of 0–6, of the childhood emotional pattern, both for the individual and his society.

It has been said that man himself is the "missing link" between the ape and the human being. It seems to me that the mature part of man is what makes him distinctively human: this is his capacity for social cooperation, for living identification, for adapting, for constructive repression, i.e., for virtue, morality and ethics, for responsibility. If the childhood emotional pattern is too strong, too hostile, too fixed, then the person is more unconscious and automatic, more a rigid mechanism that can only function in limited ways, hence more like the animals but at the same time not so naive and unpretentious, and therefore not so attractive.

It should be glaringly obvious that in today's world unlimited reproduction is senseless, especially when we are threatened with a population explosion. Too many of any species upsets the balance of nature. Perhaps two or three thousand years ago it was desirable to increase and multiply; today what is needed is not *more* people, but *better* people, better in the sense of "more mature." Maturity is only achieved in physically healthy individuals by properly rearing children, from conception to age 6 or 7, and this means with love, understanding and respect for their personalities. We need not quantity of humankind, but quality.

"You can't teach an old dog new tricks." Children reflect the homes in which they were raised. Even in the vegetable kingdom, "as the twig is bent, the tree is inclined." If all children were raised with love, understanding and respect for their personalities we would have a world of relatively independent, cooperative, loving spouses, parents and citizens of good will—and a world with much less crime, cruelty and war, wickedness and evil.

REFERENCES

Freud, S. (1924): The economic problem of masochism, *S.E.* 19.

_____ (1930): Civilization and its discontents, *S.E.* 21.

Horney, K. (1937): *The Neurotic Personality of Our Time.* New York: Norton.

Kubie, L. (1943): Relation of the conditioned reflex to psychoanalytic technique, *Archives of Neurology & Psychiatry* 32:1137.

Leakey, R. and Lewin, R. (1977): *Origins.* New York: E. P. Dutton.

Lorenz, K. (1952): *King Solomon's Ring.* New York: Crowell.

_____ (1966): *On Aggression.* New York: Harcourt, Brace and Jovanovich.

Saul, L. J. (1976): *Psychodynamics of Hostility.* New York: Jason Aronson, pp. 166–174.

Staub, H. (1943): A runaway from home, *Psychoanalytic Quarterly* 12:1.

Waelder, R. (1941): *The Living Thoughts of Freud.* New York: Longmans.

7 | Sexuality

This chapter is not a comprehensive review of sexuality, but only a discussion of its relationships to development and regression. For this purpose two aspects of sexuality will be distinguished in accordance with clinical observation: (1) sex as a biological and psychological force and (2) sex as a mechanism and a pathway for the expression and the drainage of all kinds of emotional impulses and tensions. But first, a few general observations.*

SEX—A BEARCAT OF A PROBLEM

There is the physical, sensual sexuality that culminates in orgasm, whether via normal coitus, masturbation or perversion. There is mature, true, unselfish love. Then there is the instinct to mate, to have the long steady, reliable companionship and loyalty of one of the opposite sex. And fourth, there is all of the devotion, responsibility and effort to spouse and young (the family) as seen in many species besides man. Obviously no species would survive more than a generation if its newborn were helpless. Egg laying species make other provisions. Mankind would become extinct in one generation if its newborn were not cared for, since they would die in a few days if they were neglected. Mating and family is as essential to the survival of the species as sex and reproduction—in some ways, more so, as man will learn if he does not pay attention to the *kind* of adults we rear as well as their numbers. The young of the sea elephant can survive independently after three weeks; therefore, there is no need for sea elephants to find permanent mates and establish nests or homes. But in man, there are problems if the sex, the mating until the young are mature, i.e., for life, and responsibility for the young, fail to fuse or do so temporarily and then break apart from each other. For sex in man is not so firmly, intrinsically

* For a fuller discussion by this author see *The Childhood Emotional Pattern and Corey Jones*, New York, Van Nostrand Reinhold, 1977.

integrated with monogamous mating and the rearing of young as it is in some other species. (*See* Carrighar, Sally (1965): *Wild Heritage,* Boston: Houghton Mifflin Co. This book contains a comprehensive bibliography.)

With sufficient maturity the adolescent tolerates the pressure of sexual desire, and if he gratifies it, does so in ways which injure no one. The emotional life of man is very imperfect and plagued with conflicts for which there are no fully satisfactory resolutions. Conflict results from the normal access of full sexual drive, potency and fertility at puberty, at about 12 to 14 years of age, when the rest of the organism has not yet reached its full growth physically and is still very much a child emotionally. Marriage at this premature age is a doubtful solution. But also questionable for future adjustment is sex without the other three components: love, mating and responsibility. For sex, love, marriage and parenthood are all parts of the great mechanism of species survival. Sex without love, *sans amour,* we feel to be somehow not wholesome, to be "cheapening," i.e., in some way injurious to love, marriage, parenthood. For powerful as these instincts are, yet everything mental is delicate, sensitive (in animals as well as man) and easily deranged, as shown by the irregular recurrent turmoil of the streets, campuses and the world as well as in the rates of abortion, illegitimate births, and divorce. Some cultures try solutions by toleration of premarital sexuality and even of marital infidelity. But no cultural sanction can withstand the personal biological reaction of jealousy and hurt pride and the resulting rage, turbulence and crimes of passion.

Another conflict is between monogamy and promiscuity, for every human, no matter how loyally and devotedly married, reacts to attractive members of the opposite sex. Yet monogamy is basic and powerful in man and, as we have said, in other species also. In societies which sanction polygamy and polygyny and wife lending (and there are usually cogent reasons of economics, food supply, proportions of men to women, and so on, for this) 80 to 90 percent of the adults are nevertheless monogamous. As a further complication, a person may be enormously urged sexually to one who is otherwise in personality incompatible. Free sex, marriage before maturity or before finding a compatible mate and being established occupationally and financially, continence until then, prostitution—no solution is without serious objections. Moreover, in most people there is some disorder of the sexuality, its being too inhibited or uninhibited or perverted, or some disturbances in the rest of the personality, or both. And since sex involves not merely another body but another human being with a personality, all the interpersonal emotional interplay enters in and emotional disorders play a central role in the whole relationship, if not in the sexual act itself.

Very often the physical urge of sex brings together a couple but the neurotic (emotionally disordered) parts of both personalities interact to make each one miserable, or even to destroy each other. Normal sexual intercourse requires another person, thus involving all the problems of emotional interaction, which in turn are largely determined by each partner's childhood emotional pattern. An ethologist friend told me that if a male and female fox encounter one another by chance in the forest and have sexual relations, forever afterward they will recognize each other and have a special relationship. I do not know if this can be established scientifically, but it rings true and I mention it here because of its relevance to humans. Our "Age of Permissiveness" seems to have shown that a certain degree of control and repression are not all bad, and that too much license can be. The most workable principle is still The Golden Rule.

At best, sex is a bearcat of a problem and it takes a considerable degree of maturity to handle it.

SEX AS A DRIVE

1. Relations to Mature and Infantile Motives

First, let us consider sex as a drive in its own right. In general, sexuality seems to be allied with the forces of development rather than with those of regression. This is apparent from the everyday observation that whatever the vicissitudes of the sexual development, whatever its infantile components, however early in childhood or infancy its stirrings are apparent, still in part the goal of this complex process is biological sexual maturity, the capacity to love, mate, reproduce and rear the young. However the sexual urge may be perverted, one must not lose sight of the central fact that sex has something to do with reproduction. Nature, taking no chances on fertility, is bountiful sexually and provides more sperm and egg cells than can possibly be utilized,* and a generous bonus of pleasure. Hence, the great tide of sex, especially when restricted, as it is in human society, spreads out in many ways and forms that may seem to be remote from reproduction, but the stuff of sex is still sperm and egg cells, and its central purpose is reproduction and all its consequences in the way of responsibility for the family and the rearing of children. In the absence of definitive conclusions as to the strength of the sex urge, we might point out that for centuries men thought the urge was weak in women and only men could feel it strongly. It now appears the opposite may be true: on the average, once "awakened," it may be stronger in women. Certainly its strength often increases with age in many women, while the potency and performance, if not the lust, decrease in men.

Not only man but certain other mammals and certain birds mate for long periods or for life. Mating, reproducing, contributing to the family and rearing the young are adult functions. It is toward this end that sexuality tends, however diverted or sidetracked it may become on the way. Such sidetracking signifies an impairment of the normal sexual development, and such impairment is often the *effect* rather than the *cause* of neurosis. Freud showed the kernel of genital feeling in all loving and being loved and therefore broadened the use of the term "sex" to include just about all pleasurable feelings and all tendencies of people to come together. Eventually, he described genital sexuality as part of Eros, the basic tendency of protoplasm to build up, sociologically as well as biologically. In his early writings he was not consistent in using the term "sex" in the broad or in the narrow genital sense, and much misunderstanding and confusion resulted. In this chapter we shall keep to the narrow, common usage, unless otherwise indicated. Neurosis is often caused by frustration of the need for love, *part* of which may be

---

* An egg cell a month in the human female and several millions of sperm cells in each ejaculation of the male. It has been estimated that within a few years' time the population of India, for example, were it not for the enormous infant mortality, would exceed that of the whole world at present. But now this is only part of the world population expansion of the last 35 years, correctly termed an "explosion" and a greater threat than the atom bomb, with many national populations doubling every 30 to 50 years. Thus the effects of the Aswan dam in increasing the food supply of the Nile valley have already been obliterated by the increase in population, which as Malthus said, always outstrips the food supply.

genital feelings. The effect may be disturbances of the genital feelings and functioning.

Sexuality stands in a two-fold relationship to the emotional development. It is a force in itself and is also a channel and pathway for expressing all kinds of emotional tensions, feelings, and motives. As a force in itself, in the direction of mating and reproducing, it is a powerful stimulus toward growth to independence of the parents, toward the responsibility of family and, in general, toward all the requirements and orientations of adult life, which reflect the attitudes of the parent to the child rather than of the child to the parent. If the sexuality of the child has been too much inhibited and repressed by the parents, this stimulus is lacking, and insecurity and frustration become well-nigh unavoidable; if the sexuality has been too unrestrained, even stimulated by the parents, it may retain childish characteristics, remaining pleasurable play but nothing more—never integrated into the adult function of mating and family responsibility. Thus, disturbances in the sexual development affect adult functioning.

Conversely, although the sexual training may be very satisfactory and the sexual functioning quite normal, if other aspects of the emotional development remain problems, sexuality may be used for the solution of these and thus function in the service of infantile or childish aims rather than express the adult activities and capacities of loving and mating and a responsible attitude toward family, friends and society. For example, a Don Juan may use sex purely for bolstering his prestige and compensating by his conquests for inner feelings of masculine inadequacy. Or an insecure, grasping girl may use it for "gold digging." All sorts of sexual disturbances can result from unresolved childhood emotional problems. The sexuality affects the rest of the emotional development, and the rest of the development affects the sexuality.

According to Alexander's theoretical formulation of the "principle of the surplus" (1961), the child being essentially receptive and dependent, its biological energies go into its own growth and development. But after adolescence, when its full biological growth is reached, these energies of growth spill over for the individual to use to make his own way and take care of himself, and to reproduce, found a family and take care of them and of others.

Sexuality, then, as a force of development, is a part of the individual's total development to maturity, and maturity is characterized by independence, productivity and "object interest" in the sexual as well as in the social spheres.

A. Adolescence. From this angle, as we have already pointed out, much of the emotional problem of adolescence consists of the struggle to win independence from the parent. Much of the paradoxical behavior of the adolescent becomes intelligible on this basis. The adolescent is part adult, and all eagerness to prove his or her adulthood, strength, sophistication, independence. On the other hand, the ties and the attitudes of childhood are not yet resolved. The adolescent still may be emotionally and financially dependent on the parents. And parents often are loath to let their children go and hence often aggravate the struggle by subtly, often unconsciously, trying to keep their adolescents children, rather than facilitating their development toward independence. Parents often regard their children as sources for their own satisfaction. The capacity to waive one's own desires and to be interested in the children in order to understand them as persons, and to facilitate their development by providing the necessary security and freedom for it—this "object interest" is an important part of the attitude of the mature, independent parent.

B. Adult Love. Love, using the term in its broadest sense, is not something given in order to get, but something given as an expression of regard for the person loved, even to the point of sacrifices for the beloved. Throughout childhood it is of prime importance to *be* loved. Life depends on it. But in adult life one can be strong enough to diminish the need to *be* loved by others and to develop the enjoyment of *loving* others. This capacity to *enjoy* giving interest and love becomes the basic adult attitude toward the sexual partner, children, friends, profession, job, hobbies. The capacity for loving, for object interest, for the enjoyment of productive, responsible attitudes and activities—this is an attribute of maturity, an expression of the overflow in the adult of the biological energies which previously had been devoted to his growth and development. This distinction between the infantile need to *be* loved and the mature enjoyment of giving it is vital, as we have seen in Chapter 3.

Sexual love is so flooding an experience that we often forget other forms of love—maternal, paternal, brotherly, love of humanity and love of God (following the Greek).

2. Sex in Relation to Dependence and Needs for Love

Being, in general, allied with the developmental trends, the genital-sexual drive is usually, but by no means entirely, opposed to the regressive desires. In an earlier chapter it was pointed out that the regressive desires sometimes impel people, without their realizing it, to the security of institutions such as jails and hospitals, and that normal sexual desire usually urges them in the opposite direction—to freedom and independence. We mentioned a young man who freed himself from an overprotective mother through marrying against her will. Many persons marry late or not at all because of undue or prolonged attachments to one or both parents. In such a case, the sexual and mating urges are seen to be in open conflict with the childish dependence on the parents. This is a common conflict. Usually the sexual urges even without mature mating are opposed to this dependence on parents.

Another case was also quoted in which a young man was financially and emotionally dependent on his parents and unable to free himself so that he could devote himself wholeheartedly to his profession and marry his fiancée. He was still tempted to relinquish his profession and return to his home and his father's business and to break his engagement. Both withdrawals were manifestations of the same tendency—to give up the adult position of independent, responsible activity in the two spheres of profession and of sexuality and mating. He was tempted to abandon his adult masculine position in both fields. The equivalence of these two fields was seen clearly in this case by his having the identical conflict over both. Often a complementary rather than equivalent relationship is seen, and the person endeavors to compensate in the one sphere for inadequacies, inhibitions or like problems in the other sphere. A man with relative impotence sexually may compensate by extra drive to success in athletics, or work; while a weak, ineffectual man among men may seek sexual conquests with women.

These Passive-Receptive-Dependent (PRD) tendencies often impair normal sexual development and functioning. This is to be expected, for, as we have already seen, these regressive tendencies are powerful enough to cause severe emotional disorders. They are, in fact, more fundamental than the genital sexuality. (As we have said, Freud believed that they are themselves partly manifestations of sexuality, in the very broad sense of pleasurable feelings which existed prior to the predominance of genital sensations and came to contribute to these. Moreover, like any strong feeling, they become more or less sexualized.)

For the child, and often for the adult too, they transcend the genital sexual. Usually for the child the sexual differences between the parents or those who care for it are overshadowed by the great need for love. It is a secondary matter whether it is loved and cared for by mother or by father, for basically it is on being responsibly loved that the child depends for the animal affection, the shelter, the food and the care which are necessary to its very life. In this sense its needs for love are part of its self-preservative tendency.

The strength of the primitive, dependent, receptive, emotional demands as opposed to the sexual has been humorously expressed in the story of the laborer who admitted killing his wife and her lover. "Well, Judge," he said, "Monday—come home. Six o'clock. Eat on table. Eat. Go into bedroom. Find wife in bed with Vladek. Okay. Tuesday night. Come home. Six o'clock. Eat on table. Eat. Go into bedroom. Find wife in bed with Vladek. Okay. Wednesday night. Come home. Six o'clock. No eat on table. Go into bedroom. Find wife in bed with Vladek. Take knife. Kill wife. Kill Vladek. Six o'clock *must be eat on table!*"

It must be added that, depending on the childhood emotional pattern, the dependence sometimes does not oppose the sexuality but fuses with it and reenforces it. It is not unusual to see a man who makes excessive sexual demands upon his wife as part of his overall exaggerated dependence upon her. Such wives, although they may be highly sexed, eventually lose their desire for intercourse because they sense that for their husbands it is only another demand upon them, like the demands of a little boy upon his mother.

A. Choice of Sex Partner. The childhood desires and needs usually affect profoundly the choice of the sexual object and of permanent mate. In fact, the budding sexual feelings attach to images of emotionally charged members of the child's family, and his later objects are usually, if not always, substitutes for (or defenses against) these. This is probably one reason why sexual desire never can be completely gratified. For example, a young woman's parents had had serious marital friction all during her childhood. This young woman was an only child. The father became hostile and withdrawn in his attitude toward the child as well as toward the wife. The wife, as so often occurs, turned her unsatisfied emotions toward the child and besides having the full responsibility for its care, became overly affectionate and loving. The child thus learned to receive the satisfactions of its needs from the mother alone, with only coldness and antagonism from the father. She kept this pattern in adult life and developed strong homosexual wishes to love and be loved by women rather than by men, while her normal adult feminine sexual impulses urged her in the direction of relinquishing this homosexual childhood fixation in favor of a normal heterosexual marital relationship, for which the pattern toward her father was poor.

How early emotional attachments form a channel for the later physical, genital sexual drives is clearly seen in animals. Konrad Lorenz removed the mother of newly hatched graylag goslings who then followed his boots instead of their mother (imprinting) as he walked. When sexually mature they had relations with his boot (1952).

B. Desire, Impotence and Frigidity. The childish, dependent trends can influence the strength and the quality of the sexual current. When these trends are very strong, there is usually an overt or a *latent* impairment of the heterosexual functioning. That is, one factor tending toward impotence or frigidity in certain cases is the passive-receptive-dependent tendency; while, conversely, a strong sexual interest usually provides a certain safeguard against too great childish dependence. If a man wants sexual relations with a woman he must be something of a man and have more to offer her than sex alone. Some very weak, passive individuals dream of being very potent sexually, and some are sexually active in life. But this is usually an overemphasis on this masculine activity ("masculine protest") to serve as a denial of the infantile, passive, dependent desires. The typical unconscious representation of this is the very common dream of men of a little boy (or, where there is a strong feminine identification, of a woman) with a huge penis, "like a baseball bat" as one patient reported.

It is not unusual to see cases like the following: A rather infantile young man was supported and sheltered by his family. He felt inferior because of this, although he did not recognize the reason. He was highly sexed and attractive, and his conquests and sexual performances bolstered his injured self-esteem. Yet, withal, he admitted that he always doubted his potency and feared that at any time he might fail at the crucial moment. Fate helped him to develop and become more independent by landing him, through a series of unforeseeable circumstances, in a situation in which, separated from his parents and cut off from outside support, he had to sink or swim on his own. Moreover, being ambitious and capable, he found himself loaded with responsibilities and many daily demands. Now all his energies went into the battle of life, meeting the daily demands, holding his own among men. His self-esteem rose, but his sexual interest and activities diminished enough to worry him. When much was coming in emotionally and he was almost as irresponsible as a child, he expressed his masculinity in sexual activity—not in mating but only in play, love affairs. Now, with no parents to support him and his energies going out into adult, responsible activity, little was left for sexuality. It so happened that on a lengthy vacation he became dependently attached to some older people who took a personal interest in him and offered him an excellent business opportunity. This emotional satisfaction and support, and the prospective security and allaying of anxiety, resulted in a return of his libido in its old force. With more coming in and less going out emotionally in the nonsexual spheres, more energy (libido) was available for sexuality. This is no doubt one reason, among others, why many men lose sexual interest in their wives after marriage, when the wife no longer represents love to be obtained, but rather demands and responsibilities to be met.

These observations are generally valid only if one takes into account *latent* inhibitions of the sexual potency. For example, many men are on the surface fully potent, even exaggeratedly so, and yet will confess that they fear the opposite, namely, that at any time they may lose their potency. Heightened sexual desire and too rapid ejaculation (ejaculatio praecox) often alternate in the same man with impotence. Many Don Juans among men and many apparently oversexed women are found to feel insecure in their sexuality. Conversely, it is a bad sign, so far as therapy and prognosis go, if a very infantile, passive, dependent individual does not show a reasonable amount of heterosexual drive. It means that there is much less to work with and that he has relinquished even the powerful urgency of physical genital sexuality in favor of regression to infantile dependence. Of course, this regressive trend is only one of the factors that can disturb sexual functioning. A further complication is the fact that sexuality can also drain and satisfy the regressive trends themselves to a certain extent. An example would be the philandering, irresponsible playboy who uses sex with women to gratify childish needs for mother love. This is common among men, especially if they have plenty of money, who were emotionally deprived in early childhood by parents who had little time for them. But, in general, given a passive-receptive-dependent and a heterosexual trend in a person, these two trends point in opposite directions, the heterosexual being in the direction of development, the regressive back to infantile needs.

The young man of 30, Mr. P. D., described in an earlier chapter (Ch. 2), who married against the will of his overprotective mother, tended, as we saw, to make a mother out of his wife. He gave up his work, returned to school and depended on his wife for support. But as he did this, his sexual feelings and the potency toward her diminished. This is seen regularly. The sexual potency is usually adversely affected by the counter-current of passive dependence.

This is more readily apparent in men than in women, for normal masculine activity and forceful attitudes are in sharper contrast in our culture with the passive, receptive dependence than is femininity, which normally contains a considerable passive-receptive-dependent component in the attitude to the man. The passive-receptive dependence has the same direction and blends to a certain degree with a large portion of the normal, feminine emotional orientation toward the man; but it has the opposite direction and opposes the normal drive of masculinity. Hence, in some cases, these regressive tendencies reenforce the femininity, as seen in those women whose childishness adds to their appeal. But in women, as well as in men, this component, when too strong and not adequately compensated, can impair the sexual potency. It is in sharper opposition to the maternal urges and can hamper them seriously. However, a certain amount is normal in them. The woman with much of the child in herself often has a close identification with children on that account, and this may add to her feelings for them. If such a woman does not fight the childishness in herself, it may even reenforce her maternal feelings. But if it is too strong or too conflictful, it more often hinders real maternal feeling, giving, interest and responsibility (RPI)—"the child wife."

C. Femininity. Many reactions to the passive-receptive-dependent tendencies are seen, and many ways of dealing with them. A few of the reactions in the sexual life will be described here. We have mentioned the fact that some women handle their passive-dependent-receptive tendencies by incorporating them into their feminine attitude, and to a degree this is perfectly normal. In such women, if these tendencies are overly strong, the result is apt to be the "baby-doll" type, the "clinging-vine" type, the "play-girl," the childish type (like Dora in *David Copperfield*), who plays at being wife and mother, and so on. As is well known, such types have a special appeal for certain kinds of men. Perhaps their immaturity and weakness afford a needed flattery to the masculinity and strength of some men and in some cases stimulate the sadistic components of their sexuality. Also, for some men, such women are representations and projections of their own repressed childishness and dependence. For example, a strong, successful man feared and denied any sign of weakness or dependence in himself but satisfied these repressed tendencies vicariously by identifying with his childlike, dependent wife and enjoying her pleasure in being protected, supported and indulged. People relate to each other, feel toward each other in two major ways—by object relations (as in depending upon, being hostile to or sexually interested in), and by identification. We are usually especially attracted to other persons who are very much like ourselves in some of their emotional make-up, i.e., have similarity in some of their dynamics.

This identification is fundamental in friendships, formation of groups, good marriages, and all relationships.

If the regressive tendencies are too strong, these women, like anyone else, have feelings of being immature and inferior. These feelings may be conscious or sensed only vaguely. Their source is usually unconscious. They are apt to increase as the woman gets older and finds her responsibilities increasing and her friends developing and maturing beyond her. If she does not know the source of her feelings, she is in a sad plight, for, cast about as she will, she cannot correct the situation. She may accept it and even age gracefully. But sometimes she does not know that the adult must develop "object interest" and learn to enjoy the process of life—the responsibilities, the giving, the loving, and not only the being cared for and being loved. One result of failure to realize this is the tragic spectacle of an aging woman, ostensibly having all the world can offer, yet frustrated by the nature of her own desires and pathetically trying to cling by make-up and manner to the childishness which was once so successfully a part of her charms and is the only attitude, once workable, that she knows.

D. Oversexed Women. In an earlier chapter we saw how mothering and even having babies can become exaggerated drives. Other women try to solve their problems by heightened sexual rather than maternal activity. Sex is used in attempts to solve many kinds of problems and tensions, and as the great diversion, taking one's mind off other matters. Sometimes it is used as a means of overcompensation for feelings of inferiority which arise from persisting, infantile, receptive, helpseeking attitudes. This is one motive in the "boy-craziness" of some girls. One such girl of 18 had been reared by very restrictive parents who kept her a child. She was very pretty but was infantile in her appearance, behavior and emotional outlook. She considered sexual activity to be a mark of maturity and adulthood and tried to be grown up and sophisticated by being "uninhibited" and promiscuous. Revenge on her parents was another motive for her behavior, which had still other motivations as well. As stated previously, psychological acts are always "overdetermined," i.e., have multiple motivations.

There are circles in which sex not later than age 14 is customary; the lack of which invites a certain ostracism. Here the girl, to be fully sophisticated, has a baby at 14. Consideration for the baby and its future is not material in this egocentric thinking.

E. Splits in the Love Life. Another type of solution for a conflict between regressive and adult sexual trends is to split them and endeavor to satisfy them separately. One woman, for example, married and had a family but still kept her overstrong attachment to her parents, especially to her mother, and this was more important to her than her husband and children. The parents still contributed to her support, and she confided in them and visited them periodically. What this meant dynamically was that she kept her emotional budget in balance by receiving enough emotionally from her parents as a child to compensate for what she gave out emotionally in her role as wife and mother. She could be an adult in her marriage and fulfill her adult sexual life without too serious impairment from her infantile and childhood demands by satisfying these separately and apart from the adult sexual life.

Such a split takes a quite different form in those women who marry older men who mean to them emotionally father or mother substitutes who will support and care for them like children—and then feel dissatisfied sexually and wish for a young man as a sexual object.

Some men also sometimes seek to integrate too strong passive-regressive trends into their sexual lives and try to satisfy these trends in this form. This is sometimes a leading motive when a man marries as woman whom he looks to, usually unconsciously, as a mother figure. Sometimes this is fairly obvious, as when she is considerably older than he, perhaps has a private income of her own, perhaps is self-supporting in work of some sort, is obviously maternal in her attitude toward him and so on. Sometimes such marriages work out very well, but often there is considerable dissatisfaction. The man is apt to find that his wife is not satisfying as a sexual object, without realizing that the fault is in his own attitude toward her, in which his passive-receptive childish wishes toward her as a mother run counter to his free, masculine sexual urges toward her. The incest taboo, no sex with a woman too reminiscent of mother or sister, also usually operates. Sometimes he feels inferior to her, resents his feelings of dependence and becomes rebellious and hostile. More extremely he may feel like a "gigolo." It is a quantitative matter. To some extent, every woman supplies something maternal to her husband, and he satisifes many infantile, regressive impulses in his emotional relationship with her. Ordinarily, it is only when these impulses are too strong or too conflictful that difficulties arise.

This conflict has many outcomes. We have seen that some men feel the impairment to their masculinity caused by the passive-regressive desires (PRD) and seek to escape this feeling and deny it by exaggerating their masculinity. The exaggeration, we have noted, may take various forms—physical prowess, aggressiveness, fearlessness, accomplishment—whatever impresses the man because of his past history as "masculine." It may be a secondary sex characteristic, such as physical strength, and it is often sexual activity. This is the main motive in certain "girl-crazy" boys, who feel weak in their human relations and feel strong and masculine only in the sexual relationship with weaker women. Their sexual conquests often do not spring from any interest in the woman, let alone any love for her, but are motivated primarily by prestige—by the need to feel and emphasize and prove their masculinity and potency in this way because of the underlying feeling that it is impaired by childish, regressive trends.

Of course, this behavior is overdetermined and has other motivations as well, such as, in some cases, unconscious hostile feelings, which commonly, if not invariably, result from and accompany strong passive-regressive trends and hurt self-regard. Such men are also often spoiled children, who still expect women to satisfy their every desire, expecting to be loved and preferred by every woman as they used to be by mother, and to be given what they want, which now in adult life is love in sexual form. In some cases, there is a feeling of having been indulged and then rejected, or else pushed out of the spoiled-child role, and there remains a need to take revenge in the form of seducing women into high hopes and then rejecting *them.*

Men as well as women often try to solve the conflict by satisfying the adult, sexual and the childish, dependent desires separately. This was so in the case of Mr. P. D., the 30-year-old man whom we have mentioned several times. While he was overly dependent on his mother, his fiancée was his sexual object. To mate with her he was willing to tear himself away from his dependence on his over-protective mother and marry against her will. Thus, adult drives to sex, love, mating and parenthood, perhaps more than any other forces, separate the young adult from his parents and urge him toward independence and true biological maturity. But our young man reckoned without the force of his unconscious childish wishes for his mother. He could not cast them off by his conscious decision and will. Twenty-five years of protection, indulgence and loving care by his mother left deep desires for these which would probably never be reduced to normal proportions. Analysis could give him insight and materially help him to handle his problem, but only years of *practice in living* would diminish the intensity of these desires cultivated for so long by his mother. So after his marriage he began to turn these desires toward his wife and, as we have related, even gave up his job, returned to college and got his wife to support him, thus reestablishing with his wife the dependent relationship he had had with his mother. In so doing he sacrificed his potent, masculine attitude toward his wife, and his sexual feelings and performance toward her diminished. He became concerned about his potency. But now, with his wife a mother figure in his mind, his sexual feelings turned to other women. He would lie in bed with his wife and think of other girls. Another man with a similar reaction said directly that he needed two women—his wife to mother him and some young girl to enjoy sexually, with whom he could feel himself to be not like a little boy, as he did with his wife, but appreciated as a potent male. This psychology is one of the common causes of marital infidelity (Saul, 1979).

Such a division in the love life by no means always has the same meaning. Sometimes it signifies the opposite, as when, for example, a man takes full responsibility for his wife and family and devotes his best energies and interests to them and their support—and then one day, perhaps when he is in middle life, strays from the path. In such a case, the mature, responsible components were directed toward the wife and the family, and the other young woman represented escape from responsibility—sex as play, pleasure, recreation, diversion, sex without the obligations of marriage and family, the "useless beauty" which Guy de Maupassant has described so poignantly.

F. Promiscuity. Sexual promiscuity can have divers motivations. Another example in which it arose largely from the development-regression conflict and followed the mechanism just described is the following. A young man saw in a girl the satisfaction for himself of preponderantly childish wishes to be loved and taken care of. The girl was of a family of some financial and social standing, so that the man was attracted by the prospect of increased prestige and wealth without exertion and responsibility on his part. In other words, the girl was a "fine catch" and attracted him strongly. After marriage, however, he found himself involved in many responsibilities. His wife no longer represented all kinds of gratification but now made normal but constant demands upon him. He must work, support her properly, help with the home and the children and so on. Now that she had become a responsibility, his sexual interest in her waned. He became interested in other women, who represented to him escape from domestic responsibilities and efforts. Now even marital sexuality came to appear to him as another demand of his wife, another chore which he had to do, whereas other women to whom he felt no obligation attracted him as promises of escape from responsibility and of gratification of his own wishes. After a while, this man began an affair with one of these girls, but it soon followed the same course. He found that the relationship, instead of being only a source of pleasure, again involved him in efforts and responsibilities and obligations to satisfy the woman's demands. With this, he lost interest in her and again looked further afield for the source or image of his wishes for play and pleasure without responsibility or the necessity to satisfy the woman's emotional demands on him.

Both these mechanisms, escape from dependence to masculinity and escape from responsibility to play, may be operative in the same individual; and other motivations also, as in the middle-aged man mentioned earlier, for whom marriage meant obedience, submission and restriction, and whose turning to a young girl had both these meanings (escape from responsibility and escape from dependence), and, in addition, sprang from intense feelings of rebellion and defiance. So long as the proportions and the balance between the adult and the infantile impulses which seek expression sexually is within certain limits, the individual functions satisfactorily. But if this balance becomes upset, either because of the quantity or the quality of the infantile components, or because of other factors, such as intimidation by the parents of any sexual manifestations, then all sorts of disturbances and distortions of the sexual life occur.

3. Differences Between Men and Women

A study of psychodynamics reveals some of the details of the psychological differences between men and women. These have been touched upon above in connection with the passive-receptive-dependent trends, which, in women, more readily integrate with the feminine sexual demands while the responsible, productive, giving tendencies, more readily take a maternal form. Other impulses, such as hostility, are also usually handled differently by the two sexes. Thus, juvenile delinquency in girls is generally thought to take the form of sexual promiscuity more often than of crime as in boys, although there is far more to the problem than this. The secondary sex characteristics, as well as the form of the sexual desire, permeate the entire organism and cannot but be reflected throughout its functioning. The sexual difference lends a cast to the whole outlook and mental life. Just how it is reflected and comes to expression is a matter for observation. It can be seen in the aggressiveness of the male and the seductiveness and the motherliness of the female throughout the mammalian kingdom, as well as in clinical studies of animals and of human beings. The fundamental needs, the course of development and the regressive trends are probably independent of the sexual difference, but the way these are handled is strongly influenced by the sex. Of course, the sex difference, although usually gross and unmistakable, is in some part quantitative emotionally. Men have certain feminine characteristics physically and psychologically, and women have certain masculine ones. Apart from biological reasons, this inevitably would result in some degree from the *psychological identifications* with both a father and a mother. Every boy who respects his mother tends to absorb many of her characteristics; and conversely every little girl who loves her father tends to be like him in many ways.

In some cases, the man's masculine or the woman's feminine trends are inhibited, and, in addition, the emotional life may be handled very largely in ways characteristic of the opposite sex. In such persons the psychological differences between the sexes are not so marked as in the normal. Faced with a direct threat to life, as in war, men and women may behave in ways which are not determined so much by the sexual difference. But these are special cases and conditions.

Cultural factors are of obvious importance in differences in behavior between the sexes; but in evaluating such factors it must not be forgotten that they are themselves man-made and are to a certain extent the *results* of the sexual differences, as are the society's history and ideologies. These are transmitted through the generations and are part of the emotional influences of the parents on each individual child, making it a person of good will or of cruelty and violence.

4. Sexiness

Why some persons have more sexual feeling, why sex means more to them, why it is for them more of a mode of expression than for others is a question which cannot be fully answered at present. Apart from possible heredity, the kind and the intensity of the underlying feelings which seek expression are important in this, and also the childhood environment and experiences, particularly the degree to which the sexuality is stimulated and aroused in childhood.

Moreover, the personal relationships in childhood often determine whether or not sexuality is the main emotional outlet. For example, a young man had lost his father by divorce and had been brought up from infancy by his mother and three older sisters. With no male in the family except himself, all his strongest feelings were bound up with his mother and sisters—all his needs for love, his ambitions, his dependence, his rebellion, his rivalries, his loyalties—all were toward these women. And, following this pattern in adult life, he sought to work out with women all his emotional problems. (The sex follows the emotional pathways of childhood and attaches to similar objects, just as Konrad Lorenz's ducklings attached to, "imprinted," his boots and later, with the access of sexuality, used them for sex relations.) Women and sex became the fount of all his gratifications, the outlet for all his tensions and the attempted solution of all his emotional problems. Men hardly existed for him. But he was always involved with several women. By way of contrast, in another family two brothers, only a year apart in age, competed intensely for their father's favor. They grew up with women relatively a side issue, and their strongest feelings were directed toward men.

Because everyone has impulses and inhibitions of them, opposites are the rule in the emotional life. Hence, one often sees outcomes which are the reverse of the two examples just given, but at bottom these can also be reactions to the forces described and so are determined by them. At least, such observations are suggestive as to a few of the reasons why some people are more highly "sexed" than others.

SEX AS AN OUTLET

We have been discussing sexuality as a biological force, especially vis-à-vis the forces of dependence and needs for love. But we have also pointed out that sexual activity is a means used by many persons for expressing other tendencies in the service of dependence, prestige, hostility and so on. Sexuality is not only a force in itself but it is also a *pathway* and a mode of emotional expression, and as such it can *drain, channel, relieve* all sorts of emotional impulses and tensions, including many which in themselves seem to bear little or no relationship to sex. This seems to be one reason why the sexual urge is so powerful (Ferenczi, 1938). Apparently, any strong emotion cannot only heighten the sexual tension but can be more or less "sexualized" or "erotized." * Needs for love in a nonsexual sense can grade easily into the sexual; infantile desires for love can assume a sexual coloring. It is as though the sexual mechanism can operate as a pathway for the *expression* or the *drainage* of all kinds of impulses, for example, those of love and affection (the hero), but also those of hostility (the villain), as seen in rape and in lust murders, or of guilt, as seen in women who fall in love with men who make them miserable; and sexual love may

* Freud put forward the propositon that "sexual excitation arises as an accessory effect of a large series of internal processes as soon as the intensity of these processes has exceeded certain quantitative limits; indeed, that perhaps nothing very important takes place within the organism without contributing a component to the excitation of the sexual instinct."

drain impulses to give and to care for (protective and maternal elements), as well as impulses to receive and get, as seen in exaggerated form in "gold diggers" and "vampires." The pattern in the adult usually follows closely that of the individual's childhood. To put it another way, behind the sexual feelings lie other feelings which are determined by the degree and the form of the individual's childhood emotional pattern. That is why so many marriages fail as the deeper demands and hostilities, leftovers of childhood, emerge from behind the unifying sexual love.

1. Content and Components

A. Love. Psychologically, then, sexuality is not something simple, homogeneous, irreducible and unanalyzable. It has a long and often intricate developmental history (Freud, 1905). Psychologically, sexuality has *content*, it has component impulses, and it serves as a means of expression, gratification and drainage for these impulses. In childhood these impulses are naturally predominantly those appropriate to childhood. With development to maturity the content of the sexuality normally changes quantitatively to express in greater proportion those strivings which are characteristic of the adult—the capacity for love, object interest, mating, producing children, responsibility for the family and so on. The maturation of the sex organs, secondary sex characteristics and sex drives urge the individual along this pathway of development to the adult attitudes. Thus, mature, adult sex when fused with mature, adult love can bring out what is best, most generous and most constructive in human beings.

B. Hostility. It is sometimes said that love and hate are the same. I think this is usually said in order to seem profound, but it only means that although they are obviously the opposite, there is an inner relationship between them. This consists partly in the fact that thwarted love causes anger and hate—a hostility which would not exist were it not that love had been there to be thwarted; and probably, in a rough way, the stronger the hostility, the stronger was the demand for love and so the more painful the thwarting. Mature, generous, altruistic, giving love when thwarted brings disappointment, but not rage and hate.

Another element in the relationship of love and hate is this capacity of the sexuality to drain hostility. "My husband no longer loves me," reputedly says the peasant woman, "for he has stopped beating me." The sexual object can be a means for satisfying aggressive, hostile impulses as well as feelings of love and tenderness. Sometimes "love," especially on the part of the man, is largely gratitude toward the woman for permitting him to satisfy, in sexual form, feelings which are predominantly hostile and aggressive and for loving him in spite of his hostility.

This is often seen in men who are weak, submissive, intimidated or ineffectual in their social lives, in their relations with people and in making their way in the world. Their aggressiveness is inhibited in life. Usually they feel their weakness and react to it with rage and hate which are never expressed directly because of fear of the consequences, although they probably always influence the personality and come out in disguised, backhand, devious, often unconscious ways. Probably the repressed always returns. In many such cases, the one most nearly direct way in which this constant pressure of anger and hostility and feelings of weakness can find relief is through sexuality. Such a man need not love the woman. He may have no real interest in her at all, indeed, may even hate her—but yet he may find her irresistible sexually because she yields to his sexual feelings, which in reality mean a hostile, aggressive attack on her, assertion of control and domination and relief of other pent-up tensions. In such a case the main "content" of the sexuality is hostile attack, exercise of power, and, perhaps also, the child's intense needs for love.

In Chapter 6, "Hostility," a young man is described who was under constant pressure from repressed rage and hostility; one of his outlets for these hostile feelings was sexual. If anything occurred to heighten his anger, then whether or not he at first became overtly angry, he would suddenly feel an access of intense sexual desire. His urge was so compelling that he usually somewhere, somehow, found a girl. If he could not, he would masturbate. (On one occasion he became so angry at a business meeting that he excused himself, went to the men's room and masturbated.) He was "girl-crazy," "sex-mad." And the basis was not love but hate. The sexual relationship also drained other feelings of his, but the driving force was hostility. His whole mental life was occupied with two main types of fantasy—being attacked or injured and being a sexual aggressor. Both were ways of dealing with his hostility.

Sometimes he thought of boys as objects instead of women, but he never indulged in overt homosexual activity. Freud has pointed out that in some cases of homosexuality the source is hostile attack which takes a sexual form with a member of the same sex as object, and that in such cases sex acts like a protecting substance which flows over the object, guarding it from the naked hostility—sex preserving the object which hostility seeks to destroy.

In lust murders, and even in the sexual excitement which apparently not uncommonly accompanies other types of murder, the sexuality, as an expression of Eros, the life-preserving and unifying tendency, tries to protect the object against naked hostility by relieving this hostility through sexuality. Rape is not basically sex but is hostility in sexual form—but it is less destructive than murder. Sex can drain hostility for women, too, as well as masochistic impulses.

1. Split in Love Life. The hostile component of sexuality can be one source of a split in the love life and object choice, and this was demonstrated by our young man. "Love" for him was sharply "sacred" or "profane," and the meaning of this to him was clear. Profane was the animal expression of his hostility, and he could vent it only upon women for whom he had no regard or respect. Despising them only increased his desire, and with them he experienced premature ejaculation. Sacred was the expression of his tender feelings and was his relationship to women usually a little older than he with whom he identified and toward whom he had a dependent, submissive attitude—mother substitutes, to whom he looked for eventual marriage and a restoration of his lost childhood position of being indulged and supported. He wanted to marry such a woman—one who was beautiful and wealthy and strong of personality, who would be a companion, a reflection of himself, and also would satisfy his prestige as well as his dependent, submissive, regressive desires. But he could not attack such a woman, who represented himself and the satisfaction of his needs, and as a result he was not only socially shy and inhibited with such a woman but also was impotent sexually. Homosexuality, impotence, ejaculatio praecox, satyriasis, nymphomania, inhibitions and perversions can all result from too intense hostility in some status which seeks relief through sexuality.

2. *Normal Zest.* It must not be forgotten that a certain amount of aggression and hostility are normal components of male sexuality. One way in which the female cat seduces the tomcat sexually is by hitting him in the face with her paws until she arouses his aggression. Women as well as men can drain hostility through sexuality. Because of the woman's part in the relationship, she is more adapted to draining the hostility in the reverse form of being attacked. Women generally expect a certain amount of aggression and mastery from the man, even with a tinge of physical attack but with kindness and gentleness psychologically.

Being attacked or punished is a large component of the sexuality for some women. It is generally recognized in the common dreams of women being pursued by a bull, by a man with a knife or gun, by snakes and so on; these are symbolic representations of the man in attacking form. It is a subject for humor. In a cartoon in *The New Yorker* some years ago, two young women are treed by a bull. One says to the other, "If this were a dream it would be significant!" And there is the old joke about the elderly spinster who is afraid of burglars and every night looks under her bed before retiring. One night she really finds a burglar there. She exclaims, "At last!"

2. Disorders

A. *Frigidity.* Powerful as the sex urge is, like everything represented in the mind, it is subject to all sorts of disorders. In general these arise in two main ways: by direct mistreatment of the sexuality during childhood, for example, by excessive stimulation or intimidation physically or psychologically; and by the effects of emotional disorders in the rest of the personality upon the whole sexual mechanism of desire, performance and choice of object. If, because of the woman's own hostility and guilt feelings, the sexual relationship means to her being *too much* attacked or punished, then instead of being thrilled by this component she fears the relationship and becomes inhibited.

In a woman with nymphomania (exaggerated sexual desires of women toward men), one important cause was her insatiable infantile needs for love; but the strongest force driving her sexually was her repressed hostility seeking relief in sexual form.

Sex, as we have said, can drain all kinds of emotional tensions and impulses, and if these have not developed sufficiently to adult orientation, they can cause all kinds of sexual inhibitions, exaggerations and deviations.

B. Homosexuality. Passive homosexuality in both men and women is often a direct expression of infantile, passive, dependent, receptive, submissive tendencies. One such young woman dreamed repeatedly of her mother, of breasts and of eating; for her the homosexuality was an almost direct expression in sexual form of her longing for her mother. Normally, much of this childhood longing for the mother gets turned to a man and satisfied heterosexually. But if the father is of little importance during childhood, and if the mother makes the relationship to her daughter excessively close and intense, by overprotection, control and domination, demands or whatever—and in whatever combination—so that this becomes the central overpowering relationship in the child's life, then, when grown the daughter may be unable to break out of the feelings toward her mother into a healthy relationship to a man. Like the geese reacting sexually to the boot that they imprinted as goslings, the daughter erotizes her image of her attachment to her mother and turns it to other women as homosexuality.

In an earlier chapter the operation of too strong passive, dependent, submissive, receptive desires in a series of men was described. These often come to expression in the form of passive homosexual trends, either latent and appearing only in dreams and in manner or else overt. This is a part of folk knowledge, which has long recognized that parents who indulge, restrict or dominate their children, or by any means make them too dependent and submissive and too much tied to their apron strings, impair their development in a way which often results in the girls being boyish, and the boys girlish, and both remaining childish. Calling a boy a sissy equates the results of his overprotection with femininity.

Feminine trends in men, whatever any congenital or hereditary tendencies (which have not been proven), are certainly commonly produced, developed or exaggerated by such infantilizing treatment. To put it differently, the childish passive, regressive trends which are developed thereby become "erotized" or "sexualized" and come to expression as feminine trends (in the boy), which may be latent as character traits but may even result in overt homosexual behavior (in both sexes).

An example is a young man who was the son of wealthy parents. He was considerably restricted as a child and raised in close association with a sister two years older, many of whose activities and attitudes he shared. He lived at home until he was 28. He grew up in the realization that he would always be secure because of the family fortune, and he enjoyed a large allowance all through school. As a result of his upbringing and of his financial security, he never felt the need to exert himself in school or work. He followed the path of least resistance and escaped or avoided hard work, unpleasant situations and independent decisions, thought or effort. He never found it necessary to take any responsibility but always went to his parents. He felt that something was wrong and that it was somehow connected with his attachment to his home. Finally, at the age of 28, he summoned up enough push to leave home. He made a special point of finding a position in a different city and, unlike his previous positions, getting it through his own efforts and without his father's help. But with all his education and his excellent intelligence, he dragged along at an unskilled job at $95 per week. His attitudes were internalized by now—a part of his make-up—and not simply "reactive" to the temptation of being at home. Geography no longer could make much difference. Moreover, he continued to accept his allowance, which was much larger than his salary.

C. The Sexual and the Social. Knowing this much, we would not be surprised to find that such a young man reacted against his passivity, which caused him to feel weak and ineffectual in his work and social relations, by emphasizing his sexual potency, that is, compensating in the sexual sphere for passivity in the social and occupational sphere. In other cases the reverse is true, and social aggressiveness compensates for passive dependence or particular inadequacies in the sexual sphere. For example, a man was very dependent on his wife, whom he looked to as a mother, and had very little sexual activity with her but was very aggressive in his business. Other persons are normally active in both spheres, although the distribution of energies between home and work is a common problem.

In the wealthy young man we have just mentioned, the passive, dependent trends pervaded his whole make-up.* They came to expression in his sexual life even more clearly than in his social and occupational relationships. The passive trends, through early and long pampering and overprotection, were so strong and pervasive that his masculine drives were too weak for him to care about girls. His masculine drive was impaired too much for him to react against this even by *active* homosexual impulses, as is common, but he disliked his passive feminine homosexual desires and resisted them. When they appeared in his dreams they were associated with being protected, supported and cared for, escaping from adult masculine independence, activity and responsibility—they represented the wish to live on his parents or parent figures and not to work and make his own way.

Passive receptive desires eventuating in feminine trends in men (or masculine trends in women) by no means always result from overindulgence and overprotection but are very frequently a result of heartbreaking *deprivations* during childhood. We are not interested here in various sources of homosexuality nor the many mechanisms of its formation, by direct erotized attachment, identification and so on, but only in its relation to the main developmental and regressive forces (Saul and Beck, 1961).

D. Castration Complex and Penis Envy. As might be expected, the trends causing feminine wishes in men cause unconscious self-castrating tendencies, and masculine trends in women motivate desires to have a penis. Because of the tendencies of all kinds of impulses to be drained sexually, and possibly for other reasons as well, castrative tendencies, whether directed toward the self or others, are common and important. We have seen that fear of castration is very often a reaction to hostility, which is sexualized and

---

* The reader is reminded that the term "passive" in this connection connotes an absence of responsible, constructive activity, of work, of productive accomplishment, even if there is kinetic motion. For example, a husband who shunned work and the tasks of home life could be called a passive character, despite his considerable activity in frequenting gymnasiums and bars.

takes the form of cruel sexual impulses to castrate other males, causing retaliation fear, guilt and hence fear of being castrated; that it is often a reaction to sexual impulses which cause guilt because of simple repressive conditioning or because of hostile components, whether against the woman herself or against a rival. And, just as the phallus is typically symbolic of masculinity, strength and independence, so opposite desires to be weak and dependent often assume a feminine coloring, are more or less sexualized and lead to impulses to be castrated—which also cause castration anxiety. Hostility of women to men also often takes the form of castrative impulses, and the sexual act for these women comes in some part to have this meaning.

We have discussed "the punishment fits the source," and the punishment is logically directed to the organ that does the deed.

3. Erotization

The concept of "erotization" and that of sexuality as a drain or pathway for other impulses are closely related but not identical. In the latter, the impulses find expression in the sexual activity, which is central. But, conversely, an impulse can obtain sexual coloring and cause sexual excitation and sexual sensations without resulting in genital sexual activity. An example is "sadism" or pleasure in cruelty, so called after the Marquis de Sade, who obtained sexual pleasure from his various cruel practices upon his victims. He did not satisfy his hostilities by sex relations but venting them directly in cruelty (e.g., luring a woman to a barn loft and there beating her with a rope) gave him sexual satisfaction. (Of course he was severely ill mentally and many of his writings were done in a mental hospital. Most criminal behavior is a symptom of serious emotional disorder. This is evident today in so much of the widespread destructiveness, breakdown of law and morals, and disregard of others.) Perhaps this, too, is only quantitative. The degree of erotization or sexualization of the hostility did not go far enough to substitute sex for naked cruelty and destructiveness. It could only short-circuit a certain amount of the hostility into sexual excitation but not enough to drain it as coitus and thereby prevent harm to the victim. Erotization probably plays a part in the process of adaptation—not only getting used to a situation, however distressing, but also gradually learning to make the best of it, and even to derive a certain pleasure from it.

4. Sex Appeal

An interesting question is why some persons are generally more attractive sexually than others. One must qualify such a statement by the term "generally," because the individual who is most sexually attractive to one person may not be to another—and an individual to whom most people react but little may be most stimulating to certain others. There are highly individual factors in "sex appeal." Nevertheless, some persons are generally agreed to have much more appeal for most people than others, and the question is whether any general statement as to why this is so can be contributed from a knowledge of psychodynamics. A few thoughts on this subject may be of interest.

A. Perfection in Biology and Art. In the first place, there seems to be the biological factor of perfection of form. People vary in size, shape, complexion and so on. Probably everyone has some human defects and aberrations, but we all have a feeling, whether innate, from experience or from our own defects, for what a perfect being would be—and this sense of perfection would seem to be a component of sexual feeling. This is so in part through the love of that perfection which we all wish were ours and want to identify with; in part perhaps from biological tendencies to mate with members of the species who have such perfection to produce more perfect progeny, and maybe for other reasons also. Of course, in speaking of this perfection, a certain leeway must be allowed for individual and cultural variations. In Turkey, for example, fat women were reported to be regarded as most appealing, while in the U.S., slimness is the ideal, and different countries and times have different tastes and standards, within limits, as to perfection and as to beauty in humans, animals and art. Is not esthetic perfection of form, balance and proportion, in the arts, a representation of that perfection of form which each of us desires in ourselves, our mates and our children, who are parts of ourselves; and is this not what biology strives for in the species, so that the "ugly" is always a sign of pathology? In the artist's creations we find that perfection which human protoplasm so rarely achieves. This is no place to muster the reasons for this thesis, which have been formulated many times before. The important thing for us is that it relates art to biology and to sex; and sex is notoriously important for artists and for art (Arieti, 1976).

B. Intensity. A person's sexual desire appears to play some part in heightening his or her sex appeal. Because of it, even some persons who are sexually inhibited, but not too deeply so, and therefore under great sexual tension, consciously or unconsciously, arouse powerful sexual responses, as do persons whose feelings are very strong and free. Many a man who strongly desires a certain woman does not realize that his urges are largely in *response* to her conscious or unconscious seductive longings for *him*. This often occurs the other way around, also.

C. Freedom. Further reasons are the freedom of certain of the component impulses of sexuality, for example, the free giving and receiving of love. We have seen elsewhere how inhibitions in receiving can affect the receiving of love and sexual interest. Free, receptive wishes often appeal to the woman's maternal giving impulses and to the man's giving and protecting impulses. Hence, adults who were spoiled children and are warm and crave affection very often have considerable sex appeal.

Freedom of aggressive impulses is also important in many cases. We have seen the converse—women in whom guilt and fear of being attacked, arising from repressed hostility, inhibit the sexuality. But when in women the wish to be attacked (the "masochism") is not too strong and only adds a "thrill" and is a free, accepted desire, and when in men the wish to attack is properly tempered and is free, these trends can heighten the sexual desire and apparently also the sexual appeal, whereas inhibitions decrease it.*

---

* There is a juvenile ditty that goes something like this:

> Treat me rough, kid, treat me rough,
> What I want is lowdown love,
> Heavy knock-down caveman stuff.
> Yank me wildly to your breast,
> If I struggle, break my neck.
> I'm no soaring turtledove,
> Treat me rough, kid, treat me rough.

No one really meant it, but they thought the lyrics were cute.

D. Sex as Funnel. Another factor, and a most critical one, is the degree of erotization of the component impulses, the extent to which they seek satisfaction in sexual form. This, in turn, may be determined in part by the early personal history, for example, by an overly demonstrative or seductive parent or other important figure during childhood. When a woman or man promises gratification of all kinds of desires through sexuality, the sexual appeal is thereby heightened. Individually, people love those who fit their emotional needs, and as all feelings tend to be erotized, this fit increases the sexual appeal. These remarks are, of course, tentative and are meant to show that the psychological factors in sexual attractiveness are susceptible of analysis through a psychodynamic approach.

Love, passion, infatuation are terms which describe feelings and states of mind which are mostly end-results. They tell little about the "content" of the feelings and the many, often conflicting impulses that compose them. "True love" is generally considered to be an attribute of maturity. It implies that an important part of the content of the sexual feeling is unselfish interest in the loved person, with impulses to give to her or him of one's own energies and even to make sacrifices and take on responsibilities for this loved one. This is the kind of love the hero has for the heroine. The content of the villain's "love" is much more selfish, inconsiderate, hostile, infantile—to take, to attack, to consider only himself and not the happiness of the girl.

In this connection, reviewing remarks earlier in this chapter, let us differentiate clearly (1) sex, (2) romantic love, (3) mating in marriage, and, for completeness, (4) parental urges; and let us bear in mind the important distinction between loving and being loved. Sex without love is exemplified by sexual attacks on women and by the transient conjugation of a man and a prostitute. A man may be a great lover, a Don Juan, but never mate, never marry, and if he does, may remain poor husband material. Happy then the man or the woman who finds a mate who is passionate sexually and fervid romantically and also able to mate maturely and to be a good breadwinner and parent—to fuse sex and romance with love and responsibility for mate and offspring (Saul, 1979, Chap. 3). Women more than men seem to mistake sexual advances for love. Reputedly, sex, romance and mating are more often closer, more intimately interwoven, in women than in men. *No doubt sex should be in a setting of mutual love. It is one of life's problems that it so often is not, that sex, romance, love and mating touch and overlap but are not always united.*

5. Idealization

The idealization seen in "being in love" has many sources, which vary in importance with the content of the "love." It springs from the gratitude, or something akin to it, which one feels toward the source of so great and manifold gratification, and this gratitude is sometimes anticipatory; it springs from the anticipation of pleasures even if these are not actually realized, and this anticipation is usually in large part for the satisfaction of the infantile impulses; strong receptive-dependent satisfactions, or anticipations of them, are usually accompanied by idealization, often repeating the idealization of the parents and one's own feelings of weakness as a child in comparison with them; it springs from the projection of one's own self-love, loving the other as part of oneself, and giving rein to pride in the object—one's affianced or spouse—which would be crass vanity if directed to oneself; it can spring, too, from over-compensation for hostile feelings and probably from other sources as well. (A girl sees her fiancé in her child image of her father—all-powerful, all-good—but after marriage finds him an imperfect, childish mortal like herself and then tends to project her father's image upon other men whom she now idealizes at a distance—reminiscent of Somerset Maugham's *The Unattainable.*)

6. Battle of Sexes

A considerable portion of the "battle between the sexes" in marriage often originates in the development and regression conflict. To the man who feels burdened by the efforts, the responsibilities and the obligations of the adult male in our civilization, the woman's lot seems to be a much easier one. He must be the breadwinner, live up to masculine ideals, hold his own in the world and take the responsibility for his wife and his family, while it so often seems to him that the wife merely accepts this support and has nothing to do but the light, easy task of running the home. Thus, one man who had great difficulty in working and taking responsibility and yearned to withdraw from his adult obligations and thought only of getting out of his job and going away on vacations could not stand it to see his wife relax for a moment in the home. If she took things easy and simply read or "wasted time," he would become infuriated. He envied women this. He saw no truth in the old proverb, "A woman's work is never done." In most cases, the man's pride does not allow him to admit to himself that he envies women their role. It is a very educational experience for a husband to have the full responsibility of the home for a time—and for a woman to get a taste of the burdens of breadwinning, as increasing numbers of women are doing by working outside the home.

One very often sees women who envy men. For example, one of these women, who was an excellent wife and mother, nevertheless resented carrying the manifold responsibilities for the thousand details of the house and children and at the same time being an emotional support to her husband, listening to his many recitals of his personal problems and successes. In her outlook, she carried the whole burden of responsibility for the family, while her husband enjoyed his variegated adventures, experiences and successes in his occupation, where, it seemed to her, he had little in the way of responsibility and much in the way of fun and satisfaction and could gratify his needs for esteem, while she got no prestige from her labors and successes in the home. (Me slaving in this hot kitchen all day, and you down in that nice cool sewer.) This woman had a strong wish to be a man, not because she wanted to be masculine but indeed just the opposite. She really wished to be not a man but a little boy, since this meant to her escape from her feminine and maternal obligations and responsibilities, and she envied men because their role in life seemed to her easier than her own. It is not uncommon to see men envying women and women envying men for the same motive, namely, escape from adult interests and responsibilities. Each thinks the other is nearer to the Garden of Eden—escape from RPI to PRD (see Chap. 25). Sometimes one of them is. Sometimes both are far too overburdened realistically. When this is so it is apt to put a strain on their mutual love.

A previous observation is pertinent here. A man and a woman are attracted to each other because, for example, both had deprived childhoods and therefore sense a similarity in each other, understand each other in the deeper feelings; but after marriage their needs for love and sense of deprivation turn toward each other—and the frustrated love needs that brought them together, by enabling them to identify with each other, now become a source of growing frustration and hostility.

7. *Libido Theory*

A. Problems of Normal Development. The child's dependence on its parents may be a manifestation of Eros in the broad sense and is an impulse which can come to expression in sexual form. Freud, as we have noted, eventually considered sex, whether pregenital or genital, as but one manifestation of Eros, which term he used to signify all the life-preserving tendencies in cells which build people up and bring them together, even in the formation of societies, indeed, all the unifying forces which tend to build up, increase and preserve protoplasm. Sex in this perspective is one force in the service of Eros. The life-destroying impulses, whether outwardly expressed as "hostile aggression" or inwardly as masochism or as a wish to die, Freud saw as manifestations of Thanatos, the basic trend in protoplasm to revert to the inanimate state. Life would then appear as a struggle between Eros and Thanatos (Freud, 1920).

As stated at the opening of this chapter, our purpose has been a review of sexuality only in relation to developmental and regressive trends. Hence, we have not gone into its origins and evolution. Freud saw that other bodily stimulation than genital was connected with sexual feelings and described the synthesis of other pleasures, especially of sucking and of excreting, with the dominant genital feelings. Later workers added a dynamic component to this description, showing how hostile giving, receptive, retentive or other impulses could take anal, oral or genital form, and so on, and hence influence sensation in these areas (Alexander et al., 1934).

Freud considered the infantile pleasures, whether in being nursed, snuggled, diapered or otherwise loved and tended, to be sexual in nature, using the term in a broad sense. Such pregenital pleasures gradually come to contribute to genital sensation, when, beginning at from three to five years of age, these begin to predominate. Hence, oral, anal, skin, muscle and other components come to contribute to genital attraction and sensations. If they persist too strongly and demand satisfaction directly rather than as part of genital sexuality, they provide the bases for the sexual perversions later.

Before birth, the relationship to the mother is largely through skin contact within the womb. After birth, the great event of the infant's day is suckling, whether at breast or bottle, and its demands for satisfaction through the mouth, by eating, sucking and biting, are imperious and dominating. Then come the new problems of weaning, walking and coordination and bowel training; then of comparison with others, concern with one's adequacy, concern with the difference between the sexes and the size, the presence or the absence of the genital organs, especially in the phallus; and then, with increasing predominance of genital sensations, the problems of masturbation and of rivalries based not only on dependence and infantile needs for attention but also on sexual feelings and mature powers.

Freud was impressed by the early age at which children's feelings become erotically toned, apparently passing a peak at from three to five years, and then subsiding somewhat (latency period) until the great surge at puberty. The attraction to the parent of the opposite sex and jealousy and rivalry toward the one of the same sex, Freud called the "Oedipus complex," after the tragedy by Sophocles, in which Oedipus, the king, seeking the slayer of his father, discovers not only that he himself unknowingly did this deed but also that he has married his mother. We have seen that the feelings toward the parents are also determined by other factors, such as spoiling, deprivation, domination and so on.* There is always attachment to the parent of the same sex, too, and jealousy toward the other ("inverted Oedipus"). The term "oedipal" has also come to be used in a rather loose fashion for all the attachments and rivalries in relation to the parents, affected as they are by how the parents feel toward the child and treat him.

---

* "I do not wish to maintain that the Oedipus-complex covers entirely the relation of the child to its parents; this relation can be much more complicated. Furthermore, the Oedipus-complex is more or less well-developed; it may even experience a reversal, but it is a customary and very important factor in the psychic life of the child; and one tends rather to underestimate than to overestimate the influence and the developments which may follow from it. In addition, children frequently react to the Oedipus-idea through stimulation by the parents, who in the placing of their affection are often led by sex-differences, so that the father prefers the daughter, the mother the son; or again, where the marital affection has cooled and this love is substituted for the outworn love" (Freud, S., 1916).

All these developmental phases and the problems and emotional experiences during them leave their marks on the growing child and influence powerfully the ways in which it will handle its later feelings and problems. These phases and these persisting trends in persons, called by Freud oral, anal, phallic and oedipal, are, of course, overlapping and by no means sharply set off from one another. Special difficulties in the course of development cause "fixations," which not only influence the personality throughout life but also determine the kinds and the degrees of regression and the nature of the neurosis and the symptoms if a person develops these. In other words, all these influences shape a specific emotional pattern in each child.

B. Causes of Warped Development. What retards or warps the development is a *traumatic situation* which forms the nucleus and the core of the neurotic manifestations, not usually a single overwhelming event, but the long term, unrelenting influences, such as overprotection, spoiling, seductiveness, ambition, restriction, domination, deprivation, rejection, harshness and hostility and other emotionally injurious influences, singly or in various combinations, acting upon the growing child. For example, for the unwanted child, being unwanted can be the central trauma, overshadowing the problems arising from the difference in sex between the parents and similar problems. Without traumatic situations the normal problems of family life and growing up are solved and only a normal amount of neurosis remains. Without traumatic influences no child, so far as is known (always excepting organic damage and the extremes of psychoses, of which little is known), develops serious emotional problems only because he has a mother and a father—or siblings.

The pine tree grows straight of its own nature. If it is inclined, then it was bent as a twig. The infant matures of its own nature into a responsible, productive, relatively independent spouse, parent and citizen, an adult of good will, if it is reared with good feelings and respect. If the adult is emotionally disturbed, with neurotic, psychotic, criminal or criminoid behavior or pathologically hostile acting out then something was seriously wrong in the influences upon him from birth (or conception) to about age five, six or seven—from 0–6. Analytic treatment is designed to correct the after-effects in the adult of these early injurious influences during his childhood. Its effectiveness depends upon how early, strong and constant the trauma was, how uncompensated by positive influences, how severe and deep-seated the effects; and on the competence of the analyst in comprehending in detail the patient's basic psychodynamics and in using this understanding therapeutically. (Saul 1972). Since treatment on a mass scale will probably never be practicable, the only hope lies in prevention. Not until children are better reared can we possibly get a better world. As Thoreau said, "There are thousands hacking at the branches of evil to one who is striking at the root."

REFERENCES

Alexander, F. (1961): *Scope of Psychoanalysis*, ed. by T. French. New York: Basic Books, pp. 167–169.

_____ et al. (1934): The influence of psychological factors upon gastrointestinal disturbances, a symposium, *Psychoanalytic Quarterly,* 3:501.

Arieti, S. (1976): *Creativity, The Magic Synthesis*. New York: Basic Books.

Ferenczi, S. (1938): *A Theory in Genitality*. Albany, New York: Psychoanalytic Quarterly Press.

Freud, S. (1905): Three essays on the theory of sexuality, *S.E.* 7.

_____ (1916): Introductory lectures on psycho-analysis, *S.E.* 16, p. 303.

_____ (1920): Beyond the pleasure principle, *S.E.* 18.

Lorenz, K. (1952): *King Solomon's Ring*. New York: Crowell.

Saul, L. J. (1972): *Psychodynamically Based Psychotherapy*. New York: Science House.

_____ (1979): *The Childhood Emotional Pattern in Marriage*. New York: Van Nostrand Reinhold.

_____ and Beck, A. (1961): Psychodynamics of male homosexuality, *International Journal of Psycho-analysis* 42, Parts I & II.

8 | The Grasp of Reality

INTELLECT AND EMOTION

The grasp of reality is a sense and a function which develops slowly and gradually as the individual matures. Only little by little does the infant and then the small child become aware of its surroundings and of the significance of the inanimate world around it and of the persons who enter its life. This comprehension of the outer world depends in part on the intellectual development, the intelligence, and in part on the emotional development and orientation. These two components are interrelated. For one thing, emotion influences the operation of the intellect. It is common experience that when a person is greatly upset emotionally he finds that he cannot think clearly and often notices some confusion and difficulty in concentration. Sometimes the effect of the emotions on the intellect is extreme; for example, a boy of eight was considered, on the basis of observation and special tests, to be seriously retarded mentally and unable to do ordinary schoolwork. This child was embroiled in a most distressing relationship to a brutal father, toward whom he seethed with rage, which, out of fear, he kept pent up within him. When he eventually was removed from his home and placed in a setting in which he was happy, he gradually brightened and before long was doing excellent work in school. The more one observes, the clearer it becomes that not only the level of intelligence, the I.Q., is strongly influenced by the feelings, but that the sense of reality, the processes of reasoning and the conclusions reached, are all colored, shaped and even determined by them. The needs, desires, urges, the passions, the emotional forces are what is primary and the intellect is at best their servant, at worst their slave. The intellect is to this extent the computer which serves the motivations and reactions, the emotional forces.

REALITY SENSE AND MATURITY

Impairment by Dependence

But whatever the relationship of the emotions and the intellect, it is obvious that a grasp of reality is an essential characteristic of maturity. Lack of experience with reality impairs the emotional development, and, conversely, lack of emotional maturity interferes with a grasp of reality.

One of the commonest ways in which the development of a sense of reality is impaired is through excessive dependence on the parents. When one or both parents have so sheltered the child, being its eyes and its ears so to speak, the child never learns to use its own powers of perception and comprehension. In some cases, this does not hinder the development of the intellect itself, and the result is something like the brilliant but absent-minded and impractical professor. In other cases, the interference with the reality sense is so serious that the individual may not be able to get along in life at all in spite of a very superior intelligence.

As an example of the contrast between intellectual development and emotional immaturity, a bright, attractive young man, Mr. G. M., came to see me a few weeks after obtaining his Ph.D. in chemistry. His academic record was one of outstanding brilliance. He had attended a university of standing and had won every prize and honor in his field. He had been awarded a fellowship, and several excellent jobs in industry were offered him. He had accepted one in a large city. With what complaint did he come for help? He seriously told me that although he had this brilliant record he really did not know anything about chemistry and simply could not hold such a job in it!

Now it is a rule that the patient is always right in the sense that what the patient believes represents the truth somehow to him, however strange this may sound to another. It is part of our task to discover in what sense the patient's belief is true. In this case it was not difficult. What he sensed was that he had been passing courses, making A's, writing brilliant examinations and winning approval, but he had not been learning chemistry as a reality.

This was an exaggeration of an experience which, I suppose, many students have, of passing an examination with very little actual interest in or grasp of the subject, so that a week later most of it is forgotten. It represents an intellectual exercise, a tour de force, and has little to do with grasping the reality of the subject. This boy was capable of remarkable intellectual gymnastics, but they had little to do with reality or with emotional *interest in the realities* with which chemistry deals. He was an only child. He had been extremely restricted, pampered, overprotected. He was still a babe in arms so far as making his way in the world was concerned. He was a caricature of the impractical professor. He could memorize symbols, he was a virtuoso in the wiles of logic, and he could pass examinations and win the praise of his parents and teachers, while living at home and being supported and cared for by his family. But to take care of himself in the big city, to understand people, their emotions and motivations, to hold his own with them, to make his way by productive work, by his interest in and his ability to solve the real chemical problems encountered in his job—this was beyond him, not intellectually but emotionally. His emotional immaturity hindered his intellectual grasp of reality. His intelligence quotient was very high so far as abstract intellectual processes were concerned, but very low so far as his grasp of reality was concerned. His intellect was a fine instrument, but it lacked the emotional base for adequate operation and comprehension in the real, practical world. His thinking was an abstract intellectual exercise rather than an expression of a sense of reality, an absorption in reality. He illustrates how extreme childhood emotional dependence on the parents and interest in oneself and in one's own wishes, thoughts and fantasies, rather than independence, interest in reality and in other persons and capacity for social productivity and responsibility, can undermine a career, despite personal charm and unusual intellectual gifts.

Such overprotection and dependence on the parents form only one of the tendencies which can impair the grasp of reality. Any strong emotion can influence a person's outlook, what he sees and how he evaluates it.

Before coming to a more detailed discussion of this topic, let us consider for a moment the possible origins of reality testing. Freud's idea was that the infant freely fantasies for itself whatever satisfaction it wants and cannot distinguish between its fantasy and the reality. In other words, if it wishes to suckle, it hallucinates the breast, which it does not distinguish as an object but feels to be part of its own body. Gradually, however, from the lack of real satisfaction afforded by the hallucination, in contrast with that derived from the actual breast, it begins to distinguish the reality, and in a similar fashion, through pleasure and pain, gradually learns to discriminate between its own body and the rest of the world. Most pathological mental phenomena in adults turn out to be the recurrence of the mental processes of very early childhood. Thus, the hallucinations of psychotics and the dreams of normal people may well reflect a resurgence of mental processes which predominated before language was learned, therefore before thoughts could be expressed verbally, and while feelings could come to expression only in the form of visual images. However that may be, and our primary concern is not theory, although normal adults do not hallucinate except in their sleep as dreams, yet their wishes and feelings strongly color, if not determine, their views of the world about them.

Excessive dependence on the parents, as we have said, tends to atrophy the reality-testing functions. It does this in at least three ways: (1) it makes their use unnecessary; (2) when the individual has not been sufficiently on his own, he is unable to identify with and understand those who have; hence, he has no firm basis for understanding them psychologically; (3) if his emotions are bound up with his family, he does not have sufficient emotional concern with, absorption and interest in other persons and in the doings of the world to have these mean much to him. He lacks interest, involvement and *emotional investment* in things and therefore lacks a grasp of them. Lack of understanding of reality is often used as an excuse for asking help and thus satisfying the underlying dependent wishes. The innumerable questions of children, prompted by curiosity and other motives, often have the meaning of getting attention and help from the parent. This is a common experience in psychiatric work; the dependent patient seeking gratification of some kind wants direct attention and help from the doctor and endeavors to obtain it by making him answer all sorts of questions. Consciously he may want help in becoming more independent, but unconsciously he tends to use the relation to the analyst, the transference, for direct knowledge, advice and help, that is, to serve and satisfy the dependent desires.

We have been speaking of intelligence in general. Seen in individuals, it is a very specific capability. My neighbor's daughter, for example, scores in the ninety-eighth percentile or above in math, but does poorly in the verbal tests. She can do integral calculus but struggles for hours to write a paragraph. A man who is so talented in music that he has absolute pitch, plays the piano and composes, cannot read or write down music. A friend gave him a score and he had to take it to someone else to play it so that he could listen and then play it by ear himself. Where special talents are involved, as for music, drawing, math or writing, a person sometimes becomes interested and deeply involved emotionally, and this emotional charge works toward further development of the specific talent.

EMOTIONS AND ILLUSIONS

So greatly does dependence hamper and do other emotions warp an individual's grasp of reality that hardly any two persons agree fully in their views. Indeed, often each party to an argument believes the other to be deluded, or at least to have illusions, or at the very least to have strong prejudices. As we have said, people's emotions influence radically their grasp of reality, and the more dominated the person is by childhood emotions, especially over-strong, warped, pathological ones, the more distorted his view of reality, especially psychological reality, is apt to be; while, conversely, the freer the individual is from his infantile and childhood emotions, the less colored and prejudiced is apt to be his view of the world. Thus, realism is something which is an attribute of healthy maturity and is a quality gradually achieved through a long process of emotional development.

1. Childhood

Childhood illusions, that is, the interpretation of reality not objectively but in terms of wishes, are considered a charming attribute of early life. Here the role of wishes is clear. Let the child believe in Santa Claus and fairy tales and his imaginary companions, one says, let him enjoy his wish world while he can, for all too soon he will have to face harsh reality. This may be referred to, as Groddeck suggested (1928), in the story of Adam and Eve, who lived like children with everything provided until they tasted the fruit of the tree of knowledge. With maturity comes sexuality, knowledge and eviction from the shelter of the home into the work and the struggles of the world. "When ignorance is bliss, 'tis folly to be wise," is Thomas Gray's famous line.

2. Psychoses

In the illusions, the delusions and the hallucinations, one sees the extremes of distortions of reality by the emotions. Apparently, almost any emotion, if strong enough, can cause an individual to alter his grasp of reality in accordance with his needs. Thus, a severely frustrated young woman, left all alone in the world and abandoned by her lover, believed that he was communicating with her by telepathy and often would hear his voice and carry on conversations with him. In fact, so pregnant was her imagination, as Professor Macfie Campbell once said in presenting this case, that she soon believed herself to be the mother of a whole brood of children.

3. Distortion by Projection

In other cases, not love, or rather needs *for* love, but hate alters the person's picture of the world. Thus, an inadequate young man could not tolerate his younger brother's success. This brother had outstripped him in every way in life—in looks, in income and now in achieving marriage and establishing a happy home. The weak older brother now became dependent on him emotionally and financially. This hurt his pride more than he could bear. He built up an implacable hatred for the brother and began to think of ways of killing him, being partial to poison. Then he broke down with a paranoia which centered about the delusion that the brother was poisoning *him*. As this example indicates, not only can the primitive impulses of love or hate alter one's perception of the world but also the conscience reaction. One of the commonest methods by which this is accomplished is, as we have seen, "projection." The delusions of the frustrated girl mentioned in the preceding paragraph were based upon a direct wish, her longing for her lost lover, but the paranoid young man attributed his own hostility to the brother.

One's judgment of oneself can also be projected. In the play *The Informer,* to which we have already referred, the protagonist, after betraying his friend, feels so guilty, that is, self-accusatory, that he interprets the most harmless remarks of other people as accusations.* An example of shame projected rather than guilt is afforded by a powerful young man with an intense pride who felt deeply humiliated at having to come to the hospital because of an anxiety attack. He could hardly bear to ride on the bus when reporting for treatment, because he felt sure that the other passengers were all thinking it a disgrace that such a strong, healthy-looking young fellow should be coming to a hospital. This illustrates a very common reaction—people tend to expect other people to judge them as they judge themselves, that is, they project their own evaluations and conscience reactions toward themselves upon others.

4. Neuroses

In the neuroses one encounters the same distortions of reality as in the psychoses (Freud, 1924), but in lesser degree. The distortions are often more subtle and are usually well rationalized, but since everyone has some degree of neurosis, that is, some domination by childhood patterns which are not yet fully outgrown, the interference with the grasp of reality is often of about the same dimensions as in the average person, in whom we do not usually consider the matter in this way. We merely think of each person as having his particular views and outlooks. Thus, in the anxiety neurosis, one may note only a certain worrisomeness, but if this gets to the point of the individual's being unable to sit in a theater or go above the first floor of a building, then the lack of reality becomes noticeable. However, let us remember that severe paranoids with full-blown delusional systems, for example, of being persecuted by organizations whose members they believe are everywhere about them, may go many years before being detected. They often do not betray overt symptoms until an advanced stage of the disorder has been reached. It is not surprising, therefore, that "an average normal" person's views and outlooks may not have a rational, realistic

* But they whose guilt within their bosoms lie
  Imagine every eye behold their blame.—Shakespeare: *Rape of Lucrece*

basis as appears on the surface but may express considerable emotional disorder. A man in a good position over-identifies with underdogs. In his outlook every, or nearly every, poor person is good while all the affluent are selfish, hostile, dangerous. The poor have all the virtues, the rich all the vices. Therefore, he associates almost entirely with the poor and unsuccessful. He himself was deprived emotionally and financially, and envies the affluent to such an extent that he cannot stand close association with them. The next man can only identify with the well-to-do and hates the poor and deprived, because they represent his own childhood of poverty and deprivation, which he now despises and denies. It is these inner personal dynamics, formed in childhood, which determine their social and political views and behavior, and not their knowledge of reality. Another man, strictly raised, with a strong temper which constantly threatens to break out and must be constantly under control, sees lack of discipline in children and adults as the source of just about all of our nation's ills. His views may coincide with reality but their origin is within, formed in early childhood.

It is hard to escape the conclusion that the views of reality of most people are more or less extreme distortions, emotionally, i.e., irrationally determined, that they are mostly rationalizations, and that it is not reason and reality, but rationalization, which rules in all human affairs.

HEIGHTENED PERCEPTION

Libidinal Desires

In some cases, emotion heightens the individual's perception (Saul, 1938), as is always evident when one treats, for example, a man with a homosexual problem and learns that he can perceive this tendency in another man through the faintest hint that the average person would never notice.

We do not have to seek far for examples of how libidinal desires can alter one's perception of reality. There is the repressed woman who loves to gossip about the sexual doings of others, and there is the man who looks to his wife as a goddess while other people comment, "What does he see in her?"

DISTORTION

Hostility

Hostility plays its role in innumerable situations in coloring one's grasp of reality. For example, the overanxious mother exaggerates every danger to her child. In the manic-depressive reactions one sees a caricature of the everyday tendency to have ups and downs and of some people to see the bright and others to see the gloomy side of life. The world looks bright or dark, depending on one's own emotional make-up and feelings at the time. In the compulsion neuroses one sees the exaggerated fear that harm will befall unless one goes through certain rituals which he himself considers to be silly; nevertheless, they have for him so magic a potency that he develops panic if he does not perform them. One man was convinced that if he did not spend many minutes each morning arranging his underclothes to perfection he would certainly develop a chafing of the skin which would lead to an infection that would injure his genitals. The more rational part of his mind knew perfectly well that this was fantastic, but the other part believed it to such a degree that he simply could not take a chance. We all know better, but how many of us can utterly disregard knocking on wood when we have mentioned some good fortune and how many studiously avoid walking under a ladder, taking room 13 or breaking a mirror?

Some details as to how a person's emotions affect his perception of reality are afforded by a few incidents which occurred during the treatment of a young man. During a certain interview he was feeling very friendly toward the world, for he had just achieved a minor but satisfying success, and also toward me, for I had just had occasion to pay him a compliment. His associations consisted chiefly of very pleasant memories. One of these was of sitting at a luncheon, some years back, with three classmates. He mentioned the names of two of them and to his surprise was entirely unable to recall the name of the third. A few days later we found the reason for this. I had had to cancel an appointment, and he was angry at me, although not entirely conscious of how angry he was over this minor frustration. He told a dream of the previous night; he had seen in it the face of the classmate whose name he had forgotten. Now it came to him at once, along with a flood of unpleasant episodes connected with him; in fact, this boy was the one dark spot during those times, the one person the patient thoroughly disliked, a man who justified the patient's resentment. Thus, when the patient warmed with friendly feelings toward me, he could not bring into his stream of thought this man's name, which was to him a symbol of justified hostility; but when he was angry at me, this name and the memories associated with it and the resentment that it symbolized came spontaneously.

A further incident with this young man is also illuminating. During an interview when his anger at me was acutely mobilized by my proposing termination of treatment in the near future, he launched a variety of accusations against me, designed to show how badly I treated him, dwelling particularly on the inconvenience of the times we met for his new schedule. He soon saw that he was projecting his resentment to me, feeling that I was hostile to him, rather than the other way round. And when, after seeing its real sources his anger dwindled, he suddenly realized that we were waiting for *him* to find out what his new schedule would be, so that we could change the appointment to fit it. He had excluded this fact, which conflicted with his wish to prove that I abused him. When his anger gave way to reason, the span of his reality sense widened.

IMAGO AND REALITY

Freud attributed Goethe's optimism and self-confidence in part to the fact that he had won out over all the other members of his family in gaining the central position in his mother's love. Others are not so fortunate. The following is an example. A young man was brought up by a father who, on the one hand, was charming and exerted himself to hold his son's affection while, on the other hand, he was cruelly perfectionistic for the boy and merciless in his criticisms of him, even in front of others. This young man was unable to tear himself away from the father's emotional grip on him, but at the same time he harbored an intense resentment against him. He was conscious of this resentment and at times was tempted to attack his father physically, but he did not know how automatically he transferred this pattern toward every man whom he unconsciously put psychologically into his father's position. A soldier in World War II, he was constantly embroiled with his officers, for he did not see them as they were but rather as a class, or category of person, to which he reacted as he did to his father, with a combination of attraction and hatred. Thus, his childhood emotional involvement with his father, the *imago* of his father, formed in childhood, ever afterward impaired his perception of psychological reality and warped his view of every man who was older or in a position of authority over him.

Everyone forms during childhood composite images of the persons who are emotionally important to him. These "imagoes" may be sharp or blurred, fixed or easily shifted, fused or discrete. The kindly ones, the hostile ones, the rivalrous ones may be grouped in this way. These imagoes are largely what forms the superego. Each person, with these composite images in his mind, tends to project them onto other persons, onto groups, onto fate, and thus sees the world through them. Psychodynamic therapy operates largely by correcting trouble-making imagoes. It is a great handicap to go through life hating all authorities and always being in trouble with them, because one hated one's father or mother as a child.

Every individual, then, emerges into adult life with a picture of others which is largely a continuation of the picture he has of his own family. He does not yet know that the world is any different or will treat him any differently from the little world of his home which is all he has known through these years of childhood. Then, as an adult, he begins to learn how different from home life really is. " 'A tragedy with a happy ending' is exactly what the child wants before he goes to sleep: the reassurance that 'all's well with the world' as he lies in his cozy nursery. It is a good thing that the child should receive this reassurance: but as long as he needs it, he remains a child, and the world he lives in is a nursery world. Things are not always and everywhere well with the world, and each man has to find it out as he grows up. It is the finding out that makes him grow and until he has faced the fact and digested the lesson he is not grown up—he is still in the nursery" (Waelder, 1941). His illusions, whatever they may be, sooner or later, rudely or gradually, become painfully shattered. But nevertheless, although perhaps freed of any extreme illusions, his view of life will remain *colored* by the emotional patterns of his childhood and by the way these have caused him to react to the vicissitudes of later life. That is why the huge majority of people believe in simple causes, simple answers, panaceas. Certainly few can face the fact that most people are emotionally ill, their hostilities turned against themselves as addictions and ruined careers and against others, against spouse and children and innocent members of society, as personal, political or criminal behavior. Probably the most sinister source of distortions of reality is the hostility of man to man. Turned against himself it uses greed to make suckers for gamblers and failures in the stock market. Turned against others it uses any convenient rationalization to justify cruelty and violence, often undisguisedly criminal, but always rationalized in some way.

REALITY AND EDUCATION

In general, our education has failed in preparing the young for life; for it teaches intellectual knowledge alone, but in no systematic way does it acquaint the developing child and youth with his own make-up, his own dynamics and how they were formed and with what life is really like, what it can expect, how different real life is from its daydreams and from the fantasies of Hollywood. Shakespeare held the mirror up to nature, but his plays are rarely taught as portrayals of the realities of life. Knowledge of life is left to the back alley and to chance, and few institutions give the child any preparation for it in their teaching. However, there is a growing recognition of this need—so I once thought but now it would be hard to substantiate this optimistic view. We see all kinds of therapy groups mushrooming across the country, each based on some fragment of psychodynamic knowledge, revealing the extent and depth of emotional disorder and the need for therapeutic help; but there is a dearth of systematic knowledge of psychodynamics offered by experts that could help prevention.

Sometimes a person feels that his childhood attitudes somehow keep him from being like other people and from actually participating in life. We have mentioned a young man, Mr. G. M., intelligent and personable, who had been unduly sheltered by his parents. He became a respected scientist but he felt that he had never emerged into the stream of life like other men; he felt as though he were in a shell and vaguely sensed that this had something to do with the fact that he had never really had to be out on his own and make his way in the world through the use of his own powers. (As Goethe put it, *Ein Talent bildet sich in die Stille, ein Karakter in der Strom des Welt,* and to repeat Freud's words, "Necessity is a hard master but under him we become potent.")

SOCIOLOGICAL IMPLICATIONS

1. Disillusionment

The social manifestations and effects of the emotions in impairing the sense of reality are ubiquitous and part of the tragedy of humanity. The child is apt to think of its parents as omnipotent and omniscient, so great is the gap between the little child and the adult and so great is the child's dependence upon parents. In adult life, people tend to repeat these childhood patterns not only in their own small circles but also toward society as a whole, treating other individuals in their groups like siblings, and reacting to the leaders and high officials as to fathers, mothers and older brothers. It is usually a disillusionment to find that the world is run by infantile or childish human beings and not by omniscient figures on a sociological Olympus. Sooner or later, one realizes that other adults are not godlike, or even parentlike, but underneath are insecure, disturbed, hostile children, themselves craving help and support. Insofar as this enforces self-reliance and stimulates self-confidence it is a milestone on the way to maturity. For out of childhood attitudes and misconceptions spring much grasping and envy and much of man's struggle for power.

The advice never to discuss politics or religion testifies to the recognition that here the emotions play so predominant a role that they, rather than reason, will dictate the argument. Perhaps now more than for some decades, the irrational and emotional seems paramount and one searches the scenes of streets, cities, campuses and politics for some signs of reason, reality and maturity in the face of preconception, dogmatism and rationalization which leads to the corruption and violence that erupt every so often.

2. Fads and Prejudices

A suffering soul craves some sort of help, and if he cannot get it from the doctor then he may turn to all sorts of fads and fancies because of his terrible need to feel that somehow he is getting help and becoming freer and stronger. To discuss the matter with such a person is hopeless, for his belief in the particular food or exercise or pill stems from his emotional needs. In the case of the alcoholic, the person may even realize that he is ruining himself and his family and may not attempt to offer any rationalization. The same for cigarette addicts. One man, a heavy cigarette smoker, in his mid-thirties with a wife and four children totally dependent on him, developed emphysema and was threatened with removal of a lobe of his lung—but still he could not stop. Usually this is because the hostilities directed against the self are too strong and unconscious and unreachable by conscious awareness and will. Fads, prejudices—such as race prejudice and all sorts of emotionally de-termined convictions—are like alcoholism or other addictions; they do not yield to reason, for they gratify powerful emotional needs which are all too ready to turn reason into rationalization (Saul, 1976).

Adults never get over being children and needing parents. The child persists in every adult and seeks substitutes for father and mother (Parens and Saul, 1971). *This need is so intense that people tend to put themselves in the hands of others, including quacks, with but little discrimination.*

3. Hope from Science

Here we come to the possibility of man's being realistic about himself. Science is one of man's proudest achievements and of itself a manifestation of maturity and an expression and refinement of man's striving to grasp reality. He has turned it freely toward the physical world and toward his own body, and great have been its accomplishments; *but will man be able to tolerate turning its light on his own true motivations and reactions and the workings of his mind?* If so, he may yet solve the problem of resolving the conflicts which are in everyone and may achieve a degree of inner psychological and outer social harmony as yet undreamed of.

Within himself lies that truth which, if he can hold to it and use it maturely, will make him free. The essence seems simple: most children are so reared that they do not love their parents and develop good, warm feelings toward them, but react to them with a large amount of anger, hate, hostility; they grow into adolescence and adulthood with these patterns which they then transfer to others. Thus are raised men of hostility rather than men of good will. It is a quantitative matter, but there are enough such people and they are hostile enough to keep our country and the world in constant threat of turmoil and violence. Can this be dealt with scientifically? It is a challenge to science and to education, to religion and government. As we have said, "Every child a wanted child" is a good first step, and also, "What kind of world is this in reality wherein anything else is thinkable?" It has also been said that "all that is needed for evil to triumph is for the good to do nothing."

REFERENCES

Freud, S. (1924): The loss of reality in neurosis and psychosis, *S.E.* 19.

Groddeck, G. (1928): *Book of the It.* New York: Nervous and Mental Disease Publishing Co.

Parens, H. and Saul, L. J. (1971): *Dependence in Man.* New York: International Universities Press.

Saul, L. J. (1938): Telepathic sensitiveness as a neurotic symptom, *Psychoanalytic Quarterly* 7(3):329–335.

———— (1976): *Psychodynamics of Hostility.* New York: Jason Aronson.

Waelder, R. (1941): *The Living Thoughts of Freud.* New York: Longmans.

9 | Persistence of Childhood Patterns

NUCLEAR EMOTIONAL CONSTELLATION
MOTIVATIONAL FORMULA

We have mentioned the fact that the persistence or recurrence at a later stage of development of emotional reactions, particularly warped ones, which developed at an earlier stage, is the nucleus of emotional disorders, from psychosomatic symptoms through the classic neuroses, to the acting-out manifestations of personal and political cruelty and violence. Again and again we have seen that in each case there is a *central traumatic situation* which provides the key to the emotional problem. Every person has his own individual emotional constellation arising out of his reactions to the emotional influences and experiences of his own childhood (always including the effects of congenital, physical, social and other related factors, whether we have stated them explicitly or not). In other words, each child is born into this world with all the potentials for development and reaction that genes provide. It is born into a specific life situation that exerts a variety of emotional and physical influences upon it. This highly conditionable, formative, shapeable human baby and small child, from the moment of birth, begins to interact with all of these influences; some of these facilitate the child's inner potentials and forces of development to maturity. But because childrearing is so often atrocious, many of these external influences, by omission or commission, inhibit, block, deform or otherwise warp the child's emotional development. In any event, the interaction produces an emotional pattern of outlook and response to other individuals that is spread from family members or substitutes to other persons outside the family, and this pattern lasts for life. This "nuclear constellation" is at the core of every personality. The entire constellation of motivations and reactions includes all that is developmental and mature, but also residues of childhood emotional forces, the healthy ones and also those which have been exaggerated, inhibited or otherwise disordered by the traumatic deprivations or pressures. If this childhood area is relatively healthy then it only colors the adult personality. But the more disordered this childhood constellation, the more it forms a nucleus of emotional problems of every degree of intensity and severity. It determines the *vulnerable emotional points*—the emotional Achilles' heels—and thus what stresses in life a person is most sensitive to and most likely to break down under. These effects on the personality and on the mental and emotional life depend on the nature, the intensity and the extent of the emotions in this nuclear constellation or "emotional core" * and on the integrity and the health of the rest of the personality, including the strength of the forces of control, intelligence, judgment and so on (the strength and the health of the "ego"), on the environment and its influences in which the person is functioning and often on other factors as well. A simple example will make this explicit. A young man, successful in his profession, was rather a "loner" and had difficulties with his wife because he could not confide in her and be close to her. He was an only child and his mother had permitted him no privacy; even when he was old enough to receive letters she continued her close supervision and would open and read his mail before he saw it. Over his early years he built up a resentment of what he considered "spying" by his mother. In marriage he repeated this pattern toward his wife, in part wanting to be close to her, but also feeling his privacy threatened and unconsciously rebelling by being aloof, as he was during childhood. Thus his mother's unrelieved interference formed a neurotic pattern in him,

---

* "Nucleus" and "core" are excellent descriptive terms. As used here, they do not in the least imply rigidity or unalterability. Although not easily changed it is, of course, to this basic area of the sources of the person's problems that causal treatment is directed. "Neurotic" is loosely used to cover all non-psychotic emotional disturbances, but also it is frequently employed narrowly in distinction to all those forms of disorder that grade from psychosomatic through addictions, perversions, behavior disorders and other symptoms, to criminal forms of acting out. Therefore, for accuracy, it is usual to use more cumbersome expressions such as "emotional disorders," to be sure that what is referred to is the whole range of manifestations of psychopathology. The correct term for this whole range is *pathological*, the only objection to it being its relative unfamiliarity to most ears. It would add clarity and definition if it were in common usage.

a way of behavior he did not like in himself. Except for this, he was a mature young man who enjoyed working and loving. He could have these qualities because his mother was basically loving and responsible toward him. His "ego," his official conscious personality, was relatively healthy and mature, but his mother's hyper-supervision created an emotional problem. She had not only helped him mature into a fine husband, father, professional man and citizen, but she had also created a neurotic problem.

The highly individual childhood pattern can be seen in all the cases we have quoted. Sometimes it is quite simple, sometimes quite complicated. *No personality, no patient's emotional problem is understood unless this nuclear constellation is clearly seen and comprehended.* Even where the emotional disorder is precipitated in very strong men or women by enormous external emotional strains and pressures, to understand the patient one must know his nuclear constellation, that is, his emotional make-up, how he functioned prior to his symptoms, his emotionally vulnerable points, and just how he reacted to the stresses to result in this present condition. There is a *motivational formula* for every personality, for every emotional disorder. For understanding and treatment, it must be found as quickly as possible.

1. Examples—Find the Formula

In an earlier chapter we have seen examples of young men who, in varying degrees, resisted or gave in to their passive, dependent needs. These tendencies and some combination of reactions to them, whether in the form of rationalizing indulgence in them, resisting them or compensating for them, formed an important part of the "nuclear constellations" or "basic formulae" or "childhood emotional patterns" in these cases. In Chapter 7, a young woman was mentioned whose love-starved mother had enmeshed her in such a close relationship that in adult life she longed for the love of a woman rather than of a man, and then struggled against these homosexual wishes. These trends and her various reactions to them formed the "core" of her emotional problem. Then there was the woman whose central problem had been rejection and deprivation as a child; she longed for love but was unable to make any demands for herself and reacted against these cravings by exaggerated maternal activities in having babies, mothering and giving. These results of deprivation and rejection, her hurt self-regard, her longings and her various reactions—this constellation of interrelated emotions formed a major part of the "nucleus" of her personality. Other women, because of different balances of forces in their personalities, reacted to similar longings in other ways, for example with increased sexual activity, and showed variations of this constellation. There was the young man described in an earlier chapter whose central traumatic situation had been domination and over-protection by his father; he longed to be submissive to and dependent on his employer and became intensely jealous of his co-workers and hated to work, but at the same time could not stand his own desires for submissiveness and dependence. He reacted with a rage which he dared not express openly, and he sought to relieve it by sexual promiscuity toward women whom he despised, while being impotent toward women whom he respected and idealized. These were the major emotional trends which formed the pathological part of his nuclear constellation. We are focused upon what impairs the development to healthy maturity which proceeds, like all sound growth, from its own inner drives, its *elan vital,* the "life force"; in each case we make no effort to describe in complete detail the dynamics of the total personality but *only the central pathology producing these emotional patterns.*

2. Relation to Libido Theory

Freud's libido theory is a first attempt to outline the course of the *normal* libidinal development, as we have noted in Chapter 7. The child goes through problems of suckling, of toilet and other interests and training, of exploring the differences in sex, of handling the feelings toward parents and siblings. With kind understanding, respect for him and his dignity as a person from birth and with guidance that is sympathetic, understanding, patient and gradual, with parents who enjoy him and their home, identify with him and are on his side, the child grows up through these stages and handles these problems to become a secure, happy spouse, parent and citizen. It comes successfully through these normal vicissitudes of growth; but if the child is not reared properly, if he is subjected to injurious commissions and omissions during his most formative years (0–6), then it reacts to these harmful influences, these traumatic situations, with impairments and warpings of development. This is the way patterns of personality and pathology are formed. This point is repeated here to clarify the relationship of this concept to the libido theory. Freud himself succinctly expressed analytic therapy as an *"after-education of the neurotic;* it can correct blunders for which his parental education was to blame."

(In one of those interesting incidents in the history of science, Freud discovered trauma but then all but abandoned it. He was studying the role of sex in the neuroses and described the injurious effects of sexual experiences in childhood. Then he found that some of these experiences that his patients related never really happened, and were only their fantasies. This may have played a part in turning him away. His doing so had tragic consequences for the future of psychoanalysis and, through it, of all psychiatry. His influence as the outstanding pioneer and explorer of the emotional life swayed attention away from trauma and its effects, which is of the most vital central importance theoretically and practically. Attention was directed instead to seeking the primary source of emotional pathology in the vicissitudes of the libido, as though these were not passed through as normal growth even though there was no trauma. In this view, the basic emotional problems arise from within, uninfluenced by how the child is treated. This pessimistic blind alley is completely unjustified. There is no proof that the genes determine psychopathology—with rare exceptions, possibly, however much they affect temperament. Therefore, the quotation from Freud on "after-education" has special significance. Every dynamic psychiatrist today knows the role of trauma and uses it in the office, although it has not achieved the central position in analytic theory that it warrants. It is an indispensable necessity for understanding, for causal treatment and for prevention. Franz Alexander was attacked for saying the same thing in almost the same words as Freud, describing analytic treatment as essentially a "corrective emotional experience." It is largely a method of reconditioning to correct the effects of trauma and reopen the emotional development.)

(It may be that the failure of psychoanalysis to fulfill its promise in theory and therapeutic effectiveness is largely, perhaps chiefly, because of its preoccupation with libido theory to the near exclusion or de-emphasis on the results of childhood traumata, their therapeutic correction and the possibilities of prevention. Therefore, Freud's great breakthrough in the ability to reach unconscious motivations, reactions and processes, even the understanding of dreams, their formation and meaning, one of the few outstanding advances in the whole field of science, has not realized its potential.)

Every person is motivated at the core of his personality by a constellation of emotional forces which are formed by his interactions with physical and emotional influences on him during infancy and childhood.

3. Degree of Consciousness

Some persons are quite conscious of many of their motivations. However, probably no one is much aware of his childhood pattern, the essential nucleus of emotional forces within himself, the variety of his reactions, the interrelationships between them or the ways and the degrees to which they are organized. Like the tip of the iceberg, some motivations may show in consciousness but the main mass is hidden. The true core of the personality is usually remote from the person's consciousness. The main trends usually are better seen by discerning outsiders than by the person himself. Probably the dynamically-trained, long-experienced psychiatrist with a grasp of unconscious motivations and processes can dissect, observe, describe and appreciate these constellations in their flow, detail and dynamic balance more directly than any other professional. To do so is the greatest thrill in psychiatry. It is to come face to face at the deepest psychological level with what really makes people tick. *It is the core of psychology.* Moreover, it is the *sine qua non* of any rational psychotherapy—and base for prevention.

One reason our childhood emotional patterns are remote from our consciousness is probably to save psychic energy, because so long as we are well-adapted to ourselves, to others and to our life style our minds are able to work smoothly and automatically without the distraction and effort of conscious awareness. It is when we suffer emotionally that insight is required to help fix what might be causing the trouble. So the central role of therapy is an understanding of the childhood emotional pattern. You cannot fix a squeaky door or trouble in your business or suffering in yourself without first understanding what is wrong. Knowing as we do that the childhood emotional pattern is the most common source of trouble in the personality, it is incredible that even today ultra-naive individuals will say that a child's early experiences can do no harm because the child is too young to be aware of them! We know that the reality is exactly the opposite, as both clinical experience and experimentation with animals tell us.

Have you ever had an exciting experience and felt a strong urge to tell someone about it? Have you ever been buttonholed by an individual who just has to tell about his or her operation or the "cute" thing little Willy did? When a child is very young and pre-verbal, it lacks the grasp of reality and the means to understand and express its feelings. Its inner emotional tensions and pressures, so much less comprehensible and expressible than in an adult, are consequently more traumatic to the tender, immature organism. As Freud summarized it, "It is not to be wondered at that the ego, while it is weak, immature and incapable of resistance, should fail in dealing with problems which it could later manage with utmost ease" (1940).

4. Treatment

Dynamic psychotherapy must be based upon an understanding of the major forces in the traumatic situation and in the patient's current difficulties. In the vast majority of cases the central features can be discerned in the first visit or after a very few hours. Only when the interplay of the main forces in the patient's emotional life is understood can therapy be planned rationally, soundly and scientifically. To begin any type of treatment, from shock to classic psychoanalysis, before the patient is well understood is to neglect to make full use of psychodynamic knowledge and to operate in the dark. The paramount dictum in psychiatric treatment is: *There is no substitute for understanding the patient.* Through *psychiatric accuracy*, understanding the central dynamic forces in the patient and dealing carefully and consistently with these, treatment becomes more flexible, brief and effective. Psychotherapy is psychological surgery. The danger equals and the delicacy and the subtlety exceed that of any physical procedure.

5. *Degree of Organization*

Although in everyone there are many independent and often conflicting impulses, the childhood pattern always has certain interrelationships and a certain degree of *organization*. Thus, the woman
who had been rejected as a child reacted to her longings for the love
she missed with fear of risking further rejections and with shame
and guilt about any "selfish" demands she might make; hence, she
could only give to others and denied her own longings. These feelings and motivations, and many others in this woman, were all
closely interrelated; and in this followed a certain logic. One motivation is often a reaction to another; they reenforce one another,
conflict, overcompensate, serve to hide one another and so on
(Alexander, 1961). These interrelationships are as important, both
for scientific understanding and for psychotherapy, as are the
motivations themselves. Without a thorough comprehension of
them one is faced in every case with a confusion of emotions and
impulses, without seeing in perspective what are the *major* motivations and reactions in the person, what are secondary and sub-
sidiary ones, and how they are integrated in the personality; and
treatment then misses the fundamentals, gets side-tracked in
minutiae and is apt to leave the patient more confused than when
he came for help.

6. *Major and Subsidiary Motivations*

Of course, some persons are much more integrated than others.
Some are impelled by many relatively independent and only
loosely related motives, the "impulse-ridden personalities," while
in others the emotional constellation is so organized and integrated
that in a detailed analysis the interrelationship of almost every
impulse with the whole pattern is apparent. Often certain interrelationships are reciprocal, as seen in emotional vicious circles such
as those described in connection with competition and frustration.

In general, the relatively normal well-integrated person does not
seem to be any more aware of his nuclear motivations than the
more neurotic individual; indeed, in some pathological conditions
the individual is more aware of them than can be considered nor-

mal. In perfect health one is not aware of his vegetative organs or their functioning. He "does not know that he has a stomach" or a heart or any other organ but simply lives. Probably the same holds true, to some extent, for the functioning of the mind. So long as living goes on fairly smoothly, one does not notice one's deeper emotions and motives.

MENTAL HEALTH—IS THE AVERAGE PERSON NEUROTIC?

Mental health, Freud is reputed to have said, is the ability to love and to work. Some do this but only barely; they keep going while "living lives of quiet desperation." If we attempt a dynamic definition rather than the descriptive one, it seems correct to say that in its essentials mental health consists of adequate emotional maturity plus adequate adjustment. Complete maturity and perfect adjustment to our cruel, turbulent world can only be ideals. How much is adequate? Measuring scales aside, perhaps adequacy lies in the *enjoyment* of loving and working, of the functions of maturity, as well as of "playing," i.e., of a balanced life.

The average person who passes for normal (in the sense of healthy) is one who is able to function and carry on in the adult role but nevertheless usually carries a considerable degree of emotional tension and conflict resulting from a core of persisting childhood reactions. There is only a quantitative difference between the individuals described in this book and very many, perhaps the majority, of the persons whom one meets in all walks of life.

As an example, there was a certain husky, healthy engineer, known as an "extrovert" and a devoted family man. Gradually, it became apparent that as his profession took him to new places, at first he would be very popular. Then it would be noticed that he was always either talking against people or else being so piously considerate of them that there was obviously some lack of sincerity. Also, he would look out for himself in many petty ways. He was less interested in his job than in getting away with all he could. He would become known as aggressive and piggish. He would not notice this but think of himself as superior to his colleagues. Although well-to-do, he would pinch pennies with poor people. He kept his wife restricted and was bad-tempered with her. He had been "spoiled" and over-indulged in childhood in a way that had left him self-indulgent and grasping and tending to get out of work and responsibility. He reacted against this with emphasis on his masculinity and by a dominating attitude toward his family. He so dreaded any dependence or submissiveness in himself that he also could not stand it in his son with whom he over-identified; and constantly and unconsciously pressed him to masculine accomplishments beyond his years, which resulted in the boy's becoming depressed and a behavior problem. This, then, was a man who was considered a model of normality by himself and others. In him were the same emotional forces and mechanisms as in any of the persons described in this book—or as in anyone else—only their influence *pervaded his life instead of expressing themselves as frank neurotic symptoms of behavior.*

As we have said, in every adult there persists the child he once was, with his needs, impulses and problems. Scratch an adult and find a child, and scratch a child and find an animal.

An attractive young woman was the wife of a lawyer and the mother of two young sons. They were a vivacious and popular couple. But underneath she was an infantile personality, extremely dependent on her husband in a little-girl fashion. Because of this childish dependence, she felt inferior and unconsciously reacted against it, to hide it from others and deny it to herself, by trying to be superior socially and by trying always to be in what she felt to be the superior position of giving to others and never in the inferior position of receiving from them and having to be grateful. But she was demanding toward her husband, whom she wanted to be too much of a father to her, and continually urged him to make greater efforts to earn more money—in order to give her more and to help her compete on this basis with her women friends. She was angry at him for not satisfying all her demands and even jealous of his close relationship with the boys. Because of her infantile dependence and her guilt from her anger at him and from her competitiveness and envy toward her friends, she felt insecure and anxious, and to reassure herself she would test her charms on other men. As her dissatisfaction and tension mounted, her social drinking became a little excessive. The children felt the emotional tensions and developed behavior problems. The husband was of an easy-going disposition without much drive, and her constant demands and her ambitious urgings irritated him to an exasperation, from which increasingly he too found relief in drinking.

Such persons as these do not regard themselves as neurotic; in fact, they would indignantly resent any such implication. They pass as average people, with their own particular problems. They are not aware of the core of their motivations. Even their close friends may notice little. And the psychiatrist, who may have heard how well-adjusted they are, may be surprised at what he finds.

INFLUENCE OF THE PATTERN

The childhood constellation may be severely pathological, with feelings toward self and others badly deranged and full of hate, as toward members of the family in childhood; or it may contain good, warm, friendly feelings and only be immature because of too strong love needs, as in the person we refer to as "like a friendly puppy."

These infantile emotional cores influence some persons more than others, and in different ways. Some individuals are less mature and more dominated by these trends than are the more mature, more independent persons who have more successfully outgrown and overcome their infantile emotional attitudes, fixations and patterns; and some generally more infantile people get on better than more mature ones because of the *nature* of their infantile impulses and how fate has treated them, and perhaps for other reasons also. Thus, a childish girl married a man with a similar outlook, with similar tendencies to social and financial exhibitionism. But he also had the intelligence and the practical sense to make the most of the opportunities chance cast his way, so the two could satisfy these immature desires. By contrast, a very mature man, a real contributor to society, suffered from guilt for a certain leftover resentment toward his father, and despite his inner maturity and great worldly success, was an unhappy person. Lincoln is an example of a very mature man who suffered.

PATTERNS AS SEEN IN DREAMS

In addition to the life history, current behavior, and associative material, the dreams are regularly of great assistance in revealing the basic emotional constellation. A series of dreams of a given person will be found, if one goes beyond the manifest content (the simple dream as it occurs in its fantasy form) to the real feelings and life topics with which it deals (latent content), to represent from various angles a relatively small number of subjects and emotional constellations (Saul, 1977). The person's basic motivations come to expression again and again in varying forms in his dreams. His dream may be stimulated at different times by innumerable circumstances—meeting an old friend, getting a raise, marrying, an injustice and so on—but it is always this particular individual, reacting to his life experiences in his own characteristic ways. And these ways are determined in his deepest feelings by his nuclear constellation of emotions and motives. Thus the dreams of the woman who was always deprived in childhood and could not make any claims for herself but only give to others reflected this constellation and her desires for romance, which were always frustrated. If a series of, say, 50 or 100 dreams is studied, it will be seen that even the manifest topics and main themes are limited. And if the dreams are analyzed, that is, traced to the drives, the thoughts and the desires which created this fluid imagery, it will be found that the basic emotional reactions of the individual repeat themselves, now one, now another, partially or together. In cases under analytic treatment, the first ten current dreams are usually enough to reveal the major emotional forces and conflicts in the individual, and from analyzing them alone it is usually possible to formulate the basic emotional pattern of the personality, which then unfolds in its varied facets and details over subsequent months.

Thus, dreams are highly intimate, personal and individual creations which express the essence of each person's emotional life. Moreover, *they correlate directly with the person's life.* They reflect what the person is striving for or against and how he handles the powerful underlying forces which motivate him. They reveal how effective his conscience reactions are, how much he will give in to his primitive impulses and in what form and how much and in what ways he will punish himself. In this sense, dreams in their real meaning come true. This is probably the kernel of truth underlying the abuse of dream prophecy. If a patient threatens suicide or murder, the dreams will tell whether or not this is a serious intent or an empty gesture. In such cases, what the patient says consciously is of little importance compared with the force of his deepest, mostly unconscious feelings and motivations. It is these which must be understood. And the dream is one of their clearest modes of expression. Again it must be emphasized that we are speaking not of the apparent or "manifest" dream, but only of its true meaning, the thoughts and the impulses that form it, the "latent content," as revealed by careful dream analysis.

Dreams (Saul, 1972) offer the clearest expression of the interplay of the forces in the emotional life. In fact, *it is not possible to understand the interplay of emotional forces and motivations in a person without knowing his dreams and penetrating their meaning* and understanding how these feelings, forces and motivations express themselves in these remarkable psychological formations.

A man beginning treatment dreams that he is given a free trip. In life he tries to get things free and has a history of not paying his bills, and immediately finds rationalizations for not paying my bill. One person can never dream of any sexual freedom and is very much inhibited in reality. Another is very free in dreams in this regard, and also in reality. A man's hostilities appear in his dreams only as directed against himself. In life they are so inhibited that he denies any such feelings, and he exposes himself to attack by others. A young man dreams that his mother helps him provide food for his wife and child and that when he eats it he becomes nauseated. In life his central problem is his unsuccessful struggle to free himself from dependence on his mother, which part of him enjoys. His chief symptom is nausea. A man dreams of jumping out of the window but not being killed. He later makes an ineffectual attempt at suicide. A man dreams of older, established men being attacked; he runs in fear to a woman but then flees until he is caught alone at the end of an alley. His major problem is hostility to his father and to father figures. His attempts to get along with women fail. His chief symptom is anxiety and being lonely and isolated from people. A man who is a gentle soul, on the surface, but acutely anxious, and filled with repressed anger because he still feels deprived as he was in childhood, has dreams filled with violence, all of which is projected, none of it perpetrated by himself—fights, explosions, outbreaks of war, and so on. Lincoln dreamed of his own death shortly before his assassination, stubbornly refusing the adequate personal protection which might have prevented it (Sandburg, 1939; Wilson, 1940).

Dreams reveal our psychological mechanisms of defense and the key to the meaning of many of them is "Not that painful reality, but only this trivial matter." For example, a man has a gall bladder attack and learns that he must have an operation. That night he dreams that someone is cleaning the motor of his car. A woman who has been divorced by a neurotic, philandering husband repeatedly dreams that she has lost relatively minor replaceable objects, such as her pocketbook or a ticket.

The best account of the psychology of dreams is still Freud's *Interpretation of Dreams*, one of the world's fundamental books. The best popularly written exposition is in his *A General Introduction to Psychoanalysis*.

A person's very *first memories*—the few little scraps prior to continuous memory, dating often to age two, and sometimes even earlier, little scraps one is not certain he truly remembers—also are remarkably revealing of the basic motivations of his personality and therefore of the pattern of his inner feelings and his life (Saul et al., 1956).

It must be reemphasized that the illustrations given above aim only to make clear the nature of the nuclear constellation, its formation and its expression in life and dreams. Hence, relatively simple examples have been selected, and only the central figures of each case are given. In every personality (and this is reflected in dreams) there are many ramifications, details and complications. But these are always manifestations of the major issues. The most lengthy and detailed descriptions of each of the briefly mentioned cases would only add other mechanisms and reactions to the central emotional constellations. If it is borne in mind that our case illustrations are *simplified by concentrating on the main issues and omitting the many details and peripheral themes*, then they will more clearly exemplify the phenomena we are describing and will not give a false impression of simplicity in the personality and of the emotional life.

FACTORS FORMING PATTERNS

In all cases, we see a repetition in the adult's mental and emotional life and behavior of patterns of reaction which were formed in childhood by the congenital endowment interacting with environmental influences. Probably (1) the stronger these influences, (2) the more continually they operate, (3) the less the counterbalancing forces, and (4) the younger the child during this time, the greater will be their effects on development.

As stated previously, psychoses aside, there is no cogent evidence that heredity, except in rare instances, determines psychopathology, the emotional disorders. However, it seems to play an important role in *temperament*. The term "congenital" signifies that with which one is born. It not only includes heredity, what is in the genes, but also the effects of external influences from conception and from long before it, directly and indirectly upon the egg and sperm cells—for how far back? The unborn and the new-born child are so delicate that the strongest heredity is like a frail reed in a hurricane against the abuses the child can be subjected to. We have mentioned René Spitz who showed that babies deprived of maternal affection at five months of age, although otherwise perfectly treated, reacted with emotional and physical deformities, and some died.

A little boy of three and one-half years had terrible temper tantrums. Four times now these tantrums had increased in violence and terminated in epileptic attacks with loss of consciousness. The surmise could not be avoided that the rage had mounted in intensity until it produced the attack. The tantrums at first had occurred only when he was with his mother, but now they occurred on other occasions and with other persons as well. The mother was young and of a very simple-minded, direct peasant type. She frankly and unhesitatingly related the story of her childrearing—a story which a more sophisticated mother might have never admitted. This was her first child. He weighed not quite six pounds at birth, she said, which was considerably less than the babies of her friends. Therefore, she tried from the very first days to make him gain by forcing him to eat. She forced the feedings down him, and when he screamed and finally vomited them, she forced them down again. She believed that babies should be toilet-trained by six months and tried to accomplish this by beating him severely every time he soiled his diapers. Her husband neglected her, and she admitted freely that she became fed up with the house and the child and often hated the child for being a nuisance to her and a handicap in her growing resolve to get a divorce and remarry. She was quite conscious of these motivations but also overprotective and overanxious, lest harm come to the child. She smothered him with hugging and with endearing attention—unconscious overcompensation for her hostility to him.

She was a rather infantile person. Her father had not liked girls and had neglected and mistreated her while favoring her younger brother. This caused a jealous rage and revenge reaction which persisted in her and was the deeper, unconscious cause of her hostility to her son (and an important part of her nuclear emotional constellation). She reacted to her husband and child with the pattern of hostility engendered in her by her father and younger brother.

TRANSMISSION VERSUS HEREDITY

What childhood influences determined her father's hostile rejection of his daughter in favor of his son I never discovered, but such observations as these show *how neurotic reactions, psychopathology of all kinds, are transmitted from generation to generation,* and they caution us against jumping to the conclusion that because neuroses appear in generation after generation, they are hereditary. Perhaps some *tendency* to emotional disorder is hereditary, but these two factors must be evaluated independently. It is similar to tuberculosis. Because it "ran in families," tuberculosis was thought to be hereditary. Then the tubercle bacillus was discovered, and it was found to be transmitted. But some hereditary weakness which increases susceptibility to tuberculosis may also exist. Such observations also encourage the analytic therapist, who usually spends more time with his patients than is required in other specialties but effects major alterations in the personality and can reopen the process of development (Saul, 1972).

Sometimes no great change is noticeable during the treatment itself, which reveals the nature of the basic problem and forces and mobilizes them so that they can be dealt with. In many cases this means the difference between being on the way "into" emotional difficulties and being on the way "out." Often, as with the two lines which form a narrow angle, only a slight deflection at first gradually leads the two lines as they go further from the point of contact to diverge widely from each other, like two trains leaving the station on parallel tracks, but one eventually heading north, the other south; so a slight change in the emotional freedom, capacity for development and attitudes toward life leads, with the passage of time, to the person's being very different five, ten or fifteen years later from what he would have been had he not branched off from the old track to the diverging one. The effects of the help usually go far beyond the individual to his family and to his children and to his children's children. Had this woman's father not so aroused her hate and revenge during her childhood, she would not have vented this on her little son and so caused him to react with tantrums and to warp *his* development, so that he will certainly be severely disturbed, perhaps criminal, and will certainly hate women and be himself a bad husband and father, who may well cause further pathology to the fourth generation and beyond. (Psychodynamics is far enough advanced as a science so that such a prediction can be made with confidence.)

Enough has been said to indicate the thinly veiled hostility and the gross mistreatment to which this little boy had been subjected since birth. Small wonder that he reacted to this with temper tantrums. Severe emotional traumata probably produce much more deep-seated effects on the development of the personality when they are experienced during this early formative period than they do after the third year. Some authors are convinced that the first year is the most important one (and there is much support for this), and further, that up to one year infants cannot tolerate frustration and rage without permanent ill effects (Ribble, 1943). The nerves of the brain are in a state of growth and do not obtain their fatty coverings (myelination) for as long as six years after birth. It is even possible that the finer organic structure of the brain area can be affected if it must mediate intense emotion before it is well developed, and it is not impossible that this will show up later in the shape of the individual's electroencephalogram (Saul et al., 1937) (a tracing of the amplified electrical activity of the cells of the outer layers of the brain, just as the electrocardiogram is a record of the electrical activity of the heart).

INTERNALIZATION AND FAILURE OF DISCRIMINATION

Leaving these speculations, an important fact about this little boy is that his temper tantrums were no longer exclusively reactions to his mother. They occurred in other situations also, whenever he was thwarted or whenever a sensitive spot was touched. He did not *discriminate* between his mother in particular and other persons. His sensitivity to domination was already a characteristic of his make-up which went with him wherever he was. It was no longer merely "reactive" to his mother and her treatment of him but was now "internalized" and felt toward, projected on, anyone he could fit into this pattern.

PATTERNS AND ADAPTABILITY

Everyone has an internalized nuclear constellation of infantile motivations, but, as stated, this varies in kind, extent, intensity and degree of pathology from person to person. Sometimes it merely colors the personality, while in other cases it forms a fixed pattern of reaction. The result, apart from specific symptoms, is a degree of rigidity of reaction, a lack of flexibility in adaptation. This part of the personality has not achieved maturity and the adaptability of adult attitudes but goes on reacting in accordance with the set childhood patterns. Everyone's personality and behavior are colored and affected in a large degree by the childhood emotional constellations, but the *more* these interfere with adult behavior, the more disordered and hostile they are, the *more rigidly* they determine behavior, the more "neurotic" (in the broad sense of emotional disorders, including the acting-out forms, as criminality) is the individual. Again it is a quantitative matter: how much of the personality has developed with basically good relations to the emotionally important persons of earliest childhood up to age 6 or 7, and how much has been fixed into pathological patterns.

A simple example is a certain career woman, no longer young. Her father had been away a great deal while she was a child, and, while at home, he was partly very indulgent toward her but also partly irritable and neglectful. She reacted with longings for him but also with a deep resentment against him. This became a fixed pattern in her relations with men. She repeated it in her marriage and in position after position. She longed to be a favorite of the head of the firm but would never admit this. She would start off doing very well and making an excellent impression. But gradually her hostility to her employer would become so open and intense that it would be only a matter of time before some incident would precipitate her departure.

In one firm she became good friends with one of the junior members. He left later to go into business for himself and asked her to go with him. She was by this time openly hostile to the boss and gladly accepted the offer. Things went well for a time, but then the old pattern reasserted itself. So long as this man was a junior partner, himself somewhat rebellious against their boss, she got on with him famously, for she unconsciously identified with him, as a child hostile to his father, like herself. But when this same man had his own firm and was in the father position himself, then she could no longer identify with him as a rebellious child, and she developed toward him the hostility that she was destined by her inner reactions to have toward all men whom, for one reason or another, she looked to as fathers. She attracted passive, dependent young men who, because of this weakness in themselves, had an exaggerated envy and hostility of successful men in superior positions, to whom they looked as fathers. The same pattern repeated itself in her marriage. As soon as her husband became established and could give her the things she wanted, she reacted to him as she had to her father, became hostile, tried to turn their children against him and finally sued for divorce—to his relief.

Such an unconscious tendency to put certain men into a category is a failure to discriminate them from the original object, in this case the girl's own father. Often the men were in reality totally different personalities from her father, and they were usually amazed at her reactions to them. But, because of her *imago* of her father in her emotional pattern she saw them as a class and not as the individuals they really were. Her thinking in these stereotypes and not perceiving reality clearly was dictated by her pattern of feelings. She must revenge herself on all men in superior positions for her father's treatment of her, instead of being angry only at him and treating other men as different individuals. This reaction against her father became a *set pattern,* carried with her years later after her father was long dead and she herself was a grandmother.

REPETITION OF PATTERNS

One's constellation of desires and impulses always seeks and always finds ways in life of choosing individuals and situations in its efforts to be gratified. It is *this complex of desires* pressing for satisfaction which, more than anything else, seems to account for the *persistence and the accuracy with which everyone repeats in adult life the emotional patterns of his childhood.* And it is these patterns which cause one to fit other people into classes, categories and stereotypes formed by these desires. Perhaps mother was kind and sister a bitter rival—hence, an exaggerated tendency to look for love from older women and to fear and compete with women of one's own age. To put it another way, the person becomes "conditioned" to hating, loving, competing and so on, in relation to certain individuals in childhood and then fails to discriminate between them and others but reacts to whole classes or categories of persons of his own making.

Some people do not emphasize whole categories of people so much as they select a few actual persons in life with whom to repeat their family relationships. One young woman reacted to her husband just as she had to her slightly older brother and always established a relationship to her employer similar to the one that she had had to her father. Her marriage was rocky because she increasingly repeated toward her husband the envy and the competitiveness she had toward her brother.

The degree of rigidity with which a person reacts to categories of people varies greatly from person to person, as we have already pointed out. The man who, because he had a cruel father, cannot get along with authority figures or with older men may yet get along with a certain older man, whom he may react to as he did to his mother—that is, because of this older man's kindness or other qualities, he makes him a mother rather than a father image. The imagoes are not necessarily bound by sex difference. A man with a stern but loving mother may love his wife and transfer his hostility to his mother's sternness to certain men.

If a child has good relationships with most members of his family, then he has enough such models and imagoes for later life so that he probably will get along well with almost everyone. But if most or all his childhood relationships are bad, then he lacks the models for good relationships and almost certainly will have serious difficulties with people in later life. Probably no one can live long without developing serious difficulties of some sort, if he has not had at least one good emotional relationship during his 0–6.

We have focused upon the effects of external influences such as deprivation, spoiling, cruelty, domination and many others, in forming the patterns. In some cases, internal factors are also of importance, as when the development is impaired not so much by these environmental emotional influences as by long illnesses, severe shocks or congenital deficiencies, be these physical, intellectual, or emotional. The end-result always depends on an interaction of the congenital and the environmental factors. These physically internal factors are still external to the mind. The paranoid tends to be hypochondriacal, i.e., he feels other people or forces are malignant to him and also often that he is threatened from within by diseases. It is only a matter of where he sees the threat as originating.

One regularly sees patients *bring upon themselves in adult life situations in which they suffered as children.* For example, a girl who was rejected by her parents refuses men who are steady and devoted and is repeatedly attracted only to men who reject her, so that she never wins the love she craves and could have. Again, a child harshly treated grows up with a tendency to provoke such treatment by others. One mechanism in such cases is this: Whatever the unhappiness—rejection, harshness or any other—this comes to have the significance of punishment for guilty impulses or behavior. This guilt usually arises chiefly from anger and hostile aggression generated by the traumatic situation itself. For example, the rejection causes anger, which causes guilt. This guilt, in turn, causes a need to be punished, and the rejection, the source of the hostile impulses, is at hand as the form of punishment—a vicious circle. Guilt from other sources may also contribute to the need for punishment, which has been cast in this form by the sufferings of childhood. We have referred previously to this as *the punishment fitting the source of the hostility:* if deprivation causes hostility, the punishment for the hostility takes the form of more deprivation. Another dynamic which produces nearly the same effect is simply that the anger for the deprivation or other trauma continues as part of the pattern and of itself antagonizes others who, therefore, naturally reject the person.

SOCIOLOGICAL IMPLICATIONS

Certain elementary patterns are more or less universal. Both the relations to the parents and sibling rivalry are seen in adult life in practically every group or organization of human beings, both between individuals and between groups. There is always the hostility, out of envy and competition, toward the man at the top and also the sibling competition for the love of those in authority. All this is seen on a national scale in the relationship of various groups to the government and to the figure of the president. Each envies and resents the authority and the power of government, and at the same time seeks favors for itself in competition with other groups. The whole struggle for power, so central in human affairs (Russell, 1938), bears, as does the struggle to *get,* the mark of childhood. Overemphasis on power reflects emotionally something of the child's envy and rivalry of the father (and the mother) and reaction against his own feelings of weakness and powerlessness. The person who has outgrown this and has achieved adult orientation and identification has inner security. He no longer requires power for itself but only for reasonable needs for himself and his family and can use the surplus to make a better, safer society for all.

One of the greatest difficulties in a program of preventive psychiatry based upon a true mental hygiene of childhood arises from the fact that the parent tends to repeat toward his spouse and his children the treatment which he received from his own parents, and also his reactions to this treatment. Thus, even when parents know intellectually how to provide a proper emotional environment for the child's best development, yet they usually have difficulty in doing so because of the operation of these unconscious fixed patterns within themselves.

Much has been written and much remains to be formulated concerning these universal patterns of childhood which persist so powerfully in adults, both as to their sources and their manifestations in individual, social and political life, but our purpose is to describe only the central phenomenon. Its applications are a challenge to the future.

It may be well to point up much that has been said about the relationship of childhood patterns to the struggle, turmoil, cruelty and violence of life. A young man, R., an only child, had been much neglected because his parents were not sufficiently patient and loving with him. They were out a great deal participating in somewhat revolutionary activities, to which they soon took R. His anger at them for neglect was thereby given direction, away from them and toward the Establishment; and the meetings became for R. companionship and purpose, replacing empty loneliness. Thus was shaped a fervent, but relatively non-violent, revolutionary who identified with professional and violent revolutionaries.

V. was savagely beaten as a child by his father and less so by his mother, but he endured her special antagonism. His mental stability was saved as there was still some love from his parents, but principally because of that which he received from a devoted sister nearly ten years his senior. Both parents, full of hate, blamed "politics" for everything wrong in their lives and V. learned that by agreeing with them he could keep the peace and even win some approval. Thus, as with R., the treatment to which V. was subjected built up his hostility to his parents and this was directed, through identification with them, against the Establishment. But, in V. the intensity of the rage and the overtness of the violence made open violence a part of his pathodynamic (short for "pathological psychodynamic") pattern. Grown up, he burned with hate and was a potential murderer. He turned this destructiveness on society, rationalizing it in all sorts of ways. So much is wrong in all human relationships that there is never a lack of good reasons to mask the real reasons. For what is wrong lies at bottom in the pathodynamic patterns, as residues of childhood mistreatment, in so many individuals. While R. was a sympathizer, not a participant, in open violence, V. became a full time, rabble rousing, violence advocating, organizing revolutionary.

F.'s relationship to his father, during earliest childhood, was such that although subjected to his excessive discipline, with corporal punishment, he came to identify with his father. Grown up, his hostility toward his vigorous father was directed through this identification to those weaker than himself (the "bicycle rider" type, who bows his head to the one above but presses his feet on those below). He became a right extremist; an ardent advocate of repressive discipline, including corporal punishment.

Of course socioeconomic and other factors influence childrearing to some extent but all roads still lead to Rome: Whatever the external realities, the nuclear emotional constellations—more specifically, their pathological parts, their pathodynamic patterns—are bedrock causes of social problems. The adult turns toward society, in some degree, the emotional patterns developed toward his parents during childhood. The child so reared that he hates his parents becomes a potential violence-prone disrupter, not a builder of society, whether in criminoid, criminal or political guise.

REFERENCES

Alexander, F. (1961): *The Scope of Psychoanalysis*. New York: Basic Books, pp. 116–128.

Freud, S. (1940): Outline of psychoanalysis, *S.E.* 23, p. 183.

Ribble, M. (1943): *The Rights of Infants*. New York: Columbia University Press.

Russell, B. (1938): *Power, A New Social Analysis*. New York: Norton.

Sandburg, C. (1939): *Abraham Lincoln*. New York: Harcourt.

Saul, L. J. (1972): *Psychodynamically Based Psychotherapy*. New York: Science House.

——— (1977): *The Childhood Emotional Pattern*. New York: Van Nostrand Reinhold, Chap. 8.

——— et al. (1937): A correlation between electroencephalogram and the psychological organization of the individual, *Transcripts of the American Neurological Association* 63:167.

——— et al. (1956): On earliest memories, *Psychoanalytic Quarterly* 25:228–237.

Wilson, G. (1940): A prophetic dream report by A. Lincoln, *American Imago* 1:3.

PART THREE

The Nature of Neurosis

10 | Specific Emotional Vulnerability

Psychiatry is hard to grasp and hard to teach partly because it began historically with the most abnormal manifestations and only gradually has it come closer to an understanding of the normal. World War II afforded psychiatry an opportunity of seeing on a large scale the effects of unwonted strains on average persons. (The more neurotic men had been screened out of military service long before the unusual stresses began.) What one learns about the effects of these on relatively healthy personalities deepens our understanding of the development and the functioning of the mind of man. The war provided psychiatry with a vast laboratory in which was concentrated within a brief span and under one roof every kind of personality from every sort of background, and these were subjected to every kind of stress and experience of life. Although the immediate purpose of military psychiatry was to help those who had broken down, a further goal was to glean from wartime a body of knowledge which would be as effective in combating the misery man causes himself and his fellows as medical science has been in combating diseases such as smallpox. Millions of dollars and years of research are devoted to discovering the causes and the cures for cancer, tuberculosis, infantile paralysis and other dread scourges, but thus far little or nothing is expended on a phenomenon which is a hundred times more costly and destructive, which kills and maims the body and mutilates the spirit—man's hostility to man, or, more correctly, man's *neurotic, pathological hostility to man*—nor are public opinion and popular pressure alerted to responsibility for preventing its continuous operation.

Work on the war neuroses mostly in World War II, but confirmed by Korea and Vietnam, dealt with five main aspects of the problem: (1) the kinds of stress to which the individuals were subjected; (2)

the mechanisms by which some degree of adjustment to these stresses was achieved; (3) the types of neurotic reactions resorted to as satisfactory adjustment failed; (4) the nature of individual susceptibility to stress; and (5) general formulations. (Throughout, the term "neurotic" is used in its broadest sense to mean emotionally disordered, psychopathological, pathodynamic.) In Vietnam, the relatively short tour of duty was probably the single most important factor in the low incidence of war neuroses.

The essence of the war experience can perhaps be summed up in three words: *specific emotional vulnerability*. How an individual will react depends on the violence of the stress bearing on his specific emotional vulnerability. Thus, one would see a man who, after many months aboard ship, developed anxiety and depression in reaction to the restrictions of the service and actually found combat a therapeutic relief and a release. This man had been unusually independent throughout his childhood and had reacted to emotional problems at home by going off on his own. Bold, hyperindependent, he could tolerate combat but not restrictions. Another man was the opposite. Coming from a well-ordered home, his aggressions severely repressed by a dominating mother, never hunting, fighting or participating in rough sports, he enjoyed the neat, well-ordered life aboard ship but was plunged into desperate anxiety at the first sign of violence. Another man seemed to be completely of iron, taking every hardship, restriction, danger, bloodshed and loss of buddies in his stride, until he learned accidentally that his wife had been unfaithful and he was thereby plunged into a serious depression.

Thus, in every case we find one or more emotionally vulnerable spots. When pressures and frustrations bear upon these spots, neurotic reactions may occur. Many men endured combat and broke down for other reasons. But when the stress was prolonged, as in the infantry divisions, man's primitive fear of mutilation and death overshadowed all other fears. If the stress is sufficiently intense and prolonged, eventually everyone will break down. But some break sooner than others. Although there are basic similarities in what men feel and can stand, there are individual differences in kind and in degree of sensitivity. But everyone has vulnerabilities and breaking points.

The traumatic neuroses and recurrent nightmares about the

traumatic situation turned out again and again (at least in the sub-acute cases) to represent latent anxiety and neurotic tendencies, which were mobilized when the traumatic experience struck the vulnerable spot. The onset was precipitated by the unusual trauma, but the dynamics are apparently the same as in other anxiety states.

This condensed formulation is, of course, somewhat over-simplified; for example, a man who breaks under a specific stress would not always do so unless he had been sensitized and his controls weakened by his other experiences. Moreover, the clinical pictures varied with the nature of the stresses and the possibilities of dealing with them. For example, the picture differed among the combat crews of the air corps in contrast with the crews of a naval vessel at sea for many months without touching port.

Various terms were used by the military services for emotional breakdowns precipitated by the unusual stresses of war—anxiety reaction, flying stress, situational neuroses and so on. In the Navy these were called "operational fatigue" and "combat fatigue"; the latter term came to be used very broadly. "War neurosis" is an overall term which conveys the fact that, although the symptoms are those of neurosis, they are the reactions of relatively normal persons to abnormal situations. The picture varies from man to man, depending both on the individual's make-up and the particular stresses to which he was exposed; it is quite different in the acute cases fresh from battle and overwhelmed by harrowing experiences, from the picture seen in soldiers in their own countries months after their symptoms have developed. Hence, these terms are all comprehensive and include a vast variety of conditions. In themselves they reveal nothing of the true nature or severity of the emotional strain or disorder. A certain man was first looked on with suspicion and partly ostracized in his community because it was known that his medical discharge was for "combat fatigue"; yet, if he had had an injured ankle, that would have been the diagnosis, and no one would have been concerned with his psychiatric symptoms. On the other hand, some men with lifelong emotional problems carried on well for months or years in military service before breaking down with so-called "combat fatigue." In the vernacular of World War II, combat fatigue meant only, as the men themselves, always so direct and colorful in their slang, put it, "fed up with the set-up" and hence, "nervous in the service."

The following study is limited to a group of men seen at a convalescent hospital in the United States. These men had been in military service from two to four years, averaging 22 months overseas, and had had their symptoms from one to two years, although they may have been on the sick list only a few weeks or months. Their symptoms are perhaps a little more numerous and diffuse than in the "subacute" cases (seen a few weeks or months after breakdown, some of which also reached this hospital) and, for purposes of differentiation, they may be called "subchronic."

These symptoms appeared with almost unrelieved regularity and are well worth listing.

Tension is evident in their restlessness, insomnia, nightmares, irritability, belligerence, startle reaction ("jumpiness" at noises), stomach disorders and difficulty in concentrating. They also dislike crowds and noise. They complain of anxiety mostly in terms of "nervousness" and worry over minor matters and of their loss of interest in people and things. They dislike talking of their experiences, but most can do so if pressed. They tend to put this resistance in the general class of getting away from anything that reminds them of the war at all. Most have become very sensitive about taking orders. Headaches are extremely common. There is often loss of weight.

Easy fatigability is not infrequent. Profuse sweating and moderate tremors are seen in a considerable number. Stammering of varying degree and duration occurs often. Moods of depression are seen, differing in intensity and sometimes dominating the picture. Disturbances of sexuality are frequent and vary, sometimes in the same man, from excessive activity to loss of interest and relative impotence. Recurrences of bed-wetting, nail-biting and many other major and minor symptoms and idiosyncrasies of childhood, apparently overcome years ago, are also seen. These reactions and symptoms add up to a feeling of being different from formerly, that is, to a partial personality change. This feeling is an accurate subjective observation of an actual, we hope only quantitative and reversible, shift in the functioning of the personality.

The men we are discussing were selected with considerable care as to both diagnosis and suitability for treatment. Therefore, they must be typical of what we call chronic or subchronic combat and operational fatigue and, moreover, must represent the more treatable forms of these conditions. Yet one is immediately struck by the seriousness of these cases (just as one is struck by the seriousness of the disorders in the students who come to see the college psychiatrist). Although the disturbance is much less uncontrollable than in the acute and the subacute cases, it is no longer primarily an immediate, intense emotional reaction to external trauma, which anyone might have, which will subside with distance, security, rest and desensitization. Now there is more involvement and disturbance of the whole personality, like an infection which is quiet but pervasive rather than fulminating but transient. The more severe cases, even of this selected series, not infrequently reveal alarming depressive, suicidal, delinquent, paranoid and schizophrenic trends. One man is in danger of losing all interest in life, another feels that people are talking about him, another fears his own impulses to attack others, another has turned against society, and so on. But these severe disturbances are in the minority, and it is unlikely that they ever will develop to serious proportions or persist for any length of time in men who were previously stable and had not shown such tendencies in marked degree before enlistment. We deal, then, at least in this group, not merely with transient emotional reactions in relatively healthy personalities but also with men whose whole emotional organization is affected.

A second striking fact in these cases is the actual role played by the combat experience. A quiet, pleasant young officer comes to the hospital because, after three and one-half years on board ship with participation in numerous engagements, he developed acute anxiety, with trembling of his whole body, as well as irritability, insomnia and loss of appetite.

He presented the typical symptoms of combat fatigue. In talking with him, it soon appeared that his tremors, so strong as to cause him to fall down, had developed suddenly at the end of a leave, in the railroad station after seeing his wife off and turning to report back to his ship. Apparently, he could not face the return to combat—but this surmise turned out to be incorrect.

Actually, although normally frightened during combat, warfare did not unduly upset him. On the contrary, it even caused a certain tingling of his blood, a sense of freedom and a certain zest. In a way, it was to him like the pleasure of hunting. True, his emotional tension during these long months on the cruiser mounted continually, but not only because of fear.

Upon exploring further the sources of the increasing stress which he felt, he said that what he found more and more intolerable was being told when and how to get his hair cut! This was symbolic of all the restrictions of life aboard ship in wartime, which he found eventually to be unbearable—changing his clothes for meals, standing inspections in whites after a night of enemy action, and similar infringements of his personal liberty.

He could discuss all his combat experiences freely and with little if any discomfort, but even the memory of these minor impairments of his personal freedom enraged him. He himself deplored his reaction as foolish, but he could not help it. As the months and then years passed, his resentment increased until, at the last moment before returning to his ship, he literally trembled with rage. But he did not understand this at that time. He did not realize the intensity of his feelings and was only terrified by these mysterious symptoms. Why should this man have reacted so violently to the military routine? To answer this, we must know something of his personal make-up, and so the interview turned to his past history.

He had been raised high in the Canadian Rockies. Even before his parents' death, he had enjoyed such personal freedom as is almost unknown in the cities and even on the now vanishing farms. When he was 13, his parents died, and he went to live with an aunt. He knew in advance, and his parents had known, that he would never get along with this well-meaning but somewhat rigid relative, but hers was the only home to which he could go.

A less independent boy might have succumbed to her restrictions rather than leave her protection; but our patient, at age of 14, without further thought, went off to a small town in the mountains with which he was well acquainted, and set himself up alone in a cabin. Living here alone, and working in his spare time, he saw himself through high school. He did all his own cooking, mending and housekeeping. Self-reliant and loving the freedom of the mountains, his was the personality of the independent frontiersman. It soon became clear why he could face danger and violence coolly but could not stand four years of supervised haircuts.

It was this to which he was sensitive. He would not have broken under fear alone. Indeed, in civil life he had similar, although much milder, symptoms. Generally good-natured and easy-going, yet he had a violent temper when his freedom was impaired. Now, like the typical combat-fatigue patient, he suffered from insomnia and nightmares, but his dreams were not of battle. Instead, they were repeatedly of being "held down." For example, he dreamed that he was driving his car but it got stuck in the mud. Again, he would dream that he was back on the cruiser, but that the ship could not move because it was on rocky land. The mud and the rocks in these dreams always reminded him of the mountains, where he had so much enjoyed hunting, fishing and paddling his own canoe. Thus, his mind, when asleep as when awake, was occupied with anxiety arising not from combat but from feeling, as he put it, "fenced in"—immobilized, like his car in the mud, or his ship ashore.

This man reacted with tremendous relief to two one-hour interviews. He quickly learned that he was not in the throes of some mysterious mental malady which would wreck his personality and his life, but simply that, through his past experience, he was a hyperindependent young man who therefore had difficulty in adapting to military life and naturally reacted to the constant irritation with mounting anger and anxiety. To understand his hyperindependent needs, and to learn to handle them, meant the ability to return to duty. He was eager to finish the remaining two years of his enlistment, and, although at first he had been considered as probably hopeless for further service, he showed such improvement in a few weeks that it was possible to return him to limited duty.

This briefly sketched case illustrates several generally valid points:

1. Despite the onset of typical symptoms after extensive and intensive combat experience, combat was found to be only one factor among others. None of these particular cases should be accepted at face value as being combat-induced without thorough investigation. If we do not fully appreciate this fact we are in danger of being misled into thinking of these conditions as essentially transient anxiety reactions to the unusual stress of battle rather than as the more complex personality problems which they so often were.

Obviously, however, combat is a very different experience under different conditions. On a battleship patrolling an area for interminable months, an occasional skirmish can relieve tension, while for the infantryman, combat looms as a horror, under which in time nearly every man will crack.

2. The cause lay in a specific emotional trend, which impaired the man's adaptation to life in the service.

3. In this group, the men had had their emotional tensions and symptoms for at least a year before giving in and going on the sick list. War experiences affected different men differently. They stirred up certain tendencies which had always existed in the man and were important to his emotional life. In the past these had merely influenced the emotional life and personality functioning and had caused only minor, insignificant symptoms. Now they had become so intensified by the stresses of war that he could no longer control them adequately. A little tendency to temper became belligerency, occasional bad dreams became nightmares, a little nervousness became acute anxiety with startle reactions (jumpiness, especially at sudden sounds), and so on. The latent tendency had erupted into full-blown neurosis. Childhood emotional reactions, hitherto controlled, now dominated the feelings, the thoughts, the behavior and even the bodily functioning.

It is not a question of whether or not a man is "neurotic" but a matter of adaptation. The more neurotic man, with all sorts of symptoms and peculiarities, may adjust better than the relatively normal if his neurosis better *fits* a given situation. As we have said, most of these men had given from two to three years of excellent service. As many of them were heroes and had won decorations as were to be found among the wounded men on the orthopedic ward. A random sample run on 100 of these men showed that 29 had unit citations, 15 had individual citations, and five had both. Thus, more than one third had been decorated. The man we have described as an example was a hero of many engagements and of three invasions, but he could not stand being told when to have his hair cut.

One man took over five years of almost continuous overseas duty with all kinds of action before the strain caused him to turn in sick. Even so, he turned in only after two years of being unable to sleep or eat properly. It is easy to see that he was stable and tough to stand so much. Another man had 49 months of virtually uninterrupted sea duty on combat ships and then was given a 30-day leave. As he felt himself freed of the danger, the demands and the weighty responsibilities, he began to tremble. When he got ashore, the shaking became worse. He entered a hotel bar for a drink, thinking to steady himself. He found the trembling so severe that it was all he could do, even using both hands on the glass, to get it to his lips. Within two weeks this had quieted down, and now he began to feel restless ashore. He felt really well, at ease and at home only at Naval establishments. He could not enjoy being ashore. He could not adjust to it. He was like a fish out of water. Thus one man's poison can truly be another man's meat. One man could stand only so much sea—the other only so much shore. It is not simply a matter of stability or toughness but of very specific sensitivities and vulnerabilities—the capacity both to stand and to adapt to particular stresses and situations.

4. A fourth point illustrated by our example was that rest and temporary relief from duty affected the symptoms but little. Many men thought that if they could only return home their tension and symptoms would vanish, only to find that when they did so and began to let down, their controls relaxed and the whole reaction became, not better, but much worse. On the other hand, circumscribed but carefully focused psychotherapy, aimed at the specific source of the patient's reactions, produced marked results often after only one or two interviews.

SUPPORTING OBSERVATIONS

The four points we made in the preceding section of this chapter were not deductions but, in the main, empirical observations. However, we have ventured to advance them as generalizations for this particular group, and so they require a few further examples for support.

A young officer of 30 developed acute anxiety, irritability, restlessness, insomnia, loss of appetite and other typical symptoms of combat fatigue after three and one-half years of almost continuous sea duty with repeated combat experience. But when his confidence was won, it appeared that his symptoms actually developed when he found himself in a relatively menial job under a superior who did not value him. He was an only son of parents who pinned all their hopes and ambitions on him and made attention, recognition, praise, prestige, achievement and success as necessary to his spirit as bread to his body.

Because of these powerful drives, coupled with a fine intelligence, he felt compelled to great efforts in civil life and achieved phenomenal success. But through it all he sustained a background of anxiety and insecurity, which only increased his strivings. On one occasion, prior to his enlistment, when a project of his seemed likely to fail, he developed an acute anxiety, milder but otherwise identical with his service-precipitated one.

His final break in the military service came when, after his years at sea, he was assigned to what promised to be a very big and important job—only to find himself sidetracked by an error into a negligible, routine duty which made no use of his talents and, under a cold critical superior, afforded no gratification to his needs for prestige. In this case, not independence, as in our first case, but prestige, praise and success were the emotional demands which created the vulnerability to frustration and the consequent reactions of rage and anxiety and the other symptoms.

His reaction to combat was paradoxical. He was in an engagement during a period when he was very anxious and tense under the unappreciative superior. During the engagement, and the whole time in the combat zone, he was normally frightened but also felt exhilarated, as though he were now really contributing and was valuable and important, and he felt, slept and ate better than before. Despite the first impression, he had no combat fatigue. On the contrary, in spite of the danger, combat made him feel better! His anxiety came from other sources—from frustration of his strongest needs and from the consequent rage which he repressed for fear of meeting disapproval and punishment.

Another young man had nearly five years of overseas and sea duty and finally turned in sick after the invasion of an island. His symptoms were definitely exacerbated after this action. But in this case, too, they were mounting before this and had existed in rudimentary form in civil life. During the action, in which an enemy bomber got through and scored hits on two ships, this veteran was normally frightened and was most distressed when the bombs wounded many of our men. But he viewed the action itself with interest and his anxiety was not acute. This developed afterward and increased when he reached a safe island to the rear and relaxed in the hospital. Like many men, he found that he had carried on under much greater strain than he realized at the time. Then his controls let down.

He turned out to have been spoiled by his mother and treated very strictly by his father. The family was poor, and he was never given the education in law which had always been his one absorbing desire and his chosen means of rising above the family's poverty. Now, after five years in military service, his childhood rebellion against authority was mounting, his vanity and his need to rise in the world were not satisfied, and, above all, he saw his whole life plan, his law career, with all that it meant to him in prestige, success and satisfaction, put in jeopardy. He had been just too old for the in-service training program, and now, if the war lasted, he would be too old to start on the long road to the law degree. He was very resentful of his father for his strictness and for not giving him an education, and he was ruthlessly competitive with his colleagues, although he was also very loyal to them.

His symptoms were severe. His belligerence was very hard to handle. His repetitive nightmare was as follows: He would see the wounded on the deck, as they had been in reality, but among them he would see his father and his friends. This dream led him to guilt feelings because of his underlying hostility to his father and his friends. It was this that disturbed him and caused his anxiety.

The battle experience, especially the casualties among our own men, had mobilized his hostility, guilt and anxiety, which persisted after the battle because the sources of it persisted. He hated his friends as competitors who threatened to leave him behind, although he was ruthlessly intent on rising above them. He blamed his father for not helping him with his career, which would have enabled him to rise, and also for his strictness. Now he rebelled against military service for the same reason—it held him, regimented him, threatened his career. He was belligerent and impossible even with his wife.

His egocentricity and selfishness were pointed out to him unsparingly. He was shown how vulnerable they made him, so that the least interference with his personal desires caused rage, which, in turn, only caused guilt, anxiety, insomnia, restlessness and impossible behavior, incapacitated him and doomed his ambitions. He was shown how childish they were, how impractical, and how they defeated themselves. Only overcoming this ruthless egocentricity in favor of an interest in his friends, his wife and his work and, in the future, in his clients would make him an effective person and a good professional man. Otherwise, he would surely fail, for he could not even study in his present state of rage. He was like a baby, demanding everything from his parents for himself. To achieve his ambitions he must relinquish some of his ruthless egotistic demands and develop some of the giving, parental attitudes. The emotions involved were clear, the interpretations focused only upon the vital points. He saw how he was defeating himself and saw the way out.

The improvement after three interviews of an hour each was striking. Before this, he had been judged too severely disturbed for further duty, and even the prospect of release from the service and continuance of his studies did not cause noticeable improvement. Now, however, this prospect aided the therapeutic effect of the interviews. His marriage, which had been almost on the rocks because of his irritability and aggressiveness, was saved by his dramatically improved relationship with his wife.

In some cases a central issue is the family relationship. A navigator had flown for nearly two years, completing 30 missions over enemy territory as well as patrols, rescues and other flights. Suddenly, during a flight, he felt dizzy and barely managed to keep from fainting before he landed. Bed rest for a week did not relieve his tendency to these spells. He could fly no longer and eventually was evacuated. His spells continued, and he believed that he suffered from an organic brain condition of some sort and wanted roentgenograms of his skull and other tests made. He was quite anxious. He was relieved of this anxiety and also of his spells and improved in his outlook in a single 45-minute interview, which went as follows.

Asked about the situations in which his spells occurred, he said that he now had them only at home when with his wife and baby. Pressed for the precise details, he said they seemed to occur in connection with his getting angry, and, following this lead, he seemed to be angry because of a certain coldness in his wife. Elsewhere he no longer got especially angry and did not have spells. He had been married three years. His wife had been most affectionate then—and now that he thinks of it, he realizes that the first spell came on shortly after his child was born. With agitation he pours out his feeling that the spell occurred because now his desire to see his first child and his wife, and their wish for him, were added to his previously normal fear of death, mobilized this fear and made death seem much more terrible than before.

But every neurotic symptom represents the outcome of child-hood reactions. Not every pilot is incapacitated by the birth of his child. While still a baby, this man had lost his father, and he had been reared by his mother and three older sisters. His dependent attachment to these women had been intensified by the lack of a man in the house and by his being the baby of the family. He was spoiled by the four women but not excessively. He developed into a relatively normal young man.

But his vulnerable emotional spot was an exaggerated need for a woman's love. (Neurotic tendencies are merely exaggerations of normal ones. The differences between normality and neurosis—and addictions, crime and even much psychosis—is only quantitative.) Now our young man continued his childhood need and complained that his wife was not affectionate enough toward him. He knew she had not changed basically, though, because she was still as affectionate as ever with the child. But when she was not warm enough toward him, he could become angry and irritable, sleep poorly, lose his appetite and develop headaches, anxiety and these dizzy and fainting spells.

His nightmares dealt with his wife and child. In one of these he dreamed they were both dead and he awoke in terrible anxiety. As we have said, many of these patients relate dreams spontaneously, and some beg the doctor for interpretations. Dreams are of great value in this work, since they reveal sharply and clearly the central feelings that are concerning and distressing the patient—the feelings which are causing his anxiety, even in his sleep. That is, the dream goes right to the point, to the central irritant. In this case, we saw the intensity of the man's rage at his wife for not satisfying his demands for affection—demands dating from childhood and intensified by the stresses of military life. His symptoms became intelligible as the results of this rage. His fainting and dizziness seemed to be primarily mechanisms of escape and withdrawal from intolerable feelings and situations.

It was now possible to show the patient, from his own story, how he had kept toward his wife too much of his childhood demands for all the attention and affection he had received from a mother and three sisters; how it was natural and biological for his wife's energies and feelings to turn to the new baby, their first, and that she would give less to the patient and expect more from him; and this was normal, biological and good for the patient's development, for he must learn to enjoy the mature attitudes of *giving* care, attention and affection and not merely *receiving* love and taking it for granted as in childhood.

Since most of these patients have regressed somewhat to outlooks and behavior of childhood, this hurts their pride. And so most of them are spurred toward improvement by being shown that their symptoms, hitherto mysterious, interesting and even somewhat valued by them, are really manifestations of childishness. But it is not enough to do this—the therapist must also show them the solution, the way out, what the mature attitudes are and the pathway of emotional development toward them. Such men as this one are most grateful.

This man responded with all the emotional force one can expect in a relatively healthy personality when one is able to touch the vulnerable spot therapeutically. He said he no longer wanted the roentgenograms and tests—he knew this was it. He became conscious of his demands upon his wife and his rage when these were unsatisfied. The relationship improved and his symptoms disappeared. Of course, he was not "cured" in these 45 minutes. But what was accomplished was rational and radical. It showed him why his adaptation failed, gave him a key to cure and opened up for him a path of emotional development which he could follow with or without future help.

The Part Played by Combat

To study the part played by combat, let us select a specifically combat-precipitated case. An electrician's mate had spent two years in the Navy, almost all the time at sea. He suffered from anxiety, irritability, anorexia, insomnia, nightmares, headaches, dislike of crowds, rapid heart, sweating and loss of interest. His symptoms became bothersome after the invasion of North Africa, but he kept going. In an action in the Pacific, a year later, he was trapped below as his ship sank and was rescued only at the very last minute. The rescuing vessel was then bombed for two days, and the patient "blew his top," yelling and crying. Somewhat later, under emotional tension which made him impatient with hospitalization, he insisted on further sea duty, which he hoped might relieve his feelings. At sea, however, he soon found that he feared to touch a switch lest he make a mistake and injure himself and others. Here, then, is an energetic fighting man, incapacitated by combat-precipitated anxiety.

In the interview he stated that when he was trapped, a thousand things flashed through his brain. Asked to recall these, he said the thought flitted through his mind of how he had once ridden a motorcycle against his parents' orders and smashed it up and had almost been killed, and how he later had changed jobs against their wishes and had an accident in which he nearly was killed, and how now he had enlisted against their wishes. His other flashes of memory were all to the same point—guilt toward his parents.

It soon came out that he had other reasons for feelings of guilt. He belonged to a bunch of boys, not a bad one, he hastened to add, only friends. Nevertheless, he had been in court more than once and had been on parole. This group gave him feelings of adequacy and toughness. For him, fighting was a great outlet and also a means to prestige. That is why he had too much drive to remain in a hospital and felt the need for action and a return to sea duty, even with his symptoms. And this aggressiveness derived, it came out, largely from feelings of weakness, inferiority and inadequacy. These were caused by a certain emotional immaturity, by exaggerated dependence and insecurity in relation to his parents, who had reared him with what seemed to be a combination of indulgence, neglect and restrictiveness, and by some intellectual difficulty in keeping up with the other boys in school, socially or in jobs. These inferiorities and insecurities enraged him and put a chip on his shoulder. He was hostile, defiant, at odds with his parents and occasionally with the law. But beneath this he was a child, craving love and esteem. And so he felt guilty for his hostile feelings and behavior and lived in an anxiety which resulted from expectations of punishment. When danger threatened, it mobilized this guilt and the feeling: "Here it is. Now I'm getting what somehow I always expected."

In this case, too, emotional patterns, previously kept within limits, were now mobilized until they dominated the functioning. Sea duty was an important outlet for this man, satisfying his aggressiveness and his self-esteem and giving him a sense of social security which he had lacked in civil life. Now he was incapacitated for sea duty, and his insecurity in civil life, already a problem, was acutely increased. At the same time, his symptoms, unquestionably sincere and severe, masked this deeper insecurity. His feelings of inadequacy were heightened not only toward civilians but also toward his associates in military service. His nightmares were of being with his friends, attacking people and then being attacked, and of his shipmates attacking him.

His symptoms were all exaggerations of tendencies he had had for years in civil life. He had always been irritable and belligerent, although less so. He feared "cracking up," by which he meant losing control of his temper. But he had always feared his own anger. His father used to beat him for his fighting, and he had really wanted to be good but couldn't.

Without going into details, all his symptoms had existed in milder degrees since his childhood. As to his losing control when trapped, he had also "blown his top" twice in civil life when he was put in jail overnight. He never could tolerate any confinement. Thus, his experience of being trapped struck him at his most vulnerable emotional spot and mobilized to the point of being overwhelming all the symptoms which he had had in some degree all his life. Aggression and guilt, crime and punishment—these were the tendencies which formed his central emotional problem and thereby rendered him specifically susceptible to the violence and the danger of combat. The men previously described had other emotional problems which made them specifically vulnerable to very different kinds of stress—exaggerated independence, egotism and ambition, rivalry with a brother, too great needs for love and so on. This man experienced considerable relief from discussing his anger, but the essential limitations in his nature which caused his belligerency probably precluded any brief methods of achieving quick and lasting results.

Whatever the dynamics of the acute combat-precipitated cases at the front, these particular subchronic cases showed the mobilization of personality problems by the combat experience. An infantryman, 25 years old, with typical symptoms, had controlled his anxiety for many months while on duty immediately behind the front line. But after a few days in a foxhole in the very front line, he yelled and broke down. All his symptoms had existed in minor degree previously, had become worse in military service and much worse after this experience. He had always been willful, high-strung, quick-tempered. This was traceable to his background. His parents were divorced when he was an infant. His mother remarried but died soon afterward. His father was a rolling stone who never remarried. The patient never had a stable home or even lived long in the same town. He went to innumerable schools. He became bitter against the world. He blamed it for not giving him a mother, a home and stability.

Being put out in the front line, in the position of greatest danger, he took as the final abandonment by the world. He saw his buddies killed and realized that this might happen to him too. This was the ultimate abandonment by Fate and man—the irrevocable sign that no one cared. Now his bitterness and anger were so intensified by this that he broke down. And he used this rage and bitterness not only as a revenge but also as a protection against present and future rejection. The only way to get along, he said, is to think only of oneself, be hard and have no feelings for others. Only so can one avoid being mortally hurt. He no longer cared about anybody or anything. His fiancée married another man and he didn't care (so he said). If a person is soft, he only gets hurt, the patient reasoned, so now he was for himself alone. But he admitted that if he thought about things he cried—for he felt that no one cared about him and no one ever would care—and this was too intolerable to face—so he built about himself a hard, hostile, bitter, protective shell and denied his deep childhood longing for love.

But this defensive hate maintained his withdrawal, his irritability, his anxiety, his startle reaction, his inability to concentrate and other symptoms and estranged him from the very love he craved.

This was a difficult man to treat, but we did succeed, largely through discussing his problem frankly, in softening the biting edge of his bitterness, which was making him a danger to himself and to society.

Probably it is the men with conflicts centering around hostility, guilt and anxiety who are most vulnerable to fear and violence and so to the stress of combat. But as this case showed, combat could be reacted to in other individual ways, such as feeling abandoned.

11 | Hostility and Guilt

We have said that generally, but not exclusively, it is men with emotional problems arising from guilt, aggressiveness and anxiety who are most vulnerable to breakdowns precipitated by combat or violence. These men are sensitive to hostility and violence however directed—whether in the form of their attacking others, being attacked by others or in the self-reproaches of their own consciences. Some examples will illustrate different ways in which hostility operates. The vulnerabilities may be to combat, to physical injury, to family problems, to separation, to discipline, to superiors and to other stresses.

INHIBITED HOSTILITY

A 26-year-old artilleryman of stable family had spent 30 months on overseas duty. During this time he had been on a long-range gun some miles behind the front lines. It was when his outfit left the combat zone for a rest and he began to relax that he lost control of himself and actually was out of his head with a psychotic episode for a period of over two weeks. He gradually quieted down and, on his own preference, tried to return to duty.

He was sent back to his battery, at his own request, but after a few weeks, because of his tension and irritability, even with his buddies, as well as a spell in which he lost track of several hours ("amnesia"), it became evident that it was necessary to evacuate him to the United States as a patient. This blank spell occurred just as he was about to fire his gun. He fully expected to return to his usual self upon reaching the States, but he was terribly disillusioned by the treatment he received. He began to relax his previously high standards and to feel that he no longer cared about anything but might just as well slide downhill and become a bum. His chief symptoms were nervousness, easy fatigability, startle reaction and gun-shyness, insomnia, anorexia and headache. His story developed as follows.

He was an only child and had always been very close to his mother. The whole family had been very peace-loving. Although solidly built and apparently normally aggressive, he never in his life had had a fight. He had become angry at times, but his whole personality was imbued with the necessity of controlling any manifestation of this. In other words, his feelings of hostility were firmly inhibited. They came out, as the repressed always does, in indirect, often unnoticeable, ways. They appeared in his occasional nightmares of violence and also in his enjoyment of taking care of wounds. He had had various jobs and connections helping in dispensaries—a socialized, useful, acceptable "sublimation" of his hostile feelings.

Upon first going overseas, he was, as might well have been expected, most distressed by any expectations of violence and bloodshed but was fortunate in obtaining duty on one of the larger field guns, 15 miles behind the lines and the more gory scenes and activities. Secretly, he felt a certain thrill at firing a gun. Gradually, his repugnance to any violence gave way to a now no longer secret but frank enjoyment of his mission. He abandoned himself to the thrill of thinking of the effect of the shells he fired and of the havoc and death they caused. This stirred up a certain guilt reaction, which led him to fear retaliation and to dream of the enemy coming at him to avenge themselves, but the guilt and the fear were not intense enough to overbalance the new sense of relief and pleasure that he felt in killing at a distance.

So long as he kept firing, his hostile drives were gratified. After two years, this became for him the usual and acceptable outlet. It was like an addiction. When he was evacuated to peace and safety for a rest, this outlet for his hostility was completely removed. Now his rage, having no outlet, built up until he lost control of it. He became utterly violent and destructive, tearing up his surroundings and attacking individuals. After three weeks he began to quiet down, but his central symptom and his chief complaint continued to be a feeling of uncontrollable violence. He would feel building up in him a terrible excitement, which he recognized as anger, and an irresistible desire to attack someone. At the least argument, his gorge would rise. These belligerent impulses gave him no peace.

He became restless and anxious and developed headaches. At night he could not relax enough to sleep, and he even feared for what he might do to someone in his sleep. When he did sleep, he dreamed repeatedly of being back in the artillery crew and firing the big gun; only now, instead of thrilling to this activity, he would wake in terror, his muscles tensed and braced, as when awaiting the firing of the gun, his heart pounding. He himself was amazed at the fact that now, even in his dreams, firing the gun filled him with such anxiety and tension, whereas in reality it had relieved his feelings. In fact, he said, during his time in the field he had felt most relaxed when firing the gun, but now it was the opposite—a nightmare in his dreams and intolerable in reality.

We see reflected here the actual state of his hostile anger and cruel feelings. During his duty in the field, they served his country and accomplished a purpose. He could accept and enjoy them. Now, back in peaceful civilization, his aggressiveness was no longer useful but only a terrible menace to others and, because of his conscious reaction and fear of retaliation, also to himself. The god of war, with superb psychological alchemy, had drawn forth from this peace-loving Dr. Jekyll the violent Mr. Hyde, who had slumbered silently within him, and now, as in Stevenson's story, Mr. Hyde dominated the scene and could no longer be repressed and chained within Dr. Jekyll's breast.

As to the source of this patient's violent but previously well-controlled, overcompensated and sublimated hostile aggressiveness and sadism, a little could be learned. As we have said, he had been very much attached to his mother and considerably overprotected by her. When the depression came, the family lost its money, and all the members had to pitch in and earn what they could. Even his mother worked hard, and the patient felt impelled to do the same, although he was only ten years old at the time. Outwardly a good sport about this, the sudden loss of the indulgence, the attention and the care to which he had been accustomed previously, and the substitution for it of poverty, uncertainty and work, filled his childhood with underlying bitterness and resentment.

In military service, as in the case of so many other young men, his expectations were colored by his wishes and exposed him to disappointment. During the whole period that he was enjoying the firing of the gun and feeling so relaxed by it, he recognized that he was intensely angry. The long tour overseas, the uncertainty, the poor food, the constant air raids, the danger—both these hardships themselves and what they represented to him emotionally, namely, the denial of all the maternal care and protection which he craved—built up in him an awful sense of frustration with a consequent rage reaction, which the firing of the gun partially relieved. This alone afforded him surcease and relaxation and allowed him to forget the gnawing homesickness, especially for his mother. As in so many cases, this longing for his mother's love was connected so intimately with her nursing him and later feeding him and cooking for him, that when he felt this longing thwarted, his stomach would tighten up with his anger, he would become nauseated and frequently would even vomit.

Civilian experience has taught us that when a person is filled with rage he often takes it out indirectly upon himself. Suffering with his hostility, this man felt that he no longer cared, that somehow in revenge he would spite the world, just as when a little child he could spite his mother by backsliding from the high standards of the family. He would no longer care, he would slip and become a bum, and this would afford him a certain secret satisfaction. We can hazard a guess that this satisfaction derived in part from the reaction of his conscience and high ideals to his enjoyment of hostility, and, as a result of this, the venting of this hostility upon himself by masochistically ruining his own life. His whole personality had been built up to control all manifestations of violence. The release and gratification of this violence caused the upset in his emotional balance.

The outlook in such a case is not so discouraging as might seem. With insight, patience, encouragement, advice, security, with indulgence to decrease his frustration and with substitute satisfactions for his hostility, it was possible to decrease his rage and to replace his now damaged automatic inhibitions of it with conscious understanding of these impulses and more conscious control of them. He showed marked progress along this path of emotional healing and development. If he should succeed sufficiently in controlling his hostility and integrating it into his conscious personality, he would become a better man for the experience—more mature and better organized than if all this frustration and rage had lurked permanently in the shadows of an overly shy and inhibited personality.

Another young man, nervous, slender, very urgent in his desire for help, shifted restlessly in the chair as he described the scene which led to his breakdown. His small vessel hit a mine while on a very dangerous mission. In the explosion, half the crew were killed. One man was split open. Another's head was blown off. The patient was hurled 30 feet through the air. Because of the spray, he thought that he was under water and drowning, but after the shock, he came to and was rescued. However, his "nerves were in pieces," and he suffered from terrible fear.

His anxiety persisted for three months, and with it stomach distress and loss of appetite. Any sudden noise made him feel as if he were being shot, and he would jump violently. When he tried to read, his mind would wander to the bloody scene he had experienced. Nor could he escape it at night, for it returned to plague him in nightmares. In these dreams, the scene was almost exactly the same, but the screaming was noticeably worse.

This young man was in his middle twenties and was married. He had been in the Navy for three years and had served for two of them on the same ship. As his confidence was won, he began to tell his story in detail. His family, he said, was poor but proud. He came from a small town in which his father held a modest position in a large factory. During the depression, the family income was meager, and their frugal living was a source of distress to him. He felt the poverty keenly in his relationships with his somewhat more financially fortunate friends. When he reached high school, he was able to earn enough to have the things he wanted. He felt more comfortable and secure and seemed to be resigned to always working hard for whatever he got. He felt that his father could have managed better, so that the family would not have had to live so poorly.

This resentment showed through as the patient talked, although he seemed hardly conscious of it and quite unable to admit that these feelings toward his father had any depth. On the surface, he felt very close to his father and also to his younger brother, although not so close as to his mother. Here again, strong though it was, his repressed resentment was veiled by his gentleness. His father showed rather marked preference for his brother, although there was outward show of complete equality. But the boy sensed it in his father's attitude and in innumerable little incidents. For example, the father would refuse the patient some request, but then the boy would find that he had granted more than its equivalent to the brother.

As the young man talked, it was evident that strong hostile feelings toward the father and the brother were checked and controlled by a very loving and gentle attitude. Where this gentleness and control of all aggressiveness came from was quickly apparent when he began to speak of his mother. She was a most kind woman and religious in the best sense. The patient identified with her very closely and developed into a very gentle and kind young man. He never had a fist fight. He was never cruel to animals. He never went hunting, although this was a favorite sport in his community. He was good, generous and kind to all. He enjoyed good music and sang in the choir. He could never stand violence or bloodshed of any kind. An automobile accident or a street fight sickened him somewhat, but he never showed this. In his reading, too, he preferred comedies.

He had no nervous symptoms during childhood, so far as could be elicited, but generally was considered to be a relatively normal member of a relatively normal family. His kind outlook and his repugnance to violence were important character traits but not so exaggerated as to be conspicuous or pathological although stronger than in most men. Hating and dreading combat from the depths of his being, nevertheless, his same high ideals had impelled him to force himself to join up in order to do his duty.

During his first year at sea, he experienced no action. He adapted well to the routine and was able to control a general anxiety. Then, in taking a Pacific island, action came. For two days his little vessel was under bombardment, as were the many ships about them. He saw ships hit, saw the boys in the water, helped pull them out with their terrible wounds and burns—sometimes down to the bone— with arms and legs all but off. All this made the gunner's mate of the patient's ship furious. His fighting blood boiled. He cursed the enemy with incessant violence and thus vented and relieved his impulses to action. Huddled against the superstructure was another young fellow, weeping and moaning. This is what the patient wanted to do but he fought against it. He gritted his teeth, kept on his feet and carried on. But it was after this that all his symptoms developed.

Again we see what has often been noted, namely, that it is hard to give an accurate history of emotional symptoms. His original story that the symptoms had begun only a few months previously when his ship was hit by a mine was false. In reality, he had felt fear and anxiety during his first year at sea from apprehension alone, without combat; and after his first combat, all his symptoms burst forth. By a superhuman effort of will, however, he managed to control himself sufficiently to keep going until a year later, when his vessel hit the mine. This control was possible only because of the understanding of the crew. His terror took the form, in part, of being trapped below decks, so that he was unable to go below ("bulkhead happy"). Knowing this, they brought food up to him and even let him sleep topside.

In summary, we see a young man with considerable hostility, but because of his love by and for his parents and his careful upbringing, this hostility had long been so inhibited that he was not even conscious of it. Nor could he indulge it in the slightest even in reading or in fantasies. He could not even imagine himself as being violent or cruel to any man or beast. If there had to be violence, then he could not perform it but only suffer it.

In his mind, his own violence could not be acted out externally, but only reflected against himself. Aroused by violence or danger to fighting and rage, or flight and fear, he was capable only of the second. Exposed to combat, he could not become aggressive, like the gunner's mate—he could not become like some of the young men who taste killing and fear that this taste will be hard to overcome ("kill happy"). All his violently aroused emotion went, not into hostility to others, but only into fear for himself (not that in danger everyone does not, of course, normally feel acute fear).

The persisting symptoms in the "traumatic neuroses" have been interpreted (Freud, 1917; Kardiner, 1941; Rado, 1942) as caused by overwhelming emotions which the man cannot control and assimilate but must go on trying to digest. Whether or not this is true, as shown by the men we have described, further and much more specific, individual and detailed considerations must always be taken into account.

In the first place, there was the intensity of these overwhelming feelings. Not every man broke down in such circumstances. Many men went through worse experiences without even being much upset, or at any rate they quieted down quickly after the action was over. This was not simply because their will power and forces of control were stronger. Many of them were men who did not seem to be especially strong in character. On the other hand, many men of strong character did break down. They reacted with more violent feelings to their experiences than did the others.

In the young man we have been discussing, violence was the sensitive point. It was this which his whole personality could not tolerate. Hence, exposure to violence produced greater mental strains and, because of his strong inhibition of all hostility and his inability to fight, caused much greater fear and anxiety than in men whose hostilities were more free. Breakdown depends on the forces of control, but also on the intensity of the emotional reaction. And the intensity of the emotional reaction depends on the emotional make-up of the man. No case can be understood without not only evaluating the forces of instinct and reaction ("id") and those of control ("ego" and "superego") but also penetrating to the emotional make-up and seeing the specific effects of the man's experiences upon this.

A second point is the question of the duration of the symptoms. Here, too, in addition to struggling to master undigested stimuli, it seemed, in case after case, as if certain powerful emotions, always of importance in the personality, were mobilized by the man's experiences, and, once aroused, they strained the forces of control—like Mr. Hyde, who each time was more easily released and eventually gained control of Dr. Jekyll.

The reaction is like that of a well-domesticated dog, which having once tasted blood is ever afterward a killer. Our young man, who for so long had inhibited his violence, could no longer fully relinquish it in fantasy, yet he sought to exclude from his thoughts such unwelcome fantasies, which he could not accept as his own nature but could feel only as horrors. Rejecting any violence in himself, it caused him guilt and anxiety. Denied by the rest of his personality, his mind still kept turning to those bloody scenes. There is an old story of an abbé who had in his office two fine paintings—one a gentle pastoral landscape, the other a bestial scene of battle. The warriors, he found, turned to the pastoral scene, while the gentler souls were intrigued by the scene of violence.

TOO-FREE HOSTILITY

A powerful soldier was in constant anxiety lest he attack one of his own men, and, after returning to the States, he suffered from impulses to injure people. The slightest provocation would be sufficient to make him want to break a man's arm, and on one occasion he knocked a man out before he could control himself. Usually he would either shake with fear lest he yield to this aggressiveness or else manage precipitously to escape. Strongly built as he was, he realized the danger of his insufficiently inhibited belligerency.

It began in combat. A buddy of his was killed. He saw red, and in his rage he fought like a demon, but thereafter he failed to regain adequate control of his desires to attack people, even his own men. His aggressiveness was now felt as a threat, and combat became horrible to him. It represented the overthrow of judgment and control and the disruption of the rational, cultivated, civilized part of his personality. (How much of this occurred in the street and campus riots which erupted in the late 1960's?)

A little quantitative shift in the handling of one's powerful emotional drives can make the greatest difference in the personality. Our man, with his muscular physique, driven from within by intense hostile aggressiveness, had the makings of a great fighter, and he was a great fighter as long as the aggression was under control and directed against the enemy. But when the dikes of control weakened and began to let the flood of murderous impulses overflow toward his own men, he developed acute anxiety lest he kill or injure them.

Some men with such hostile feelings toward their fellows give in to these feelings in a well-directed and organized way—they become murderers. Still others "project" this hostility to other persons, that is, they deny these feelings in themselves and claim that they are the innocent victims of murderous gangs or malignant forces. This is "paranoia." But our patient managed to regain control of his impulses, dreaded even a thought of violence and became acutely anxious, that is, he suffered from an anxiety state or neurosis. Thus, the reactions of the rest of the personality to even a single powerful motivation can make the difference between a great fighter, a criminal, an insane paranoid and a sufferer from anxiety neurosis. (And thus, criminality is clearly seen to take its place in the series of emotional disorders previously mentioned. In psychosomatic conditions and purely psychological disorders it is kept internal, in masochism and addictions it is acted out primarily against the self, while in criminoids and criminals it is acted out against others.) (Saul, 1976)

What determined the outcome in this man? As usual, the emotional influences and the conditioning experiences of his childhood cast a flood of light upon his personality make-up and his current reactions. He suffered under a harsh father who freely but unjustly administered physical punishment to him until he was adult, and even after that they occasionally came to blows. Children always identify closely with their parents and other intimates of childhood. The father's free venting of his hostile aggression in physical attack formed a model and sanction for the patient to do the same. At the same time, the father's harshness kept the patient's anger almost continually aroused. He could not vent it upon his father, so he tended to take it out on other boys. That he did not become a bully was due to the restraining influence of his mother, for he identified with her as well as with his pugnacious father. If his father or mother had been political extremists his hostility might have been given this direction, as in examples previously mentioned.

In civil life, our patient had been considered a relatively normal, successful, energetic young man. His hostile aggressiveness toward his father and the tendency to lose control of it formed a specific emotional vulnerability, a latent tendency or predisposition to neurosis.

GUILT

Examples of breakdown stemming from overwhelming guilt reactions are everywhere to be seen by the military psychiatrist. One man triumphantly machine-guns five of the enemy and finds himself elated because of this, but then follow devastating, depressing and terrifying self-recriminations for enjoying killing. Kill he must, but to enjoy it is to be condemned utterly. He becomes terrified and depressed. He shuns people and becomes irritable. He is tormented by nightmares, loses his appetite and soon presents the full-blown symptomatology of combat fatigue.

As might be expected, a man's guilt toward his buddies is a frequent precipitant of emotional disturbances. A young infantryman in a shellhole at night knifed one of the enemy who was infiltrating our lines—only to discover, to his horror, in the dim light of morning, that it was one of his own buddies. He vomited and went into an agitated depression which lasted many weeks.

Such tragic instances seem to be almost commonplace, but they do not tell the whole story. In some cases the guilt seems to be exaggerated. Often, in fact, the man feels guilt even though in reality there has been no word or deed to justify it. And even when there is an accidentally fatal outcome that is not the man's responsibility or fault, certain men feel it to be such. Now it is a fundamental rule of the emotional life that a man's convictions concerning his own feelings are always correct, although they may not be correct in the sense in which he presents the facts. It is the job of the psychiatrist to translate the patient's apparently false belief into psychological reality. We know from experience, not only in military but also in civil life, that when a person keeps blaming himself and takes the responsibility for something he has not done, he is usually found to be blaming himself for the wish rather than for the deed. (Sometimes his guilt is "displaced," and he blames himself for something else in thought or act.)

For example, a young man developed increasing dislike for his immediate superior, who untactfully and unwisely, it must be admitted, persisted in constantly ribbing and teasing him. The lad finally came to hate him so intensely that he frankly wished and prayed for his death.

Fate granted his desire. In the first action the superior was hit and killed. But the man's satisfaction was fleeting. Instead of rejoicing, he was overwhelmed with guilt, as if he himself had caused this completely fortuitous death. He gradually became so depressed that he had to be evacuated.

Some strong guilt often colors a man's whole feeling about life and people. It often fills him with expectations of harm or calamity. He becomes unduly anxious and fearsome. This may influence his attitude toward his superiors.

One such man came to have little or no feeling about killing the enemy. He even began to enjoy it. He felt no conscious guilt whatever. But he lived in rising fear of what might befall him, and this fear was directed mostly toward his officers, who, he began to feel, might, at any time, punish him and ruin his previously excellent record. This became his major conscious fear.

One of the most tragic facts of human social life is that an undercurrent of hostility permeates all human relationships. There is, in everyone, a secret satisfaction in the misfortunes of others and even a sense of triumph when others die. This knowledge is part of human folk wisdom, reflected in such sayings as "misery loves company." At least it is to man's credit that such base feelings are often conflictful, that people hate even to admit them, and that many persons break down emotionally with guilt and shame for harboring them. Of course, the intensity and freedom of the hostility varies enormously and there is a great gulf between the sadistic criminal killer, political or personal, and the person of good-will. The existence of humanity now depends upon decreasing the former and increasing the latter.

Guilt Toward the Enemy

An aggressive young man, after two and one-half years in the Army, was anxious and fearsome, started at the least noise, was irritable with people, would let his fists fly and would not hesitate to hurl objects at his adversaries. He slept poorly, had repeated nightmares of being stuck on a beach during an invasion and being unable to move, and also had battle dreams, in which he was pursued by the enemy. Occasionally, he experienced hallucinations of enemy soldiers whom he had killed or injured—seeing their faces—although he knew they were not really there but that it was a trick of his own imagination. (Hallucinations and delusions occur in all degrees of vividness and sense of reality.)

As a matter of fact, it turned out that he was not so much changed from the days of peace. He had always been aggressive, and now this aggression had been freed even further by his experiences. He had developed into such an aggressive youngster because of his father's behavior. His father drank, and when he did, he became violent and often beat him and his brothers. When the children were more grown, they fought back. Thus the boy's defensive anger was kept aroused, and through the example of his father and brothers he learned to vent it in action.

He had had hostile fantasies as long as he could remember and was attracted by the idea of killing. He thought it would be like hunting, which he deeply enjoyed. He was not disappointed, so far as the enemy was concerned, but he could not stand seeing his buddies killed.

His hostile aggressiveness was also motivated by a sense of pride and of frustration. Down underneath, he felt that his parents did not value him and that others did not either. This is a common reaction—feeling toward oneself, and toward other persons, as one felt and feels toward one's parents. This caused a terrible sense of rejection, of lowered self-esteem and of insecurity and weakness. For him, killing was revenge for the treatment he had received, for his feelings of inferiority and for the attitudes he felt others had toward him. It was also something he boasted of, and the expression of bravery, heroism and power became a way of compensating for his sense of weakness. He was "kill happy." His was a make-up which is frequently encountered in the courts (Alexander and Healy, 1935). It is of interest that he looked forward to some sort of job in the police system, saying frankly that his reason was a predilection for killing.

But he was also raised with certain standards, and besides his hostility to his father, he also loved him. As a result, he developed a conscience. His fight reaction was aroused readily and was all too free in action, but few of us realize the power of the conscience. Often we think that we elude the conscience, only to learn in the end that its strength, although still and silent, is inexorable.

By day aggressive and handing it out, by night he himself became the butt of his aggression and had to take it. What he did or wished to do to others by day, he himself endured in his dreams at night. In reality, he moved freely off the beach, killing the enemy, but in his dream he was stuck there, exposed to their fire. In reality, and in his fantasies, he enjoyed killing the enemy, but since he enjoyed using the sword, he lived in fear of it. He lived in constant anxiety and, after a few drinks, would go into a panic because he actually believed that the enemy was attacking him, and sometimes he thought he saw them, just as he did in his dreams. Such hallucinations, like tormenting dreams, often arise from a guilty conscience.

(This has been described classically in literature, for example in the *Phantom Rickshaw* by Kipling.)

We thus see aggression aroused in this man and, in reaction, an aroused conscience—two potent forces which cause the symptoms. It is with such powerful feelings that the psychotherapist must come to grips, if he is to be of real, effectual help, but he must proceed with the care, the skill and the surety of the surgeon, lest in seeking to help he should do harm.

Guilt Toward Buddies

Guilt toward shipmates, although common enough, was not of such primary importance in the majority of the cases coming to this convalescent hospital as it was found to be in army fliers. The bulk of our patients seemed to be more similar to the ground-crew personnel, observed by Grinker and Spiegel (1945), who had been overseas for long periods and had developed emotional problems much more on the basis of the attrition of military life. This again demonstrates the caution that must be exercised when one speaks of the psychology of the war neuroses.

One patient was a well-built, handsome young Marine who presented the usual symptoms of combat fatigue. He was extremely nervous, had terrifying battle dreams, startle reaction, tremors, headaches and occasional nausea and vomiting. In the interview, he at first admitted no emotional problems of any kind, either in regard to military service or to friends or family. He was reluctant to tell of his repetitive nightmare, saying always that it was merely a repetition of what really had happened.

What really happened was that, while making a landing, a large percentage of his companions were killed, including two buddies. However, dreams are never precise repetitions of reality. No matter how faithfully they seem to repeat the actual situation, yet, if one examines them carefully, it is usually possible to find some alteration, however slight. Moreover, the endings of dreams are of special importance. The dream is merely an expression in pictures of the dreamer's feelings. In waking life, he would express such feelings, if conscious of them, in words. Because the feelings are conflictful, the scenes in dreams are usually distorted. The end of the dream shows something about the outcome of the patient's conflicting feelings, or the kind of solution he seeks for his emotional problem (French, 1939).

In this case, the patient's dream usually ended with the patient himself being caught in machine-gun fire. Except for this detail, the dream merely repeated the scene of the invasion, which in reality the patient came through completely unscathed physically. To be in a terrible situation in reality and dream that one is safely and pleasurably at home is readily intelligible; but to have come through the battle untouched, to be safely, and indeed quite comfortably, ensconced in a hospital, and yet to dream oneself back into battle and then heighten the horrors by having oneself machine gunned, is not so easy to understand. However, it is well established that the dream is an expression of powerful feelings and impulses. A dream of killing and being killed is certainly apt to represent primarily hostile feelings toward those who are killed, and guilt can be so great that one feels that he deserves in his turn to be killed.

Without going into the course of this interview in detail, the patient brought out the fact that in reality he did wish to be killed himself and that the reason for this was that he felt so terrible about his buddies' having been killed. The interview then developed as follows:

Apparently, the patient never had been entirely at ease in his relationships with people. This seems to have been, for the most part, on an emotional basis, a result of overprotection by his mother, which had impaired his masculine freedom and security. And, although of average intellectual and emotional make-up, his feeling of not being fully equal and accepted was perhaps increased by his difficulty in keeping up with the above-average people with whom he desired to be associated.

In military life he did not achieve the promotions he desired. He felt inferior to his shipmates but, of course, did not see the underlying reasons for this. He laid it to discrimination against him. This heightened his resentment and increased his difficulties in getting along with the group. He thus developed an intense underlying hostility toward his buddies but kept it under control and hidden even from himself because of his needs for recognition by them, his wishes to be accepted as one of them and his actual real devotion to them. The result was a vague feeling that people were somehow against him—a paranoid tinge to his outlook. When the buddies were killed, this secretly satisfied his unconscious and unacceptable hostility toward them. Now he, who felt himself inferior and unaccepted, was the one to be left alone on the field. This secret satisfaction of his hostile feelings toward those with whom he had to identify himself and whom he loved caused the guilt which overwhelmed him and, in addition to the symptoms listed above, caused feelings of depression and a tendency to withdraw from the contacts and activities of life. He gave up pleasures, and his mood became one of mourning.

In such a case, the physician must move with great care. Rash interpretation of his unaccepted, repressed hostile feelings can increase his guilt and depression. But discussing guilt is apt to help relieve it. In this case it was possible gradually to talk about it, with considerable relief to the man.

Guilt Toward Family

Another example of combat as a specific mobilizer of emotional reactions which then persist was furnished by the following quiet, modest, young electrician. In this case, guilt was the central cause of the condition. His interview went somewhat as follows:

His worst symptoms, he said, were a pervading sense of anxiety and dizzy spells, severe enough to cause him to fall if he did not sit down. He also suffered from headaches, insomnia, battle dreams and nausea. He had become shy with people, had come to dislike crowds and suffered from a general sense of inferiority and a tendency to withdraw emotionally. At a dance for servicemen, where he knew with his intellect that no girl would refuse him, he would hesitate to ask anyone for a dance because of the feeling in his heart that he might be refused.

In the Navy he had had sea duty almost continually, working below decks. During the first submarine attack, he was not especially frightened; but the second occurred suddenly when the men were at chow. As they scrambled for the ladders in rushing to their battle stations, the patient, unable to get up the ladder because of the crowd, felt trapped and developed his first dizzy spell. This was a vague sensation, which he could describe only as his head feeling "loose," his vision being somewhat disturbed, and the room seeming to spin, or rather roll, like a ship at sea. Although he had had his other symptoms all his life, the dizzy spells dated from this incident. In large part, because of his devotion to his ship and his wish to stay with her, he managed to hide these dizzy spells by sitting down on one pretext or another so that he never actually keeled over.

During the invasion of an island, the patient being below decks in the engine room, our air cover turned to meet the threat of an approaching enemy task force, and several enemy planes, sneaking in over the mountains, bore in upon the patient's small vessel. One crashed on the bridge, killing the officers and half the crew and tearing a huge hole in the deck.

The patient, wearied by 48 hours without sleep, was shaken by the blast and expected the ship to sink, but as the bloody waters slackened in their flow about his feet, he guessed what the situation was. One propeller was gouging the side of the ship, but the only hope was to keep moving. Although shaking like a leaf, the patient was able to keep the engines going. The following morning, he and an engineer kept up sufficient power to creep into a newly captured port. But instead of receiving hoped-for repairs, they lost certain guns and other equipment because they seemed too badly damaged to have further use for items which less damaged ships sorely needed. To their distress, it became necessary to make a long trip over a vast stretch of the ocean with a hole in the deck so huge that a moderate sea would have swamped the now barely seaworthy craft.

Eventually, as it turned out, the whole crossing was made, and a United States port was reached. The patient was granted a ten-day furlough. He traveled home across the continent by airplane. Here he had no complaints, but his mother noticed that his appetite was not quite up to normal, being somewhat impaired since his days of eating from tins outside the mess hall, which, just after being hit, was used as a morgue for his shipmates.

This young man was, as he had always been, shy, retiring and unobtrusive. He was not the type to win medals, nor did he feel that he had done more than his duty. Yet, he had not only done it in the face of terrible physical and emotional hazards but had accomplished his job in spite of quaking with fear and retching with nausea. How hard it is to tell who the heroes are in a war!

Asked what about the Navy most upset him, he immediately replied, "The fear of seeing the dead and the injured." Discussing with him some of the other things which built up severe emotional reactions in some men, he said that he liked the Navy, although he did not plan to stay in permanently. There were various things, such as standing inspection in the morning after putting in 30 or 40 hours during attacks, but he accepted these as part of military life and had no strong feeling against them. His feelings were in contrast with those of other men we have mentioned who did not mind occasional action but could not stand other pressures engendered by military life.

The interview was now directed toward finding the patient's reason for his specific sensitivity. It was immediately apparent that whereas he spoke freely of his battle experiences and seemed to obtain some release and relief by so doing, he now strongly resisted speaking of his feelings toward his family, and it soon became clear that it was this which had troubled him more severely than his memories of his battle experiences, harrowing as some of these were. He could pour out such episodes as how his appetite had fallen off after having to eat in the near presence and stench of mangled bodies decaying below deck in the stifling heat, but he could not stand speaking of his feelings toward his father.

Shying off questions as to his personal feelings, the patient reverted to the easier topic of his symptoms. His recurrent sleep-disturbing nightmare was a repetition of the real situation in which an enemy plane suicide-dived onto the bridge of his ship. In response to further questioning, he said that he had had nightmares all his life. Thus, only the form of the nightmare had changed. Since early childhood he had dreamed of wanting to run away and being unable to run, while now he dreamed of the approaching enemy plane. The interview threatened to peter out, although obviously he was disturbed by something he had not told. Since it would be impossible to help him without understanding the sources of his disturbance and something of the main motivations of his personality, an approach was tried which is generally successful. He was told the truth bluntly—that such dreams of fear and violence, still persisting although he was out of it with little chance of further sea duty, could arise only from some feelings in himself which he hated to admit but on which helping him depended. Perhaps he was very angry or perhaps very guilty about something. The patient responded to this slowly and, with some distress, told his story.

He denied having any anger at his father, but admitted that he used to. His father used to drink, and he would beat his son terribly and sometimes would attack his mother. This had gone on ever since the patient's early childhood. But worse than the beatings were the father's threats; and the nights when he implemented these by brandishing a loaded gun, the patient almost went crazy with fear. He could never hate his father unrestrainedly with a soul-satisfying hate, because on too many occasions the father would be nice to him. Because of also loving his father and of craving his love, his hate caused a pervading sense of guilt toward him. As the interview progressed, the patient now revealed something which he had never admitted even to himself and the force of which he had never appreciated, namely, his burning rage at his father's preference for his brother. This brother, only a year younger, was always favored by the father, who made a pet of him and never beat him. He literally took food out of the mouths of the rest of the family in order to spend the money on extravagant presents for this brother. The patient told all this with intense feelings of guilt and shame. He almost interpreted his dream himself, for he said that he felt he deserved to be killed for the intolerable unfilial feelings he harbored toward his brother and father. For this he deserved to be bombed by the enemy.

Thus, his own conscience was aligned with the enemy. It was a fifth column within his own mind. He feared danger more than the man with a clear conscience did, because to him danger was not only a threat but also an actual temptation to get himself killed or injured. It was this neurotic need to get himself punished which heightened the real danger for him and hence made him sensitive to it. Danger became a flame which lured him like a moth, a maelstrom sucking him down against his own struggling to be free. He was attracted to violence for the satisfaction of his own hostile feelings, but also for the satisfaction of his guilt and need for punishment. Therefore, he also dreaded it. In the balance of these forces only a slight quantitative shift could make the difference between a coward and a hero.

The danger, the hardship, the overwork, the horror and other traumas sustained by this youngster were probably sufficient to cause symptoms in the average man. Certainly under stress severe enough and prolonged enough everyone breaks down (Appel, 1946). But it is still of great practical as well as theoretical importance to know why some break before others, and just what are the mechanisms of resistance to stress and of vulnerability to it. Being concerned with therapy, our attention focuses upon the problem of breakdown and of a rational approach to its treatment and, eventually, to its prevention so far as this is possible—which is very considerable. Therefore, we shall not have occasion to study the fascinating subject of heroism. But certainly it is often a matter of masochistic, sometimes even self-destructive trends as well as of maturity of personality and strength of ego.

Now, in the interview the cards were on the table, and the patient spoke more frankly. He told how all his life he had wanted to escape from the fears and the hostilities in his home but was too dependent on his family to leave, too insecure about taking care of himself. He wanted to go away but did not want to be without a home. He thereby revealed the meaning of his repetitive nightmares of childhood—wanting to run away but being unable to do so.

Adults generally maintain with amazing exactness the emotional patterns of their childhood relationships to the members of their families. Since early childhood this man had lived in terror in his own family, wanting to leave but staying and enduring the fear. Then he did the same thing in the Navy. He came to join the Navy because of an especially heated episode at home. Now he admitted that although his father had improved noticeably, yet he could not be around him without arguments occurring, emotional tension developing, and the patient's symptoms becoming worse. It was this emotional situation at home that caused the patient's symptoms to become worse on his trips home and made him prefer remaining at the hospital.

This discussion of the major emotions which disturbed the patient, of his central conflicts that were the core of his troubles, served noticeably to decrease his guilt and anxiety. Insight tends to turn vague unknown threats and difficulties into conscious problems, to replace a mysterious unconscious or only partly conscious "neurosis" with conscious problems, however difficult these problems may be. Even this patient's deeply rooted, pervasive guilt and anxiety were perceptibly relieved by his understanding of how inevitable these reactions were to the treatment he had received. Now, in addition to discussing his own emotional reactions, it was possible to discuss thoroughly, on the basis of our understanding, the advisability of such practical steps as going through with his engagement, marrying and setting up his own home away from his father and the inevitable tensions in this paternal relationship. This interview lasted nearly one and one-half hours.

There is a great therapeutic advantage, and much time is saved if it is possible to take so long for an interview when this is necessary; for in many cases when the interview is interrupted before penetrating to the core of the problem, the golden opportunity is lost, and again to bring the man to the point of revealing the essence of his emotional problems, which usually involves the core of his personality, the psychiatrist must start from scratch. It takes a certain continuous period, a certain emotional development and progression in the interview to work into the deeper motivations. They can be elicited only gradually and with a certain continuity. The emotions build up dramatically during the interview as they reveal themselves, and if the core is grasped, relief comes with the force of a denouement—the pay-off, the reward for the concentration and the emotional effort.

Rivalry with brothers and sisters is one of the commonest sources of envy, jealousy, anger, hostility and, consequently, of guilt. The following case illustrates how this frequently operates and also shows something of the operation of guilt and shame and of the relationships between these feelings. Usually, but not always, shame tends to drive the man to action and achievement; guilt causes anxiety and depression, blocks his action and makes him want to retreat.

The first interview with a 21-year-old, married seaman went as follows:

Asked how he came to be at the hospital, he said that he had been at sea for two years and had survived considerable action and a sinking. But later a plane scored a bomb hit. The patient was knocked down and was badly burned. He remembered little of the following week, but since then had suffered loss of appetite and of 40 pounds in weight, had nightmares, showed startle reaction, irritability, inability to tolerate noise or people; he stuttered and had headaches and difficulties in memory and concentration.

Asked to describe his background, he revealed nothing unusual, but in his description he spontaneously stressed how close both he and his older brother were to his father, and the success of this brother, who also was in the Navy.

Questioned as to when his symptoms began, he at first dated them to the bombing but then recalled having them prior to this, only in lesser degree. Then, satisfied that the interviewer was sincere in trying to help him, he began to pour out his story.

At first he described the bombings and his injuries in great detail and how he remained at his post, confident that the enemy plane would be brought down, only to have it get through. For his own action he was rewarded with a medal. For months before this episode he had been getting more and more tense, and these same symptoms had been increasing gradually. What irritated him most were the drills and the calls to general quarters, but, above all, the terrible fear. Just before this last bombing, though, he seemed to have reached a sort of adjustment to it, by feeling that he "no longer gave a damn."

His immediate shipmates had irritated him increasingly. Now it was so bad that he could no longer stand people at all and would leave amusements and even walk out of parties and away from pretty girls. He could hardly bear even to be with his wife in his present condition.

Then, as so many of these men do, he spontaneously told of his poor sleep and related two of the nightmares he had had recently, and these, as usual, went directly to the hub of his emotional problem.

In the first dream he was aboard a ship, injured and on a stretcher. A shipmate, who never really was wounded and resembled his brother, appeared to be badly injured and said to him, "You are able-bodied—get up and let me lie on the stretcher." In the second dream, the patient was in a harbor on his way out to sea again and felt distressed.

We discussed these dreams, and I pointed out his feelings in both of them that he should return to duty—that he felt guilty and ashamed of lying down, of being cared for here at the hospital. He started at this and heatedly said that his brother and all his friends were still in military service, and if he got a medical discharge, especially with a psychiatric diagnosis, he would be the only one to be going out. I pointed out that he felt this obligation to return to duty but that he also feared and resisted doing so.

We then discussed his dreaming that the shipmate was injured, when, in reality, he had never been hurt, and this led him, with much emotion and stuttering, to bring out his resentment of his own condition—his burns and his emotional disorder, which threatened to ruin his life. I pointed out that, opposed to his urge to return, was the wish to lie down on the stretcher, not to leave the harbor, to be out of it and let others go to face hardships and danger and be wounded. He was visibly agitated now, and his stuttering vanished in his outpouring.

This, he said, must be why he couldn't stand amusement places, parties, people. For these people had it soft and let others, like him, suffer. He started to say that he hated them for this, but then stopped, saying that that was no way to feel, that he now got mad at himself for feeling that way. We discussed this—how he couldn't enjoy himself here for thinking of his brother and shipmates out there. But this only kept him miserable and didn't help them. Nor would it help him if civilians too were doleful for thinking of the men overseas. He saw the force of his rage, something of its sources. His relief even at this point was marked and was noticed in the next few days by others. He was starting on the upgrade and now had recovered hope and the beginnings of the capacity to face and enjoy life again.

Later we went further, and the essence of this conflict, hinted at in these dreams, emerged more clearly. Without realizing it, he was competing with his more handsome, brilliant and popular brother, with whom he had always been closely associated. This situation caused an undercurrent of resentment, which, because of the closeness and the love between them, resulted in the patient's feeling very guilty for his envy and hostile rivalry. This unconscious hostile rivalry and guilt had carried over into the Navy, where the brother, as usual, was a step ahead of him.

The patient's guilt had made him feel that he *deserved* to be injured and so had created the inner anxiety, arising from his own feelings, which predisposed him to anxiety neurosis. This conscience reaction to his own underlying, intolerable hostility to his loved brother made him feel that he should be punished, tempted him to self-injury and so, through this fifth column in his own mind, added inner anxiety to real fear. Rather, the real danger mobilized this anxiety and so exaggerated the normal fear response. Hence, he lived under terrible fear. And just after giving in to it, and "no longer giving a damn," he was injured. And now it came out that the injury was in reality caused in large part by himself, since previously he had ducked behind protecting steel plate, but this time, when he should properly have done so, he did not.

Now his competition with his brother and his sense of shame and guilt at "lying down" here, while the brother was out, drove him to want to return to combat. But his fear of sea duty was so heightened by his own anxiety from guilt toward his brother for this competitiveness that he could not bear to face it. Reducing his competitiveness toward his brother through insight and discussion reduced the compulsion to go out again and also the shame at being here, and increased his capacity to act rationally rather than under the domination of his feelings toward his brother.

He showed two opposite reactions. In part, he wanted to go back. His sense of duty, his masculine pride, his competition with his brother and with other men impelled him to do so. And so did his guilt toward them and his feeling that he should not let them suffer alone. But his guilt also intensified his fear. He felt that he should suffer what they did, that he should suffer as, secretly, he was satisfied that his competitors should.

This was an entirely human reaction and a common source of guilt. Hence, he felt driven to return to duty, but also he feared and hated it and wanted to escape from it all and lie down. But this filled him with feelings of shame and of inferiority toward those who were carrying on. If he went, he feared it and hated it and envied and hated those who were safely at home. If he stayed, he felt ashamed and inferior and hated himself and envied those who went. He was in conflict in his own breast. But he began to see and understand the problem.

This man was seen for a total of less than two hours. The remarkable fact is the relief that the therapist can give and how much the patient can do with even deep motivations such as these, in a mere one or two hours in favorable cases, if it is possible to grasp accurately the core of the emotional dynamics. If some results are not achieved in this time at the most, then usually they will not be achieved at all through this method, except over a long period of time.

FURTHER OBSERVATIONS ON HOSTILITY

Because of the fact that people react with anger (the fight part of the fight-flight response) to any irritation or dissatisfaction with the outer world or with themselves, anger occupies a unique and central position in human life. How much anger is generated, the forms it takes, how it is controlled and expressed—these are of vital importance in the organization of personality, in the formation of neuroses and in man's social behavior (Saul, 1976). Because of the importance of anger in causing symptoms, the results obtainable by dealing with this anger, even without touching anything else, are often surprisingly good.

In one case, a depressed and sullen young man of 21 improved materially after one interview. At first it seemed that his symptoms dated to the loss of his buddy. If he came across his friend's name, he could hardly control his emotions and would often become enraged at anyone who innocently spoke to him at such times. He had felt his friend to be part of himself, and his loss, even after months, seemed irreparable. But there was one circumstance under which the patient felt his old self and even lost his severe and distressing symptoms. This was when he was at home with his wife, toward whom he said he felt so close that she seemed to be a part of him. When with her, he could relax, read quietly and be at ease.

As the psychologically sophisticated reader may have guessed by now, this man had an older brother with whom he had been extremely close. When the war came, our young man felt motivated by patriotism and a sense of adventure to go into the service.

In his remarks there was often more than a hint of resentment for what he had been through while others remained safely at home. His whole three years in military service were spent at sea. He saw much action, for which he rated a score of battle stars, but fortunately his ship experienced no serious hits or casualties. Apparently, he had adapted well to shipboard life. When he got home on leave, he found himself to be tense, restless and irritable. In retrospect, he could only think that he had felt the strain more than he had realized and had developed more resentment than he knew. This was a most important observation and was true of a great many men. Long after his return home he would become angry when recounting his experiences.

He was regularly on duty for long periods. He was proud to be able to take it, but it was too much, and the strain told. Then, after his leave, he went to sea again. This time he was more conscious of the strain and of mounting anger, but he was determined to keep going and not to get on the sick list. As his anger mounted, he developed pains in his joints. (One gets the impression that these muscle and joint symptoms occur most frequently in the athletic type of individual when under emotional stress, particularly anger.) Often his head would throb. His irritability got worse and worse, until he could hardly get along with anyone. He was angered by many things—the strain of his responsibilities, the comparison of his duties with those of the well-paid civilian workers who repaired his ship, the feeling of not receiving credit in the early days when his ship was almost alone in many extremely dangerous positions. Thus, for many months before his buddy was killed, he had felt "fed up with the set up," and that he could stand it no longer. The loss of his friend was the final blow. The patient felt that it need not have happened, and he boiled with inner rage.

Even so, it was only some months later, when he was forced to turn in because of a physical illness, that he was kept on the sick list because of his emotionally caused symptoms. By this time he was extremely tense, and his irritability and restlessness were so severe that he could not get along with anyone. He also suffered from splitting headaches, from disturbed sleep and from occasional nightmares which involved his buddy.

It turned out that besides his other symptoms, he regularly walked several miles from the hospital to his home rather than take a bus, because he felt that the other passengers all stared at him because he was so husky and yet was a patient at the hospital. This man was frighteningly sullen in his attitude and behavior. Obviously, he harbored a bitter resentment, which suffused his being, influenced his movements and blazed from his eyes.

In psychotherapy, it is a guiding principle to deal with those emotions which are *central,* to prevent confusion by shunning the peripheral, the detailed, the minutiae. In this case, the central emotion was clearly belligerent hostility. In such a state of rage, no wonder he was restless and could not concentrate, could not relax, was tense, could not sleep well and had dreams of violence; and when people are filled with anger, more anger than they can hold, they very often begin to feel that others are looking at them, that is, they project it into others.

In this case, we began with the simplest explanation of his feeling that people stared at him because he was so husky and yet a patient. This, I told him, was his own opinion of himself. Because he felt thus ashamed of *himself,* he thought others had the same opinion of him. But they did not. Nor was his self-criticism justified. Quite the opposite. He had served well. At this, he laughed nervously. We went on to deal directly with his rage.

The reason that he was a patient, even though physically so well and powerful, was because of rage in his soul, not germs in his body. It was this rage which caused all the symptoms, and we discussed how it did so. It was a rage which had built up over a long period, because of his particular, individual reactions to the stringencies of military life and the demands of his duties. But now fuming was unnecessary. He might as well rage against the weather. If he were a reformer and did something constructive with his anger, it would serve a purpose, but, as things were, it only kept him sick. If he could not change reality, then he might as well adapt to it and recover his peace of mind. As long as he seethed with rage, he would suffer with symptoms.

After this, the patient fell silent. It was only later that I learned he had not rejected the interpretation but had been greatly impressed and relieved. Such an interpretation ordinarily can be given only when the patient is ready and able to receive it, when it deals with feelings which the patient is close to realizing himself and when it is *accurate*. The patient must not consider it to be true because the psychiatrist says so, but because it *is* the truth, and a truth which he is in an emotional position to grasp.

He was now in a position to attack the problem of the emotional adjustment to the loss of his buddy. In the first place, his wife filled this emotional gap to a considerable extent, and arrangements were made for him to be with her as much as possible. Secondly, the recovery of his ability to be pleasant with people now made it possible for him to replace his loss with other friends. Lastly, he had now settled down sufficiently emotionally so that the resentment, which so often underlies very close human relationships, and the guilt it occasions, could be discussed quietly and safely.

This young man illustrates one of the commonest precipitants of breakdown, namely, the loss of a buddy. Often the man feels so closely identified with the buddy that the loss not only robs him of what seems to be part of himself but also shatters the common delusion that only other people will be injured or killed, not we ourselves or our close friends. Moreover, the emotional support that the friend provided is lost, as well as the outlet for so many feelings which another person close to one affords. All this often heightens a man's rage as well as anxiety to an intensity beyond his control and also very frequently arouses the undercurrent of resentment and guilt. In this particular case, the loss of the buddy also illustrates a frequently observed point—how a certain event may be not the sole cause of a man's reactions but rather the final climactic blow or only the last straw. In fact, no single event can ever safely be taken at face value as being the *sole cause* of combat fatigue.

The third point demonstrated is the importance of the rage reaction, and how dealing with it can sometimes reduce the emotional tension and thereby make it possible to deal much more safely and effectively with a man's other emotional problems.

REFERENCES

Alexander, F. and Healy, W. (1935): *Roots of Crime.* New York: Knopf.

Appel, J. (1946): Preventive psychiatry: an epidemologic approach, *Journal of the American Medical Association* 131:1469.

French, T. (1939): Insight and distortion in dreams, *International Journal of Psycho-analysis* 20:287.

Freud, S. (1917): Introductory lectures on psychoanalysis, Part III, general theory of the neuroses, Lecture 18, *S.E.* 16.

Grinker, R. and Spiegel, J. (1945): *Men Under Stress.* Philadelphia: Blakiston.

Kardiner, A. (1941): Traumatic neurosis of war, *Psychosomatic Medicine,* Monograph Series I, Nos. 2 & 3.

Rado, S. (1942): Pathodynamics and treatment of traumatic war neurosis, *Psychosomatic Medicine* 4:362.

Saul, L. J. (1976): *Psychodynamics of Hostility.* New York: Jason Aronson.

12 | Other Stresses

Many indeed are man's emotional vulnerabilities. A prepossessing young soldier had been through the thick of it. Some of the most terrible duties of this war had fallen to his lot—he was a flamethrower. Yet, apparently, he was affected but little by this grisly job he was called upon to do. Sometimes it stirred a certain amount of aggressiveness and satisfaction, at other times a twinge of conscience. Sometimes the flamethrowing appeared in his dreams, but this was only occasionally.

Then he was returned to the United States. Gradually, he became so tense and gloomy that he had to get help. In the first interview, it came out that his main irritation was the feeling that he had been exploited without credit or gratitude, that for all his arduous, dangerous, grim work of two years he received only discipline but no credit, and, back in the States, but meager recognition or appreciation.

His early life quickly revealed why he was so sensitive on this score. He was an adored only child. A great and tragic change came into his life at the age of nine when both parents died, and he was reared by relatives who now used him all they could, with little love or reward. As he grew older, the odd jobs piled on, until almost all his spare time was spent in working, yet he was never given even a quarter to go to a movie. Finally, when he was adolescent, he left home. The scar of this experience remained upon his feelings. One might say that an "allergy" to such experiences had been developed. He was now hypersensitive on the point of feeling used and exploited without receiving sufficient love, interest and appreciation for his efforts and accomplishments. A hero of repeated bloodcurdling engagements, he endured without complaining long hardship and constant danger. This did not faze him. What broke him was his hypersensitive need for appreciation and reward.

A neat demonstration of how individual these reactions are was given by two men who came to my office, one right after the other. The first of these had seen no action at all except for dropping depth charges on one occasion. But his anxiety became so great at the end of the year that he broke down. At general quarters he would shake like a leaf and often lose control of his bowels or bladder. He developed a constant state of fear, with tension, tremors, nausea and a severe startle reaction. He became unable to tolerate people or even music.

The next man had been overseas for over two years and had seen all kinds of action, including six major engagements, packed with close calls and hair-raising sights and experiences. He was irked by the restrictions of the service, the work, the hours and the heat, and he felt tired out. But he never minded combat. He had no startle reaction and no nightmares. His appetite remained good, and the fear he felt, when in danger, never continued as tension and anxiety. Thus, the man who had not experienced combat and was at sea only six months developed a severe combat fatigue, while the man who had been through repeated action for over two years did not.

How specific these vulnerabilities are is further illustrated by the following.

A 44-year-old marine developed depression, headaches, fatigue, loss of appetite, constipation and loss of 40 pounds in weight, and was evacuated. He had served as a cook at Guadalcanal through the first months of World War II. He had very little fear of action and bombings and had unusual endurance in the face of overwork, little sleep and poor living conditions. He was devoted to his work and had special pride in serving the best mess possible to the men with what supplies were available.

These were adequate until he became dependent on the Army Commissary, when the supplies became meager, and the men began to complain seriously. When he was forced to cut sausages in half and serve one and a half to each man, he himself felt guilty and ashamed and felt deeply the sharp kidding and cutting remarks to which he was subjected by the men. The loss of their good will and the facing of their resentment was what he, who could tolerate insufficient sleep, overwork and combat bombing, could *not* stand. He tried to continue, but his symptoms finally incapacitated him.

Still another example is a young man who showed little fear of enemy action but was deplorably afraid of getting put on report. In fact, the reason I saw him was that at a captain's inspection he became so frightened that he turned pale, trembled and nearly fainted.

Then there are those conscientious objectors who willingly accept dangerous jobs but, apart from religious principles, cannot tolerate being in the armed forces. Yet many of them who volunteer for medical experiments with dire diseases actually run greater risks of injury and death than if they were in the military service. It is not death itself some fear so much, but certain emotional conditions.

Innumerable are the stresses of military life. We have mentioned only some of them and have even omitted some which are of first importance. For example, there are the stresses arising from the misplacement of personnel, which is unavoidable in any vast and rapidly expanding organization. There are bound to be many men who hold jobs beyond their capacities, and many others whose capacities far exceed their jobs; some abuse their powers and some cannot bear receiving the abuse; some find themselves in duties remote from their interests, such as the young man with a passion for things mechanical who found himself doing clerical work which he despised. Dissatisfaction with a job can produce tensions, which sometimes become pressing enough to break through as symptoms.

Our aim is not to describe every type of stress but only to give sufficient examples to demonstrate our main point, namely, that the men who develop combat or operational fatigue react to the various stresses in accordance with their own particular make-ups, the emotional vulnerabilities in their childhood emotional patterns, gradually, as the months go by, becoming, as they put it, "fed up" and "disgusted," until they become defensively aroused against the situation, filled with fear and anger and wanting to flee. They become irritable, restless and anxious and show other signs and symptoms of being thus frightened and angered and turning from and against everything that is painful or even reminds them of such situations—flight and fight.

Examples have been selected in which certain particular stresses predominate. This makes it easier to observe the different stresses and their effects one at a time. However, it should be borne in mind, that in each case a *combination of stresses* operates and a variety of reactions to them occurs, and also that under the strain of prolonged combat it is the constant danger that generally overshadows all other stresses.

REACTIONS TO PHYSICAL INJURY

How a certain young man reacted to physical injury casts further light on the war neuroses and on breakdowns in general.

This quiet, slim, friendly 19-year-old submariner was sent to the hospital with the diagnosis of combat fatigue because of nervousness, stuttering, loss of appetite and of weight, irritability and nightmares, all of which began after an accidental bullet wound of the leg one year before. Previous to this, he had had intensive combat experience, so that, at first, his condition seemed to be a direct result of the action which he had been through. Gradually, however, his story came out, and the impression it gave was very different.

He had enlisted in the Navy and after a year of training went out on submarine duty. He operated in enemy waters and saw repeated action. His ship was forced under by a bomber, depth-bombed again and again by destroyers and subjected to shelling. He kindly put at my disposal the following notes on his battle experiences, which he wrote in simple, unemotional style, after the first interview.

Around the end of October we left for our first real mission. We went to the —— Islands where we were to keep anything from getting in or out of the —— Pass. The first day we were there we saw two merchantmen and a new-type destroyer. We made an attack about ten o'clock in the morning. We fired six torpedoes, but the enemy "can" (destroyer) saw them before they got to the targets, and he started after us. We were at 65 feet at that time, so we went down to 400 feet. He dropped eight depth charges on his first run over us. Then he came back and dropped eight more. He seemed to know right where we were. The next run he dropped eight more, but not on top of us—they were off our starboard beam. He gave up after that and went off to try to protect the other ship that was left. We sank the largest of the three. All we got out of it was a caved-in deck, and a sea valve was sprung. But we were still able to continue our patrol.

During the depth-charge attack I was plenty scared, more scared than I can describe. But after it was over I went right back to my old pastime of eating. I ate almost all the time I was in the submarines. I guess that's why I went from 145 to 160 pounds. I wasn't fat, and I'm not bragging when I say it was all muscle.

The morning after our attack, a two-motor "Betty" flew right over us while we were on the surface. She missed us by about 25 feet. She turned to come back to get us, and we went to 90 feet before she dropped one on us. It didn't do any damage but did push our bow down. I was sleeping until the charge went off. Then I woke up and didn't know whether to be scared or not. I was, though, when our bow went down.

I was lying with my head aft. And when we started to go down after the charge went off, my feet came up against the bulkhead and I was standing on the bulkhead. What I mean is, all my weight was on my feet, but I was still lying in bed. When I found out what the score was, I was all right. But for a few minutes, I thought we were going down for good.

A few days after that we saw an enemy cruiser. We made contact about 1900 (7:00 P.M.). We chased it for almost eight hours but couldn't get close enough to fire torpedoes. We finally lost it. That day I got up at 0700 (7:00 A.M.) and didn't get to bed until 0400 (4:00 A.M.) the following morning. I was on the sound gear for 13 hours out of the 21 that I was awake. But I minded hardly at all. I was tired but I felt all right otherwise. I got three hours' sleep, then went on the sound gear again for four more hours. But I still didn't mind it, apart from the fact that I was tired.

The rest of the time we were there we took pictures of the Islands. We did this while we were submerged, and it was my job to keep us from going on the reefs, but I could hear them over the sound gear. So I had to give them an idea of how much leeway we had. I had to make a report every minute. Taking those pictures was a lot more dangerous than it sounds, but I still didn't mind the strain.

From there we went east to —— in the —— Islands. Our first night there we picked up a freighter (enemy) and her escort. We made an attack on the surface and put one "fish" into the freighter. She must have been carrying lumber, because we bumped into some logs the next day. After the ship was hit, the escort started to throw depth charges and shells all around the area. We were laughing until we learned about the shells. Then it was a different story. We pulled away from the scene and went down out of the way.

The rest of our time there was spent eluding enemy planes and patrol boats. We made surface patrol except for when planes chased us down. We were chased down about two or three times every day. At night we played tag with the patrol boats. It wasn't a very nice pastime.

The day we were to leave that area we ran into an enemy transport and her escort. We sank the transport about 1100 (11:00 A.M.). But the escort dropped depth charges all day, off and on, until 2000 (8:00 P.M.) that evening. We surfaced at 2100 (9:00 P.M.) and started for —— via —— Island. When we got into —— in December, I was transferred to the tender. I was transferred on a rotation of crews plan that is in use in Sub Service.

My duty on the tender was the worst I had ever endured. We left Christmas Day, for —— . That trip, which only lasted three days, was far worse than the two months' combat duty I did on the submarine. I didn't sleep at all for three days and hardly ate anything. I stayed up on the boat deck almost the whole trip, just waiting for a submarine to come along and sink us.*

I got a week's rest at the —— Hotel. We worked hard while we were in port, but I didn't mind it. When the —— came in again, the skipper requested that I be transferred back aboard. And I was—about the middle of March. We went on trials, then went out on patrol. We stopped at —— Island to refuel on the fourth day of April. One day later I was wounded in the left leg.

The blow spun the patient around, but he did not lose consciousness. He was terribly upset, trembling, weeping and vomiting. He was taken to a base, an operation was performed the following day, and he slept for most of the following week.

Then his symptoms began to subside, and his mind cleared. He looked down, and with the greatest relief saw that his leg had not been amputated. With this, his spirits began to improve rapidly.

As I discussed with him at length the reasons for his first emotional upset, it was impossible to pin it on anything except the *suddenness* of the transition, which was more than he could comprehend or digest. It was not the fear of losing his leg, for at first it never occurred to him that there was any danger of this. What he could not get over was the fact that he had been standing there, feeling happy and at peace with the world, and an instant later he was seriously wounded. It was the unexpected suddenness which he could not comprehend, and he shook and wept and vomited. But after the first week, he seemed on the way to a speedy and uneventful recovery.

Then, one month later in the hospital, he asked the doctor when his leg would be well. The doctor asked him if he had ever done any running. He had enjoyed track in school, so he said, "Yes," whereupon he was told gently that he would never run again. This was a thunderbolt from the blue, for it had never once occurred to

* This account mentions a psychological mechanism of considerable important, namely, a constant, intolerable fear while on the tender, which stood in such contrast with the writer's equanimity while on the submarine. Apparently, his aggression was so identified with submarines that ingrained in his feeling (partly by simple conditioning) was the sense that submarines attacked surface ships; so when he himself was on a surface ship, his fear of submarines was exaggerated. It is true, I believe, that most men found these tenders to be good duty and thought of them as more comfortable and safer than submarines. Now in civil life, a man may be hostile to another because, for example, of competition and of envying him for his possessions or position. If the man himself now displaces the one he envies, or even achieves these successes himself, then, just like this submariner on the surface vessel, he often reacts with anxiety lest something happen to him, i.e., it is imbued in him that hostility is directed to the man who is in the enviable position, which therefore is seen as dangerous. This was discussed in a previous chapter.

him that his leg would not heal completely. At that moment, his present symptoms burst out. His appetite fell off, and his weight gradually went down from 160 to 115 pounds. He developed considerable stammering. He trembled so that he could not write a letter, and when he thought of the future, he would be overwhelmed with sobs. What was his future? To understand it, let us dip into his past.

His early life revealed little that was unusual. His home was apparently externally average and emotionally congenial. He was idolized by a considerably younger sister. The one he seemed closest to was his father, whose love of sports the patient soon learned to share, and whose tales of his experiences in World War I led the boy to an interest in the glamour of military life. From his earliest days, he thought of a career in uniform, and when, at the age of ten, a submarine sailor visited his school and talked about submarines, how they could submerge undetected beneath the ocean, rise at will to see, move without being seen, the boy was transported and lived in almost a daze for the next two weeks. Now his ambition was set—submarines were his life choice.

After Pearl Harbor, although he had wanted to finish high school, he could not resist the urge to enlist. The rigid tests, physical and mental, which he passed, while so many others flunked out, only added zest and prestige to being a submariner. As such, he enjoyed the satisfaction of knowing himself to be one of the elite in the military service.

I enlisted in the Navy on my 17th birthday. I wanted to enlist right after the attack on Pearl Harbor, but I was too young. We were sent to —— for "boot" (basic) training. I was well pleased and glad I had enlisted in the regular Navy.

While in boot camp, I volunteered for submarine duty. Out of 15 who volunteered, I was the only one who could pass the I.Q. test. There were only 25 in the whole camp who passed it. We 25 then took a physical examination for sub duty. Only three passed, I being one of the three. I was very proud of myself, because they were plenty strict in picking submarine men.

After that, we were sent to the rifle range to wait for openings at sub school.

A few days after our arrival at sub school, we were given another physical. I learned there that we were going through the final physical before entering sub school. One of the fellows who came with me was turned down there. One week later we were given the pressure test. We had to take 50 pounds per square inch. A few days after that, we were taught how to make escapes from subs. We made escapes from 50 feet below the surface of the water.

Sub school lasted for six weeks. We went out on subs two or three times a week during the school, so that we could get practical experience. After I finished sub school, I went to the submarine torpedo school. I received the highest mark in our class on the final exam. And I again felt proud of myself, because I was the only one in the class who hadn't finished high school.

After torpedo school I was transferred to the U.S.S. —— for duty. All my duty aboard her was to train me further for the combat duty that was coming. And that is what I was waiting for. The more I learned about subs, the better I liked them. "Like" really isn't the word to describe my feelings towards subs, it's more a form of "love." Every submarine man has the same feeling or he couldn't stay in submarines. Every man aboard a sub feels that it's his. And every man tries to make her the best in the Fleet. He wants to make a name for *her*, not just so he can get medals, but so that when his ship's name is mentioned it is done so with honor. I was in more than one fight because someone said that he had a better sub than mine. That may sound a little babyish but it really isn't. It is a great insult to have anyone indicate that your sub isn't the best. While we were waiting for the U.S.S. —— to go into commission we played softball for $50 a game, one sub crew against another. We won eight out of the nine games we played.

Finally, we put the —— into commission. She was and is the best ship that ever sailed the seas. Her crew and officers also were the best. Ask the crew of the ——. They doubted it at one time.

As the patient discussed the fact that his whole life plan was now in ruins, that he could never go back to submarines, upon which he had set his heart, his face flushed and he bent his head, sobbing. This, and this alone, he said, was the source of his "nerves," and this, then, was the clue to his nightmares.

The patient told of his poor sleep. His nightmares were all of one kind: he was doing the things he most enjoyed—chatting with the crew on his submarine, fishing, playing baseball—when in the midst of his enjoyment, and for no reason that had any connection whatsoever with the scene, suddenly a shot would ring out, and he would awake with a start. When it was pointed out that this dream accurately reflected his feelings about his life—his enjoyment of the present and his anticipations of the future all shattered with a single shot—he gave a little hysterical laugh and was deeply touched.

We discussed his problem from many angles—how hard it is to know what's best for one—he might have recovered fully and then had both legs blown off. His naval experience had already interested him in electricity, and arrangements would be made immediately for him to take a course in this subject as well as to finish high school by correspondence course. We figured out ways such as these of meeting the situation externally, while at the same time making clear his primary psychological task, namely, to have the courage, the flexibility and the adaptability to develop other interests than sailing on and under the sea as one of the crew of a submarine. His masculine pride was enlisted on the side of adapting and recovering; in discussing courage we pointed out that his adjusting to his present situation would take truer courage than facing the dangers of combat. What he expressed in his words and eyes furnished one of the gratifying rewards of the military psychiatrist—a satisfaction which grew as his improvement continued.

This man's reaction immediately after being wounded confirms the role in the traumatic neuroses of the overwhelming of the forces of control by stimulation more intense and more sudden than the mind is able to comprehend and handle. But *what kept his symptoms going* was not the initial shot but the incidental result of it, namely, the shattering of his plans for his career. In this case, instead of an old emotional problem being mobilized, a new one was suddenly generated.

One of this patient's symptoms was a terrible fear of all guns and ammunition, which became to him the expression not only of his injury but also of his bitter frustration. It is interesting that he tried to recondition himself by carrying a clip of bullets in his pocket, but his fear did not decrease. His own efforts at deconditioning and reconditioning were aided by letting him see, each morning, motion pictures of naval battles, in which he was given control of the sound effects. After ten showings he was no longer startled, even by the loudest noises. To test himself further, he went of his own accord to a newsreel theater and found that he was no longer disturbed and could again attend motion pictures. He fear of shells, guns and firing was now almost gone. He finally resigned himself to another career and became quite normal. Of course, such success cannot be achieved in all cases.

Here was a man whose anxiety and breakdown came not from fear of submarine duty, not from a wish to run away from it, but from not being able to return to it!

It is now some years since this man was receiving treatment, and he reports that he is as enthusiastic about his new career as he was about submarines. He believes that his recovery and his present satisfactory adjustment was made possible by the insight he achieved in those few brief interviews.

The turning against *all* ammunition, manifested by the patient just described, his inability to discriminate between a particular shot and all bullets, is characteristic of the workings of the human mind and is an important source of neurotic symptoms. A man whose father has mistreated him becomes hostile not only to his own father but also may be *conditioned* against all older men whom he considers to be of the father category; similarly, if a man has been jilted by one woman, he may turn against the whole sex and see women as a class rather than as individuals. Some men who sustained bitter experiences with one or two officers become conditioned against all officers. (Thinking in "stereotypes," previously mentioned, is a serious handicap to the perception of reality.) In some men, the failure to discriminate causes a reaction against the entire military service; in other cases, against the whole country and even against the Universe looked upon as Fate.

FAMILY PROBLEMS

This section of this book is about men and not about women (only, of course, because it was men alone who had combat duty and came under the responsibility of the author); but the emotional reactions of women were of vital importance to the men in the military service. Man is born of woman, and *any disturbances in the relationship to the mother leave upon the growing child profound effects* which will shape his personality and perhaps cause neurotic reactions *for life*. Growing up and leaving home free a man physically from his parents, but not from the emotional attitudes and feelings toward them which he has developed during the long period of growth to maturity. After marriage, these attitudes begin to emerge toward the wife, and *rarely does one see a happy marriage when the man has had an unhappy relationship with his mother.* Much in the emotional attachment to the mother repeats itself unconsciously toward the wife. Dire reactions occur in many men when this relationship is threatened. (Of course, childhood patterns to the father, siblings and substitutes also repeat in marriage (Saul, 1979).)

This is always true in life, but it becomes more striking in wartime, when men's emotional relationships to their wives mount in intensity because of the long separation and because of all the experiences and excitements they have lived through far from home in a world of men. Thus it is that vicious circles between husbands and wives are observed so often in wartime.

Under the strain of loneliness, the wife becomes more or less upset. This upsets the husband, who senses it in her letters. His reactions and suspicions disturb her still further and stimulate her worries. He becomes that much more agitated by her responses, and the whole relationship spirals to destruction.

Here one sees a man of indomitable spirit, apparently with nerves of tough fiber, who is little affected by the minor and major shocks and dangers of military life. Danger and the stench of death, blood and boredom, frustration and irritation, cannot rock his smooth-sailing spirit. He goes through the worst of it for nearly three years, unperturbed and in good spirits. Then, by chance, comes word that his wife is stepping out with another man and soon this is confirmed. His mood blackens. He loses interest in life. In the nick of time he is saved from killing himself, but his depression persists. A hero, who is unfazed by battle and the wearing months and years in the service, apparently a man of iron, may yet have an Achilles' heel by which a hundred pounds of femininity can throw him. Not only conscience but love can make cowards of us all. Perhaps he would not have been so shattered by his wife's infidelity if it were not for the three years of service.

An intrepid sailor, unshaken by three torpedoings, many days on a raft and repeated invasions, apparently did not know what fear was and had little concern about being killed. Then he married, and his wife became pregnant. Now, when his orders came to go to sea, he found himself to be a changed man. Suddenly, because of his wife and child, he became afraid to die. He who had so repressed his fear now lived in fear.

Some wives were quick to suspect their husbands of minor and major infidelities. Some seemed to get the idea that all servicemen thought only of their own good times and nothing of their families. This conception often arose from the wife's own frustrations and emotional problems.

These frustrations and emotions of the wife might be no mark of weakness in her. Often the hardships of men in the service were not so great as those quiet but wearing sufferings endured by the wives who were separated from their husbands and left alone with the responsibility for home and children. Many a wife found herself called upon to be a good mother to one, two, three, four or more children on an inadequate income, unable to afford help or to find it even if she could afford it. At any given time, one or another of the children was sure to be in some sort of mischief or trouble or to be ill with a major or minor ailment and to cause extra work, to say nothing of the strain of the anxiety. And doctors were overworked and hard to get to come and had to be paid when they did come. These responsibilities, borne by the wife all alone, while overburdened with the physical work of the home, without help, and short of funds, would be load enough in peacetime. But during the war, fuel was short and food was rationed. The friendly storekeeper had become a suspicious enemy, who gave or withheld necessities, who might say "none left" while favoring another customer. Leisure became an unknown luxury. The pleasures of keeping the home and rearing the children became slavish labor. The wife felt chained to the stove, the sink, the washtubs, worn by all these demands, and destitute of appreciation, emotional support, admiration and love, on which all humans thrive and without which everyone fights or shrivels. Of course, she yearned for freedom, for companionship, for fun, for love, and, of course, the husband's life seemed rosy by comparison with the drab and boring drains upon herself. The danger her husband was facing seemed but a small price to pay for the fellowship and the freedom from her burdens which he enjoyed—and besides, what would the death or injury to her man mean to her and the children for all their lives? The strains on the women were great indeed, and they too developed "war nerves" or "war fatigue." They too became irritable, and, as is human nature, this irritation often turned against the husband, the closest person, the one who had sworn to take responsibility for his wife and children. Of course, women reacted in very many different ways. In some cases, separation from the husband was a return to premarital freedom, which was found too enjoyable to relinquish for a return to the conjugal yoke.

Certain emotions or combinations of them, while affecting the whole body in some degree, seem to affect certain organs more than others. Rage and fear seem to affect the heart; frustrated longings of a certain kind, the stomach, and so on. Therefore, almost every man with combat or operational fatigue (in fact, almost every person who is emotionally upset at all) develops physical symptoms of some sort. Among these men, two types of physical symptoms were seen more frequently than any others: stomach disorders and headaches. Sometimes they occurred after harrowing experiences, sometimes not. But almost always they were caused by the man's emotional upset. It has been suggested that the frequency of stomach symptoms was possibly connected with the observation that our armed forces were described as "the most homesick in history." How such a connection could exist is suggested by the following story.

An affable man in middle life, with sorrowful mien, suffered a perforated ulcer after only three months of increasing loss of appetite (anorexia) and postprandial pain. Supporting his affability, and contrasting with his sad demeanor, he asserted that he had had no troubles at all prior to the development of his symptoms. He enjoyed his duties in the Navy and was eager to go to sea.

This line of inquiry proved to be fruitless, so the patient was asked whether he had any other symptoms, whereupon, bit by bit, he gradually communicated the following train of events.

One day while on the way from his duty station to take his wife to the theater, he was delayed at the station, and two or three hours later found himself in his bunk. About a week later, he suffered another similar "amnesia" (i.e., forgotten period) and again came to in his bunk. He hid this disability from his wife but confided in a buddy and for his own protection never went out about the station without this buddy. However, his wife quickly saw through the fact that the patient's excuses were flimsy. But she began to suspect that these broken appointments were caused by his going out with another woman. A strain appeared in this previously harmonious marriage. Finally, under his wife's insinuations, the patient saw that he had better tell the truth, but now it was too late. His good wife was now sure that the amnesias were only another, and a rather weird, excuse. The patient brought his buddy as witness, but it seemed obvious to the wife that the two of them had cooked up the story together.

Her suspicions were further confirmed by the fact that the poor patient, worn down by his fears of having a mental disturbance as well as by the increasing estrangement of his wife, performed his duties only with effort, so that when he arrived home for week ends he was neither in the mood nor physically fit to afford his wife much attention or pleasure and spent most of his time sleeping and resting in his efforts to keep going. This made it quite obvious to her that he now found his pleasure during the week with another woman and used his home only as a place to rest up. The more insecure the man became, the more his wife reacted, and the more their relationship was undermined. Finally, his wife decided to store the furniture.

As the patient felt his marriage drift upon the rocks, he lost his relish for food. Merely looking at a meal was sufficient to satiate him. He began to develop postprandial epigastric pains (pains after meals in the pit of the stomach), and now this decision of his wife caused exacerbation of his symptoms. Finally, his wife did give up the home, stored the furniture and took a job, so that the patient no longer had his home as a haven for bed and board. It was at this point that the perforation occurred. By now, the patient's confidence was won, and it was easier to obtain his history and to gain some insight into that part of his personality which was related to his gastric symptoms.

His home life as a child had been congenial, but he had been conspicuously close to his mother, whom he spontaneously described as a fine cook. The only boy, with two sisters, he was especially favored by his mother. Always a one-woman man, when he married, he transferred this devotion for his mother to his wife. He had never been interested in any other woman, and they had been married for nearly ten years. His occupation involved repeated moves from one location to another. His wife was his constant companion and each time cooked for him and made a home for him as best she could. Because of this traveling, he was unable to establish any continuous friendships with other persons and thus became all the more dependent on his wife.

Not only had he no other close friends, but he had very little in the way of social and recreational outlets. Except for a little reading and occasional attendance at church, his life consisted of his work, his travel and his home. He had put all his emotional eggs in one basket, and it was for this reason that the loss of his wife's hitherto complete and unswerving devotion caused such a hungering void in him; and because the patient had no other human contacts and no adequate escapes, he could find no substitute satisfactions or consolations for this intense frustration of his emotional needs.

It gradually came out that even in peacetime the patient had had difficulty in adjusting to a military organization to which he had belonged, and now in the military service, during wartime, although he put up a fine front to himself as well as to others, he actually was under intense and mounting emotional pressure.

It was explained to him that only persons under severe emotional tension develop amnesic fugues (forgotten periods) such as his, in which they find themselves somewhere without knowing how they got there.

It was when the time came for him to leave his wife and go overseas to an especially hazardous duty that his fugues developed. Very commonly one finds that a person who is extremely dependent feels inferior because of this and seeks to overcome it by gestures of independence and heroism. This patient strove to be patriotic and heroic but overreached himself emotionally and in his fugues, without realizing what he was doing, would run back to his bed.

It was possible to reconstruct the whole sequence of events—the dependence on his mother, then the dependence on his wife, intensified by the external circumstances, his efforts toward doing the manly thing, the amnesias, his wife's reactions of anger and withdrawal and his inability to find any substitutes or consolation for this loss, the continuing frustration of his deepest emotional need, the concomitant onset of the epigastric pains and the perforation when divorce was threatened.

The interview just described proceeded in rather typical fashion. First came a discussion of the ulcer history. Then the setting in which these symptoms occurred was elicited. Next, the family history, revealing some of the development of certain main tendencies in his personality, was discussed. Finally, there was a discussion of the patient's major feelings and motivations. (For a form of psychodynamic history see Saul, 1972.)

This particular patient apparently had no important inhibitions in his capacity to receive emotionally. He accepted and enjoyed the love of his mother and then of his wife, and his ulcer developed when this satisfaction was cut off. The therapeutic problem was the restoration of the satisfaction he had lost—in this case, his wife's love, or some substitute for it, should some change of her affections or the exigencies of military life render it impracticable. The longer-range problem would be to help him to fuller consciousness of his dependent demands so that he might handle them psychologically, rather than letting the tension cause amnesias and ulcers, so that he could learn better to tolerate the frustrations and even, with time, learn to reduce these demands by getting satisfactions from other acceptable contacts and from more mature attitudes.

The *treatment* followed naturally from this *understanding of the patient's emotional situation.* In the first place, through giving him insight into his central emotional interplay (dynamics), his own intelligence and his will to get well were enlisted for the solution of the emotional problem which was hitherto not clearly grasped by him. It transformed the patient's concept of his symptoms as the mysterious result of incomprehensible neurosis into a conscious grasp of a real and understandable emotional problem. In the second place, the patient's confidence had been won, and he derived great emotional support from this relationship to a physician who understood him and was obviously trying to help him. In some cases, the patient's reaction to this interest of the physician and the feeling of understanding and security which it provided was dramatic in it effects. Further, the physician could increase the patient's emotional intake by suggesting socially acceptable satisfactions, such as the development of friendships, recreation and other sources. And even in the brief time available in the military service, something of the longer-range problems could usually be discussed with profit.

Moreover, it was often possible for the physician in the service to manipulate the environment. The emotional demands upon such a patient as this could be reduced by recommending shore duty for him. At first, it seemed that it was indicated to attempt to influence his wife. Perhaps she might have her own reasons for clinging so insistently to her belief in the patient's infidelity. It looked as if the therapeutic result in this case would rest as much upon the successful treatment of the wife, as of the patient.

This is mentioned to show how flexible one must be in handling emotional problems, and how little it is possible to say that for certain symptoms or conditions certain set procedures or technics are indicated, such as suggestion, catharsis or hypnosis. The patient cannot be fitted to some preconceived technique or theory; to so many visits a week, or the use of the couch or the libido theory, or to this or that kind of therapy. In organic medicine if the patient has a pain in the right lower abdomen, one cannot apply some set diagnosis and treatment, such as "appendicitis" and "surgery" for it may be something very different, such as gas bubble or strained muscle. The only proper scientific medicine is based on *understanding the condition;* and this includes psychiatry. There is no rational treatment that is not based on *understanding the patient.* Even if one decides that it is advisable to use shock, or chemotherapy, or not to treat at all, this decision, what *to* do and what *not* to do, must be based on understanding as thoroughly as possible what it is that is producing the symptoms (Saul, 1972, pp. (113–135). The patient's ulcer represented one outcome of emotional problems, but no two persons are alike, and each must be understood individually. The case we have been discussing actually turned out as follows.

After a single interview, with the insight that he had gained and the prospects of solution which appeared, the patient brightened tremendously, and the epigastric pains he suffered since the perforation diminished. He returned a week later, wreathed in smiles. He reported that he had explained our entire interview to his wife, including my offer to see her; and she had responded with warmth and understanding beyond his hopes. During the months since then, their relationship had been back on its normal footing, the patient felt like himself again, and his symptoms had all but disappeared. Needless to say, all cases do not go so well so quickly.

Of course, an upset relationship to a wife can cause reactions of many kinds—depression, disturbances of behavior and physical symptoms in various organs. Sometimes the man reacts by not caring, or by rage, or by going with other women or in many other ways. It all depends on the man's particular biological and psychological make-up and the particular kind of attachment he has to his wife, which in turn is part of the childhood pattern.

This example demonstrates how treatment can be directed to the *causes* of the symptoms and emotional problems, even though only a few interviews are available. The difference from all-out psychoanalysis is not essentially in the number of hours; rather, the pattern of feelings is not *transferred* intensively to the analyst and its troublesome features analyzed out of this sample human relationship.

Another man reacted differently to his marital troubles. He became depressed and distraught when his relationship to his wife was threatened.

This man had been married for ten years and had three children. When he returned from overseas, he was stationed only a few hundred miles from his home. He conscientiously wrote to his wife daily. When she did not do the same, he, faithful to her and so long alone, became extremely angry. During one such period, he wrote her threatening to go out on parties if she did not care enough for him to write every day. He did not understand her life very well. She, also faithful, was lonely too. Her nerves were on edge because of the long separation, the anxiety and the burdens of the home. The income was inadequate, and she felt herself to be a slave to the children and the house. She often found even writing a letter to the husband she loved just the last straw, the ultimate drain on her overtaxed strength. She reacted with rage to further demands on her, and she envied him his comparative freedom, his liberty nights, the parties and amusements for servicemen which he could be free to attend while she drudged at home. She wrote him an angry note, threatening to leave with the children. This note was such a blow to him that he became angry, distracted and depressed. He rarely had ever touched liquor, but now he drank.

Because both were lonely and strained emotionally, they became irritable. And so, instead of supporting each other, they vented their anger upon each other. A word from each made the other angrier—one of life's commonest and most tragic vicious circles. If only one of the two could rise above the swelling wrath, soften and give love and understanding, the circle could be broken before it built up from nothing to an emotional cyclone spinning about a hollow center.

The marriage was soon actually in jeopardy over nothing between them in reality. This kind of situation illustrates the strains on a family caused by war. And these strains did not affect the parents alone. The twig is easily bent. The child is highly sensitive to emotional influences, and if these are unfavorable and prolonged, its development is bound to be warped by them. *The effects of emotional disturbances are transmitted all too easily to the third and the fourth generations and beyond.* But so are the benefits of effective treatment and, we hope, eventually of prevention.

SENSITIVITY TO SUPERIORS

Sometimes sensitivity to superiors formed a large part of a man's problems. A well-knit, pleasant marine of 32 was the eldest of five children in a close, congenial family. The children were all treated most considerately, and a point was made of equality and fairness among them.

Seeing the war clouds gather, this young man joined the Marine Corps. All he knew of the marine tradition appealed to his own burning pride and independence. After a year he liked it so much that he thought of getting in line for a commission and making the Corps his career. Not many months later the United States became embroiled in war, and he went overseas, where for two and one-half years his duties were of the most dangerous kind. During the island invasions, he was in charge of amphibious tractors, going in with the first wave, bringing the assault troops from the boats over the reefs to the beach and carrying back the wounded. Since his regular duty was bomb disposal, immediately after the beach was secured, he would move along further stretches of beach and along such roads and trails as there were disposing of mines, booby traps and unexploded shells. This work, of course, required the most refined and sustained carefulness. Thus, when a buddy started to unscrew a fuse but did not take pains to notice that the wire was rusted, it broke and he was blown to pieces. Only two other men of the patient's group survived. The patient consoled himself with the thought that such a death is so sudden, complete and uncompromising that the victim never even feels it.

He actually disposed of mines by the thousands. When not fully engaged in this work, he had patrol duty, which in these areas was apt to involve close fighting. Under all this he bore up admirably. Terribly frightened when in danger, he felt no fear when the danger was passed. Only at one time, after 24 hours of continuous bombardment during which a very large number of men in his outfit were killed, did he have nightmares about this for about two weeks; otherwise, he ate, slept and functioned as his usual self. He did have one point of irritation, namely, certain officers. He had various complaints against them—they would grab for themselves what he considered the best foxholes, would ask after an attack how many tractors had been lost, rather than how many men and which ones, would not share beer or occasional liquor equally, and so on. He was especially angry when a young officer whom he had instructed in disposal work now tried to tell *him* how to handle a bomb. He was sure that if he obeyed his orders they would both be killed, so he did it his own way, but in his anger he could barely keep himself from hurling the now safe bomb at his youthful critic. He controlled himself fully, but his hands revealed the power of his impulse by breaking into a sweat.

Finally he was returned to the United States, where he was put in charge of a group of men doing guard duty. Now the danger was gone, but so was the sense of objective, of close comradeship and of pulling together. He was ordered to clean up an area. His men did, and he did, but he received criticism and no thanks. He had difficulty in pleasing and was often spoken to harshly. He began to swear at his own men, a thing he had never done before (in spite of the tradition about marine sergeants). There were threats of the brig, which he felt were unjust and angered him. He was ordered to march his men to a class, only to find that there was no class. Tired as they were, they lost an hour of much-needed sleep. He felt the officer should have known. On more than one occasion he felt tempted to grab and shake an officer who he felt was unjust to the men and failed to treat them with full understanding and consideration. Understanding and consideration were sensitive points with him, for they were the very creed by which he had been reared through childhood.

He never did anything that was not proper, but when angered, and wanting to hit or grab a man, his hands would sweat. He began to fear that he would get into trouble and ruin his outstanding record. He began to fear that he might do something that would make this threat of the brig a reality. He leaned over backward to avoid this and sometimes even found himself cleaning up and picking up little pieces of paper when it was not really necessary to do so and might even look a little strange. Gone was the zest, pride, comradeship. Now his duty hours were long, drab and exhausting. His fine record was threatened; his whole career was in jeopardy.

Other men, he freely admitted, could adjust to this type of duty and could get on well with the officers, but for him the strain mounted. He could sustain fear of the enemy and of sudden death, but not fear of disgrace and failure. He lost his relish for food, he could not relax at night, his sleep was disturbed, and he began having occasional nightmares. As his irritability increased, he began to jump at sudden noises, and he became more and more worried, anxious, preoccupied, withdrawn. He stayed more to himself and began to avoid people, except his few intimates. However, his reaction was still reversible, for when on visits home among his family, he seemed to forget all his cares and to be his usual self again.

The essential discipline of military service, the submission to superiors in rank, is naturally one of the conditions to which every serviceman must adapt himself. The vast majority do so, of course, without difficulty. Many take to it and enjoy being members in the hierarchy. Others do not enjoy it but, nevertheless, adapt easily. Some are irked but never develop sufficient irritation for it to interfere with their ordinary functioning. But in the case we have just cited, this became a special issue. Sometimes it was not easy to tell whether the man's reactions were more or less justified by the particular officers he happened to draw, or whether the man has been rendered hypersensitive to officers by his childhood experiences with authority or by the strains of military life. A man might be venting upon his superiors irritations arising from other sources. Such displacement is a natural reaction. Children tend to blame their parents for their troubles, and every adult, no matter how much he is willing to take the responsibility for his own life and actions, yet always retains to some degree emotional patterns of childhood and likes to find someone to blame for his difficulties. In the military service there are always superiors who can attract such a reaction, those who, however proficient technically, do not have the personality to establish good feelings with the men in their charge, who provoke irritation, even rage and rebelliousness—in contrast to the born leaders who stimulate feelings of security, of being cared for, of loyalty, of a willingness to follow. Often envy of the superior enters in and guilt, which makes the man feel himself to be badly treated. Much remains to be said on this most interesting and important topic, and much could be learned and improved;

but we are interested in it only as one of the types of stress which are encountered in military life.

The young man we have just described, even though he developed difficulties, demonstrates what a man can stand and what many go through in war.

CAREER

A very tense, anxious young marine, jaundiced by many attacks of malaria and obviously worn and underweight, but withal friendly and prepossessing, had become too nervous to carry on. He was 21 years old, and during his 20 months overseas he had participated in many actions, giving a good account of himself even in hand-to-hand combat.

His symptoms were typical. He was anxious and tense, and his anger was on a hair trigger. He jumped like a cat at any sudden noise, and the enjoyment of what sleep he could get was marred by dreams of being attacked by the enemy. After being returned to the United States he did routine guard duty at a naval establishment near a large city. As his tension mounted, he began to dread it, fearing lest he lose control of himself and club or shoot someone who unwittingly irritated him. On one occasion, when he could not get a number on the telephone, he demolished the instrument with the butt of his rifle. The civilian workers seemed to be the special objects of his wrath, but the reasons for this he could grasp only vaguely.

In telling his life story, he revealed nothing which cast much light upon the growing severity of his condition. His family seemed to be in no way unusual, and he had gone into the Navy after graduating from high school three years before. No outstanding emotional forces could be discerned, nor any tendencies in the man himself which might provide a clue. He had enjoyed his studies and athletics. He had enjoyed going with girls, but in his present state they troubled him, because of fearing their jealousy and also because of being unwilling to marry while so upset.

Since his history gave no clue to his basic problem, we turned to his recurrent "catastrophic nightmares," as these have been called. At first, like most of the men, he simply said that he dreamed of being attacked by the enemy and that this was merely a repetition of reality. However, in this series of men, no dream was found to repeat the reality precisely, and the differences from the actual occurrence frequently offered a clue to the patient's problem. The generalization that he dreamed of being attacked by the enemy was a most unsatisfactory substitute for a specific dream told in detail. Therefore, on request, he said that his dream had been as follows. He was in a foxhole. The enemy was coming at him. He reached for his rifle, but it was gone. He reached for his revolver. It, too, was gone. He grabbed for his knife. The enemy was closing in, but the knife, too, was missing. He was in a panic because he had nothing with which to fight.

The most effective method of *dream interpretation* is to obtain the thoughts which are connected with each element of the dream. To do this, one forgets the dream as a whole and asks the patient to tell what comes to mind when he thinks of *each* individual item (Saul, 1972, pp. 198–231). In many of these cases, however, much can be learned from the central theme of the dream, which in this case is being attacked and finding oneself without weapons with which to fight.

Asked to talk about the dream as a whole and also to tell his thoughts concerning the various elements, the patient told very little except that he had never actually been in this position in reality. He was told the fact that dreams, however foolish and fantastic they may seem to be on the surface, never concern themselves with trifles. This dream reflected some situation, some anxiety which the patient had about his life. Perhaps it referred to some sort of situation, disguised under the cloak of a battle scene.

What of being without weapons with which to fight? The patient began to talk. He told further facts about his life. In school he was a fine athlete. He held an athletic scholarship to a big university and had an offer from a big-league baseball club. Like his father, his heart was set on an athletic career, and with his own abilities and the offers he already had, the future before enlistment was rosy indeed for the fulfillment of his hopes. Now these were dashed by the malaria. Already 25 pounds underweight and periodically racked by chills, he saw his career shattered. All his interests were practical. Because of this, and his genial personality, he had an ideal make-up for his chosen career, but he had little interest in books and little ability in intellectual pursuits. Without his athletic prowess he felt defenseless, and now he was reminded of the dream.

He started with sudden emotion. With a burst of insight, he saw that in the dream, while asleep and off guard, he had repeated the anxiety which now tormented him. This was exactly how he really felt. Without his health, he was without weapons to fight his way through life. Gone with his health was his career, his marriage, his security. In consideration of the service he had given and of his present mental and physical condition, he knew he never would return to combat. Yet his dream persisted. Probably one of its values to him emotionally lay in the fact that he now replaced a real, present anxiety with past dangers through which he had come successfully. As he slept and felt the anxiety, rather than wrestling with its true source, in his shattered health, career, security and marriage, he attached it to a past danger which was no longer real. Perhaps it even held a certain consolation, for when he awoke he would be thinking with gratification of how he had survived the acute dangers of actual combat, and he might glean some reassurance that having come through these he would find the capacity to cope with the present and the future threats. (To form a dream, one's unconscious sometimes need fabricate only a little if it can, remarkably, select and use a ready-made memory, a scene from a book or play, an occurrence of the day; whatever fits the feelings and thoughts that come to expression in the dream.)

The dream expressed not only his current anxiety but also his rage. As so very commonly happens, the dreamer's own rage and aggressiveness are represented by one or the other characters in a dream—*projected* upon them, as it were. When we dream, we believe our dreams, and when we wake we still try to fool ourselves by saying, "It was not I who did such and such, it was he or she or that animal." But let us not forget that the dream is entirely the creation of the dreamer. If violence appears in the dream, it can have its source only in the dreamer. One of the sources of this violence is usually in the man's angry rebellion against a situation which he has found to be unbearable, whether because of the danger or for other reasons.

Now the marine began to fit another bit into the jigsaw puzzle, and the outlines of his problem and of his emotions began to take shape. He was anxious not only because of losing the talent which was his chief weapon in life, but also he was enraged by this and by the consequent ruin of his hopes and ambitions. He was no longer even a real marine, with all the burning pride of the Corps. His guard duty, although safe enough, was a terrible comedown and letdown. For him, it was a mere gesture. Now he saw what he previously had sensed only dimly, that his hatred of the civilians sprang from his *envy* of them for remaining in safety, earning good money and furthering their careers, while he himself and his buddies went through dangers and, in addition to their sufferings, sacrificed their futures. Boiling with anger as he was, he of course had a dangerous temper, was unable to relax, could not concentrate, was startled at noises, had no appetite and could not gain weight.

As his insight into the nature of his problem and feelings dawned, he brightened visibly and then poured out his gratitude, his hope and his new confidence. This, he said, was the first time he had seen what his condition was all about. It had been a terrible and incomprehensible malady, and he had been secretly convinced that he never would recover, for it was a vague evil with which he could not come to grips. But now that he could understand the problem, he saw hope of solving it and of getting along in life after all.

From this moment on, he began a spectacular improvement, even though, unfortunately, very little more time could be spent with him. We got to talk over his emotional reactions only a little further. As he felt better, he began to eat and to gain weight. We discussed the possibilities of his making a career as a coach or an athletic director, even if he could not himself be a star athlete. We talked about his pride in this connection, and the fact that, although his vanity might not be fully gratified, being a coach or an athletic director might well provide as satisfactory a life and perhaps even a more stable and happy one.

He began to investigate these possibilities. Everything was done that could be done to build him up physically, and he was glad to adopt a regular training regimen. By the end of two months, his jaundice had so far disappeared as to be barely noticeable. He had gained about 15 pounds, and he began to play a little ball. Over a period of three months, from the moment his improvement began, he had only one slight chill, even though he had been taken off quinine and atabrine, and he was gradually exercising more and more.

He so far regained his self-confidence as to set a date for marriage. He resigned himself, apparently without too much difficulty, to sacrificing his athletic career because of its shortness and uncertainty and began to think in terms of a less glamorous but more stable pursuit.

Many war stories convey an exhilarating sense of freedom, adventure and colorful, self-satisfying heroism. So often the man in uniform seemed to be a free, devil-may-care young blade, to be envied and to be feared. Perhaps this built good morale on the home front, but unless tempered with stories of that dogged, unromantic heroism of the men who faced the worst of the front lines in World War II, and those who sweated out the long months and years in Korea and Vietnam with boredom, overwork, disease, danger, isolation and frustration, marking time until they would live again, unless all this too is realized, the public will have little idea of the gratitude they really owe to those who suffered in defense of those who remained at home.

Perhaps a series of cases such as we have been presenting gives the impression that it is small wonder if a man cracks under such strains. Let us wonder all the more, then, that men brought up to a life of peace and freedom can fight in military organizations and can endure these stresses.

We are describing only the men who were eventually incapacitated. The vast majority endured these hardships without breaking in any way. For each man who was torpedoed and then developed symptoms, there were others who were torpedoed three times and developed none, or only minor ones. For each man who cracked in the hell of Guadalcanal, there were others who did not but went on from campaign to campaign. For example, a light young man of 22, with an indoor job in civil life, became a marine of the First Division. Slight of physique, he went through the worst of Guadalcanal and then through the next three campaigns and carried on, moreover, in spite of severe malaria. After his attacks, he would suffer with an enlarged, painful spleen. On one occasion, after 14 charges up a hill, after two days almost without sleep, he collapsed with heat stroke under the merciless sun, but he quickly recovered from this.

The change from his sedentary civil life to the field of battle was tremendous, but he adapted to it very quickly. At first, the dead and the wounded, the arms, and legs and the entrails lying about turned his stomach, but very soon he got used to it. True, he did have a device for protecting his feelings. Although very popular and sociable in civil life, in military service he did not allow himself to become too much attached to friends in the Corps, so that whenever one was killed he could still think of him as "only another man." He felt a tense fear when in acute danger and at such times did not sleep well, but otherwise he was never nervous or anxious, maintained his good disposition and never at any time had any battle dreams or nightmares. He is mentioned as an example of those men who seemed to be able, for a time at least, to go through hell itself, suffering no doubt, but without breaking down, for their emotionally vulnerable spot had not been touched or was not sufficiently vulnerable, and so they could adapt until they were too depleted biologically.

REFERENCES

Saul, L. J. (1972): *Psychodynamically Based Psychotherapy*. New York: Science House.
———— (1979): *The Childhood Emotional Pattern in Marriage*. New York: Van Nostrand Reinhold.

13 | Weakening Self-Control

A man's control of his emotional reactions depends on many factors—the suddenness, the violence and the duration of the unbearable experiences and of the man's emotional responses, the man's own state of physical vigor, how much emotional support he gets, and so on. Some of the forces at work are summarized in the following outline. These, it is to be hoped, will be quite understandable from the descriptions of the men which have already been given, so that further examples will not be necessary here. An understanding of these factors contains important clues to mental hygiene and to the prevention of mental and emotional disorders in both men and women.

I. The intensity of the man's reaction is determined by:
   A. External circumstances such as—
      1. Being unable to express the excitement and urges by fighting or fleeing or other *activity*
      2. The violence of the situation
      3. The duration of the situation
      4. The suddenness of the situation
      5. The special experiences, such as loss of a buddy
      6. Other factors
   B. Internal make-up and emotional state of the man. The man is already anxious and tense for inner personal reasons, usually—
      1. Primitive instinctual "id" impulses already so strong as to threaten control, e.g., excessive dependence, hostility, etc.
      2. Overstrong and neurotic "superego" conscience reaction, causing excessive guilt and fear of any hostility
      3. Weakness of will, control, judgment, etc. ("ego"), causing—
         a. Lack of independence

      b. Lack of self-reliance

      c. Lack of self-confidence

    4. Emotional development, specific vulnerabilities, etc.

II. The strength of the man's forces of control and his ability to cope with the reaction are determined by:

  A. Internal make-up, including such factors as—

    1. Adaptability

    2. Strong will, control, judgment (strong "ego")

    3. Tolerance for anxiety and hostility

  B. External factors, including morale factors, such as—

    1. Impersonal:

      a. Food, shelter, physical hardships, type of boredom, etc.

      b. Training and preparation

      c. Indefiniteness, uncertainties

      d. Other

    2. Personal:

      a. Understanding of reasons for fighting

      b. Leadership—faith in officers, feeling of interest in himself, of being valued, of being appreciated, of being taken care of, of being treated with fairness and justice

      c. Relation to shipmates

      d. Other

III. Secondary reactions:

Once symptoms begin to develop, then, just as with any illness or injury, individuals have all kinds of reactions to them—from minimizing them and hiding them, struggling against them, to giving in fully and even exaggerating and exploiting them

How the controls may gradually weaken is seen readily in many young men who went through repeated actions or were exposed to long strain. One, for example, spent 18 months as a gunner on a large ship, going through 13 major engagements. He always had had a quick temper and had considerable anxiety as a child, requiring a light in his room for many years when sleeping, having frequent nightmares and occasionally sleepwalking. His sensitivity was to combat, and his main reaction was fear. Each time he controlled it, but he felt the mounting strain. Each time he expected that this action would be the last and he would be returned home, but then he would be sent into another.

By far the worst action was the first, but as the strain began to tell, his sensitivity increased, and his controls weakened. He began to feel "fed up" and that he could stand no more. The final attack, much less trying than the first, was nevertheless the last straw. After it, he became so tremulous that he could not handle his gun, while his irritability, startle reaction, nightmares, loose bowels and loss of appetite entirely incapacitated him.

This case illustrates a dilemma that was encountered frequently at the front. A man might break down with acute symptoms under enormous stresses of combat but recover relatively quickly while at the front if he was pulled out of action quickly and given ample rest, thus decreasing the emotional reaction and strengthening his powers of control. If such a man was now evacuated to the rear, he might let down and never again be able to face combat. If he was not evacuated, it might be possible for him to return to front-line duty. But we have seen the price of this. Sent back, his next breakdown might be that much more severe, and he might be as true a casualty as if his brain had been scathed by a bullet. Conversely, some breakdowns could be prevented completely if the men were sent back for a rest in time, rather than being kept until their tension caused full-blown symptoms, but this was not always practicable for the attainment of military objectives. Such objectives cost casualties.

Sometimes a man was so fatigued by controlling his reactions, as, for example, his anxiety, that he finally gave in to the feeling that he would no longer struggle to save himself, that he no longer cared whether or not he got killed, that it was easier not to care if he were killed than to wrestle with the fear of it. In some cases this meant giving in to self-destructive tendencies (which usually arose from the conscience or from hostility turned against himself). In more than one case, after the man had decided that he no longer cared, he would handle himself in such a way as to be hit. We have mentioned one aviator who always took shelter, as he was supposed to do, in a certain way from enemy planes, but failed to do this after just giving in to the feeling that he no longer cared. His plane got through, but he was seriously injured and barely escaped with his life.

Occasionally one would be amazed at a man's apparent absense of fear, only to find that this was due, as might have been expected, in part to a minimum of anxiety in his make-up or to an unusually thorough repression. But in certain cases, as might not have been suspected, one finds it due to the fact that the man had sustained an underlying unhappiness so distressing that it had produced a dulling of the passion for life and a quiet wish for death. Some men entered the service to escape from a desperation in their lives as civilians.

SECONDARY REACTIONS

Naturally, men react with powerful feelings not only to physical injury but also to incapacitations caused by emotional disturbances. In fact, because physical incapacitation is entirely respectable, while emotional difficulties carry a stigma, the reactions to the latter are often more violent. Many men improve emotionally when they are incapacitated by injury or disease. There are a number of possible reasons for this, among them the fact that they have a disability which is acceptable, both to society and to themselves. They may even be proud of the physical handicap, whereas the emotional difficulty is a source of shame. Physical disease, such as malaria, is intermediate between wounds and emotional disturbance. One does not get the Purple Heart for malaria or filariasis, as one can for a wound, and yet it does not carry the stigma of emotional upsets. What some men have sustained physically and mentally to accomplish their tasks often deserves high awards but is hidden from the world. Although everyone must take personal and social responsibility for himself, we must recognize the fact that no one can choose his parents—the family into which he is born, or how he will be treated from conception onward, especially until about age six—and no one, therefore, predetermines his nuclear emotional constellation, his basic psychodynamics.

A man's reaction to his incapacity, whether this be wound, injury, disease or emotional upset, is called his "secondary reaction." It is so called to bring out the fact that his conscious feelings are not the *cause* of his symptoms but only his reaction to the fact of having them. One man hides his incapacity, while another boasts of it. One is ashamed of it, while another tries to exploit it as best he can; and these differences are also part of his make-up.

The secondary reaction may be so strong that it dominates the clinical picture. Thus, one marine had given an excellent account of himself during four years in the Corps and two tours of combat. But then he began to become so tense and restless that he could not discharge his responsibilities as sergeant. His symptoms were very mild, but when he was turned in with "combat fatigue," his fiery pride was cut to the quick. He began to flay himself emotionally for what he considered his weakness, for turning out to be a "psycho," a "war neurosis," which to him amounted to being a failure in the Marine Corps. He could not stand the fact that he was still strong and healthy and yet too upset for duty. He prayed that he might have lost both legs instead, for then at least he would not be a failure.

He had always had a violent temper, sanctioned by the example of his father. This aggressiveness served the patient well in combat, but now he turned it against himself, launching a terrific attack upon himself for his "failure," which so hurt his enormous personal pride. In reality, with his aggressiveness, magnificent physique and catlike dexterity, he always had triumphed in hand-to-hand encounters with the enemy. Now these encounters began to appear in his dreams, but in the dreams, unlike reality, he was attacked and beaten. This reflected not only the losing fight he felt he was now waging in life because of his emotional incapacitation, but it also represented a venting of his rage against himself because of the intolerable wound which his incapacity inflicted on his vanity.

Some progress was made, even in this case, through discussing with him not only the source of his difficulty but also how he was prolonging his emotional tension by this excessive reaction to it. We also discussed the true pride of accomplishment and the acceptance of reality, as opposed to the false pride of personal vanity. We discussed more mature attitudes of interest in the Marine Corps and its welfare, of interest in his wife and child and in his clients and friends, instead of this obsession with his own prestige. He showed some understanding and began to make some progress toward reorientation, with consequent diminution of his explosive rage. He now saw a pathway out of his emotional distress.

In general, there is a difference between the secondary reactions to combat fatigue and to operational fatigue. Some men, as we have seen, were intolerably ashamed of being afraid, and yet they carried much greater than normal anxiety about combat. Such men, if they became so upset as to be incapacitated, tended to hide the fact that it was due to exaggerated fears and related it to the other difficulties of military life. Other men took the opposite attitude. For them, being upset about combat carried far less stigma than their inability to stand the gaff of military life. They used their combat experiences as the excuse, whereas in reality for them it was more the long attrition of life in a vast fighting organization.

14 | Fight and Flight

HOW HIGHLY INDIVIDUAL EMOTIONAL PROBLEMS CAN CAUSE SIMILAR SYMPTOMS

If each of several men has an individual emotional problem, then how can we account for the similarity of their symptoms? The answer seems to be rather simple. There are in all biological organisms, whether amoeba, mice or men, certain common impulses and reactions. There is the taking in of food, mating and reproduction and the self-protective reactions to any type of frustration or danger. It is the latter that concerns us here.

Basically, as we have seen repeatedly, man or mouse reacts to any and every threat or irritation in only two fundamental ways: by hostile *aggression,* to destroy the source of irritation, or by *flight,* to escape from it.

This self-preservative reaction is, at bottom, an arousal of the whole organism to action. This arousal is an automatic biological reflex.

Our lives, to a large degree, are shaped by the fact that people respond so quickly to any threat or frustration with this readiness to aggression, this quickness to anger. If the country is attacked, if little Willie breaks a window, if the coffee is cold, or the shirt button rolls under the bed, the reaction is an impulse to belligerence and aggressiveness. Of course, if it is only a mild impulse and the control is adequate, it may not be noticed. But if it is intense, then it will upset the man's thoughts, feelings, behavior and bodily well-being. If he is stirred up to action, be the direction flight or fight, rage or fear, he cannot relax and sleep well. He cannot think calmly or concentrate for long. The blood has gone from his stomach to his muscles in preparation for action, and he cannot relish his food. He is keyed up and jumps at sudden sounds. He is tensed in readiness to fight and flares up at the least remark, and these violent impulses which are aroused in him seek expression, even during sleep, through that safety valve, the dream, distorting pleasant fantasies into terrifying nightmares. In short, a man aroused to fight or flight represents the characteristic disturbances of functioning which we call the clinical picture of combat fatigue.

Therefore, it seems that these men, with their individual problems and their own particular irritations and annoyances, have shown similar symptoms in varying proportions, because these symptoms result from the reactions of relatively normal men to any threat or irritation to the organism (Cannon, 1929).

If the man is not relatively normal but has some serious disorder of his emotional life, then he may not show this usual reaction. However, few such men are encountered in military service, since the original psychiatric screening examinations have kept them out. To put this the other way round, the man who breaks down under the stresses of military life, not with typical combat fatigue but with some serious mental disorder, was not, so far as our experience goes, really "normal" to begin with, even though he may have appeared to be so on the surface. This conclusion seems to be unavoidable from the fact that the percentage of psychoses (that is, the severe mental disturbances usually with gross distortions of the sense of reality, as contrasted with the emotional upsets which combat fatigue represents) does not increase during wartime. The real problem is why the fight-flight response persists even after the threat and the irritation are past.

It is obvious that so fundamental and universal a reaction as this quick mobilization for flight or fight must play a fateful role in everyday life and human affairs. Many are the frustrations and the irritations of daily living, even in peacetime; hence, there are few people who do not endure constant frustration, constant irritation and hence constant anger. As Thoreau once said, "The mass of men lead lives of quiet desperation." The irritation may be physical or psychological, internal or external, real or imagined. It may arise from a decayed tooth, or a miscarriage of justice, from feelings of inadequacy due to prolonged and excessive dependence on one's parents, to an unhappy home life, or to years of mistreatment during childhood, from loss of a button, or loss of a friend, from living under a leaky roof, from an uneasy conscience, or from exposure to battle conditions. Whatever the irritation, man fights it by trying to attack and destroy the source, or by escaping; and his feelings are anger and anxiety.

Let us note a few points concerning hostility which are of importance in dealing with combat fatigue. In the first place, it must not be forgotten that, destructive as hostility is, it springs largely from the instinct of self-preservation. Even the most vicious sadists, insofar as they have been studied, are found to be filled with the enjoyment of cruelty because of cruel treatment which they themselves had experienced for long periods early in life, or because of some enormous irritation within themselves, such as a sense of weakness or frustration. The practical importance of this is that when we find a man's symptoms, whatever these may be, resulting from an underlying rage, we can be sure that this rage has a very definite reason for being. Rage underlies the symptoms in almost all these men and, in part, in almost all neuroses. In almost every case, in order to be of practical help to the patient, the psychiatrist must trace the hostility to its sources. If possible, the causes must be removed. "Sublimations" must be provided when feasible, that is, the hostility and the anger must be turned into socially acceptable channels, such as taking it out by chopping wood. And the patient must understand this part of his emotional problem so that his reason and judgment can be enlisted in the process of solving it (Saul, 1976).

FLIGHT AND REGRESSION

When actual flight from a threatening or painful situation is impossible, and when fight is equally so, biological organisms still have devious resources of withdrawal. The sea anemone folds up tightly, the clam snaps shut, the turtle withdraws into its shell, and some men, in the midst of the intolerable sights and sounds of battle, escape it all by becoming stuporous. In this state they suspend their usual emotional reactions and shut themselves off emotionally from what they find unbearable. In so doing, they sacrifice also their normal human contacts.

In the milder cases, the man is his usual self but feels impelled to escape from the pressures upon him. Unable to escape in reality, he may begin to develop a *biological refusal* to function under these painful, dangerous, biologically adverse conditions. This refusal often takes the form of depression, fatigue, headache, loss of appetite, loss of interest and other signs of the organism's contraction of its activities. Perhaps the tendency is something like that of the bear, hibernating and avoiding the long, cold, unsatisfying winter.

The man usually fights these symptoms. He usually feels anxious and threatened by them. He does not want to withdraw and be a quitter. He tries to keep going and lives in memories and in hopes of happier days, when his soul and body can again expand. But he is struggling against the dead weight of biological refusal.

In many patients, this tendency to withdraw involves the recurrence of long-outgrown childish traits and symptoms, such as bedwetting and nailbiting, outbursts of temper, self-centeredness, greater needs for attention and love, hypersensitive pride, greater impulsiveness, weaker controls, crying spells and a sense of weakness and insecurity.

Insofar as this is true, it suggests that part of the flight reaction takes the form of a return or "regression" to some of the patterns and the behavior of childhood. In simplest terms, when a person feels hard-pressed, then like the child, he thinks less about others and more about himself and casts about for all the help he can get. The commonly observed diminution of interest in people and things, including sexual interest, is probably a part of this same biological tendency to withdraw. The hypersensitivity to taking orders and the resentment of any demands for work or attention are probably also partly for this reason. The man wants to withdraw and becomes enraged at any prodding toward productive, responsible effort. (Of course, as always, there are other reasons also. As one man put it, it was so long since he had been able to do what *he* wanted that he could not stand orders any more.) Even the very pursuits which he enjoyed when happy no longer interest him, and he snarls when pushed. This is of obvious importance in treatment, especially as the man's feelings are usually mixed. He himself does not want to give in fully to this withdrawal and may feel distressed and even threatened by it.

Thus, *withdrawal and the regression to childish feelings and behavior cause new problems.* The resistance against taking responsibility, the loss of capacity to work freely fills the man with insecurity and anxiety as to the present and the future. The increased demands and desires for love and care expose the man to inevitable frustration, which in turn only increases his anxiety and unhappiness and starts a vicious circle; and the very facts of the relinquishment of his effective adult functioning, the loss of his mature powers, the failure, hurt his pride and self-esteem. He wants to be mature and masculine. He cannot stand himself as he is, irritable, helpless, uncontrolled. This, in turn, enrages him further. Very often he will project his intolerable opinion of himself to others. He may fear to go on a bus or into public places because he thinks that people are staring at him, and when pressed as to why this should be, he confesses that it is because he feels they are thinking scornfully of how unworthy he is.

But all this conflict is useful for treatment. It shows that the man has not given up, that he has not accepted his own impulses to escape from life's adult responsibilities. He is still fighting, and in his fight to recover, his insecurity, his frustration and his hurt pride are powerful stimuli to get well. The physician can use them effectively in treatment.

Many a man in military service managed to control himself and keep going until he was returned to his country, and then the emotional tension he had controlled so long would burst its bonds and generate his symptoms. There are probably a number of reasons for this.

One is that the man, long fatigued with the constant effort of controlling his feelings, felt at last that it was safe to relax these controls. While overseas, he had thought that on his return the emotional tension would let down. But he found that the letdown was not in the tension but in its controls.

Another factor was probably an intensification of homesickness, for although he was now closer to all that he had dreamed of while away, he still was not free to enjoy it—his situation was like that of Tantalus, to whose parched lips the lake waters rose only to recede when he bent his head to drink.

A frequent reason, too, was the intensification of envy. Misery loves company, and it was hard for the man who had been through so much, suffered so much, sacrificed so much, to look upon all the safety and the prosperity that surrounded the folks back home. Only the most mature do not have some selfish and envious thoughts in such a situation. One mildly paranoid marine, who had been through months of hell, on his return thought that people were saying to him, "Sucker." This little delusion involved him in one or two altercations. Fortunately, it is very often possible to break up delusions of this sort and relieve considerable anxiety by showing the person that what he thinks of as the opinions and the attitudes of others toward him are really his own judgments and feelings toward himself.

For proper treatment, it is essential to understand the status of the individual's psychological and biological flight reaction. In most cases, it is better to prevent this from going too far by keeping the patient active and interested. But there are some who react well to almost complete temporary indulgence of the impulse to escape. One young marine improved greatly after 30 days of a completely vegetative existence at his parents' farm. Of course, in other cases, if this were permitted, the way back to mature functioning would be all the harder. Everything depends on understanding the person concerned. Then one knows whether it is best to permit the withdrawal or not. No procedures can be applied blindly. *Sound understanding is the sole basis of effective treatment.*

THE GIVE-GET BALANCE

Something of the balance between emotional needs and emotional output is illustrated by a 40-year-old man.

When asked to tell his story, his very first utterance was a complaint that he had been put from civil life directly into a responsible position without any indoctrination and was expected to know a great deal about the Navy. Overseas he again had a responsible position. For the first months he was subjected to bombings, but this did not especially bother him. He reacted only with normal, transient fear. The strain on him was due to the attention his job demanded, the details to be met, the obstacles to be overcome, the difficulties with supplies and personnel, as compared with his faster-operating job with a large company in civil life, and to his concern for the men under him, whom he watched over with almost motherly solicitude. He was a very conscientious man in expending his emotional energies upon his job and his men but received very little emotional support himself. Much expenditure—little income, so he drifted "into the emotional red." He became increasingly tense, irritable and anxious and developed a mild startle reaction. His appetite and digestion became deranged, and he was rarely able to sleep more than five hours a night. His tension, anxiety and fatigue mounted until, after one year, he could no longer carry on.

The interview soon revealed an intense anger beneath this man's worn expression. And as he vented this anger with increasing frankness, it became evident that its cause was a bitter protest against the demands on him and the lack of emotional gratification—too much going out and too little coming in.

His history soon showed why hypersensitivity to this unbalancing was this man's specifically vulnerable spot, his particular emotional Achilles' heel. He was an only child. While he was still a baby, his father had died. His mother never remarried but clung solicitously to him. She indulged him and overprotected him, and he became excessively dependent on her. She set all her hopes upon him and was very ambitious for him. He married at 30. But the marriage did not last, for he felt that he and his wife should live with his mother. He felt vaguely that something was wrong but did not realize that it was this unresolved, untransferable emotional dependence on his mother. He felt undefinable inferiority without understanding that it arose from the fact that although he was now an adult, part of his personality was still the child attached to his mother. In middle life, he still enjoyed her sole love, care and solicitude. He also derived considerable emotional support and security from the large company in which he had been employed since adolescence, and from the personal interest of his immediate superiors. Then came his experience in military service, a new and much more responsible job, increased personal and impersonal demands, with all sorts of difficulties to be met, but less interest and support than in his civilian life and, above all, separation from his mother for the first time in his life. His frustration and rage mounted and his symptoms developed.

This man responded with relief to a single one-hour interview, in which this interplay of feelings and motivations was discerned and discussed. Of course, insight alone is not likely to enable such a man to return to full duty, but without it this man was unable to do any duty whatever. His symptoms diminished, and he began gaining weight. He had learned what it was that he found unbearable and that aroused his rage and wish to escape. A visit to his mother and the generous interest of the company in which he had worked for years helped greatly to restore his accustomed balance. He was capable of limited duty and when discharged would be able to return to his job in civil life, whereas previously he had been too upset to be self-supporting.

The balance between needs and output, illustrated by this man, is important in most cases, being a fundamental factor in biological functioning. The organism is capable of only so much output, physically and emotionally, and has certain minimal physical and emotional needs. Taxed and/or deprived beyond a certain point, the balance is too far upset, and the organism shows protest reactions. To use the terms since introduced by Grinker and Speigel (1945), the organism becomes depleted and needs to be replenished.

FURTHER RESULTS OF REGRESSION— GUILT—ADAPTABILITY

Backsliding or regressing to egocentric childish attitudes often causes guilt and shame. This is exemplified by an upstanding young naval aviator of 22 who had been in the Navy for three years. He had suffered from mounting anxiety which, a few months before, had become so severe as to incapacitate him. He was not consciously guilty or upset about the strafing he was called upon to do, but, from the very beginning, obviously he had been more anxious than the other men, who noticed the excessive care he took to see that his gun, parachute and all his equipment were perfect to the last detail. He suffered from a feeling that he was bound to be killed, and he took this extreme, minute "compulsive" * care in his efforts to do what he could against such a calamity. He also suffered increasingly from the other usual symptoms of "combat fatigue," but these were relatively mild, and the fear of death was central. This much he told in the first interview but revealed very little of the underlying core of his personality make-up. He said that he was somewhat preferred by his mother to the other children, but how this had affected him could not be discerned. He could re-

* In "compulsion neurosis" excessive attention to details is one of the prominent features. It typically results from anxiety which is usually caused by guilt due to hostile feelings, so that the person lives under a vague dread of punishment and *feels*, against his reason, that if he does not do thus and so with great care, some sort of ill will befall him. He thus caricatures obedient conscientiousness.

member no dreams, nor in any other way did he provide a glimpse beneath the surface. He added that he had been engaged but had broken it off because he no longer loved the girl.

That was all, until five days later, when suddenly, distraught, he burst into the office and asked for a few moments because of a very upsetting nightmare. He had lain down for a nap after lunch and, while dozing off, had felt a hand on his back. He felt that he was doing to die and struck out but found no one there. He dashed into the hall, searching, thinking it might have been a WAVE (Women Accepted for Voluntary Emergency Service), but no one was there. Even then he was not sure that it was only a dream, so vivid was it. That is, it was a "hypnagogic state," a dream state between sleeping and waking. It was pointed out that whether or not someone had actually touched him, which was really unbelievable, his interpretation of this as murder was entirely his own—he must want to be killed or feel he should be killed—and that he should suspect a WAVE suggested that possibly a woman had something to do with it. He was obviously struck by this, his emotions were aroused to a high pitch, but he said nothing. This had hit the spot. Then, with great effort, and bit by bit, he began to tell his story.

It was true, he expected punishment and felt that he deserved nothing but death. He had once proudly adhered to the highest moral principles. His parents had provided him with considerable religious training, and he had been a clean-cut, responsible, hardworking, steady, open young man, who represented the best of the ethical teaching he had received. He had been in love and had become engaged shortly before entering the Navy. At first he had maintained his standards. But under the great emotional pressures and temptations, he more and more withdrew his interest from other persons, from his job and from people and things generally. More and more, his resentfulness mounted, and he felt that it was all he could do to take care of himself, and that he would get what pleasure he could and think only of himself. He slipped into swearing, gambling, drinking and philandering. Thinking only of himself, he fell out of love with his fiancée and no longer loved anyone— except perhaps himself. Now, he felt, he had betrayed his parents, thrown away his career and ruined the girl he had loved, whose heart he had broken. He felt that death was the only proper and possible punishment.

His deepest feeling appeared to be his attachment to his mother, especially his need for her love. It was his mother in particular who had inculcated in him his high ethical standards, and in this his need for her love was the main lever and motivating force. Now he felt that he was betraying her and so no longer deserved her love, and this caused such sense of abandonment, inner pain and depression that he often felt that he no longer cared to live.

Now all this was discussed with him, how he had regressed from adult interest in his work and in other persons, and from the capacity to love and take responsibility, to this self-protective but nevertheless childishly egocentric, selfish, irresponsible outlook and behavior. The road back to health was then talked over in some detail. He felt somewhat lashed by the interpretation but brightened with hope—the first, he said, since this occurred. Even going only this far into his problem proved to be a turning point. Other aids were used. Because of his anxiety he could be assured that we would recommend that he not be returned to combat for some time, if at all. He was referred to his chaplain, who was a most understanding man. He began to respond to our faith in him. From then on, however hard the road, he was on his way out, not in. He began to wonder if, after all, he might not return to his fiancée. He saw the day when he again could face his mother and again take a responsible place in society.

This patient serves to illustrate a chain of emotional reactions which probably occur quite generally and often form a vicious circle, namely, emotional strain, backsliding because of this increased strain, guilt and sense of being abandoned, which indeed he was by his own conscience, his inner psychological representation of his mother. Under the demands, the pressures, the dangers and the frustrations of the military service, the need for escape was increased. Being subject to isolation, restraints and discipline and so unable to freely to indulge in the ordinary pleasures and satisfactions caused heightened desires to cut loose. But such indulgences caused guilt and anxious expectation of punishment.

Another motivation which leads to this indulgence is anger. A child learns social behavior, in large part, because it accepts training through feeling that it is loved and avoids pitfalls for fear of losing love and because it loves it parents and would not hurt them. If it is angered, then it knows how to get back at its parents by doing forbidden things. The same reaction persists in the adult. The feeling is an angry, "Why be good any more? Why control myself any more when I'm not loved anyway?" Hence, the indulgence of these forbidden desires arises both as a reaction of flight and escape and also as an expression of fight, spite and rebellion.

Such behavior itself often has a significant result, namely, the harm that it causes to the person involved. It is often obviously masochistically self-destructive and thus carries with it a self-punishment which, as we see in the above case, and as is usual, arises from the conscience—from one's feelings of guilt and shame, which cause powerful self-reproaches. These may be so strong that, as in the case just described, they cause impulses to suicide—feelings that death alone is sufficient expiation.

One not infrequently would see a young man returning from hardships and dangers overseas, feeling that all these sufferings were on the credit side of his account with his conscience, and that now he can let himself go for a time without being punished, until he had balanced off the suffering, like the little girl in the anecdote who confessed first so that she could then enjoy the forbidden book freely. This is one of the reasons why readjustment to civil life was often something of a problem for the serviceman. Another reason was that often a man felt that all he had endured and put out justified special indulgence and support. This was an important reaction in some veterans and was sometimes a source of their continuing resentment against those who were not in the service. One man, for example failed to adjust to civil life after discharge, and his symptoms persisted. He turned out to be seething with rage because, after all he had accomplished and suffered, he felt more gratitude and solicitude were owed him, and he burned with resentment against those who had not been in the service. He had given so much that he now yielded to regressive wishes to be cared for, with an angry protest against having to take up the burdens of everyday life. In yet another case a man had been in a not very responsible duty and at the same time had been able to think only of himself, his own safety and, so far as he could get them, his own comforts and pleasures. On his return to civil life he liked being one of the boys—he liked his liberties, his freedom—he resented the restraints and the standards of his house, he shied off the responsibilities of marriage and a job. He was unable to return to the adult biological and social responsibilities of the work-a-day world. But few men were seen with this difficulty in readjustment unless it had also been a problem before enlistment.

Let us not forget that regression from adult orientation and interests to more irresponsible behavior is, as we have seen, one method of flight. As such, the capacity to regress can increase a man's flexibility and adaptability and serve as a great protection against emotional stresses. For example, two professional men came into the service together. The one held to very high standards and was very adult in all his relationships. He was warmly interested in people, very much in love with his wife and children and devoted to his work and the men under him. When obstacles arose to the accomplishment of what he deemed right, he invariably sought to overcome them. He was a strong, loyal man of high type and unusually mature.

The other man, although able, was of much easier virtue. Also a family man, his eye nevertheless often roved. His interest in his work was noticeably overbalanced by his enjoyment of relaxation, and he never fought through obstacles or for the maintenance of standards if he could possibly avoid the trouble. In the service, as things turned out, both men went overseas and were subjected to considerable stress. The former persisted in his faithfulness to his family, was much afraid for their future if he should be killed or seriously injured, strove to do his jobs with the utmost effectiveness and consideration and refused to compromise on his standards. As a result, he missed his family painfully but could not forget them with other women, and he had many battles to fight on his job. At the end of a year, although he maintained full control and performed efficiently, the underlying tension had so mounted that he developed disturbances of both heart and stomach and had to be evacuated.

The second man, however, took the easier way. He freely sought refuge from the frustrations of his job and personal life in wine, women and song—in his duty did no more than the minimum, while after hours he totally forgot his troubles in the pursuit of whatever pleasures were available wherever he happened to be. A relatively lazy, irresponsible child as compared with the former upstanding, responsible, productive, independent man, nevertheless, he, through his ability to escape into play, avoided enough frustration and gained enough pleasure and surcease to continue to function on this level. His ability to regress protected him, while the former man, not strong enough to maintain his high level and unable to regress, broke down. Human nature is variegated, and while fundamental knowledge is essential, all set rules, clichés and formulations must be regarded with deep suspicion.

FURTHER FORMS OF FLIGHT

The tendency to flight can cause, among other things, relinquishing one's responsibilities and adult functioning and giving in to childish reactions. Sometimes it goes even further than this, into a general withdrawal of almost all interest, so that the individual does little more than vegetate. Such a reaction is suggestive of schizophrenic withdrawal, and, as in all cases, the tendency can be found in the individual prior to military experience and is only exaggerated by it. The following type of case is not too unusual.

This young man of 26 never had associated very much or very intimately with men or girls of his own age but had tended to feel more at home with older people. He led an apparently normal sexual life and became engaged but never had much feeling for the opposite sex. His actual behavior was normal, but the appropriate feelings were diminished. He denied any acute or painful dissatisfactions with the service or any special reactions to its manifold pressures and dangers, but it seemed clear that he had considerable feeling which he was not expressing, and of which he himself was not fully conscious.

He did fairly well in the beginning of his naval career, but then, in addition to the dangers and other hardships, he was given a job which was difficult for him because of his lack of knowledge and experience. He developed a moderate degree of tension, but this soon gave way to a general let down in his entire psychophysiological functioning. He lost all interest in his job and in his friends and no longer cared about recreation or "liberty." He felt little or no anxiety and had no anxiety dreams. He was in his middle twenties and in excellent physical condition but had lost his interest in sports, found that it was difficult for him to remember or to use his mind alertly and even lost what interest he had had in women and sex, thus reflecting a general withdrawal from life. This impresses one as an eminently biological reaction similar, as mentioned above, to that of animals that roll up and become motionless when danger threatens, such as the opossum and the turtle, and the animals which do not reproduce in captivity and those which do not even live in captivity. It seems related to schizophrenia. (Schizophrenia means, very roughly, not "split personality" but a splitting off of the normal feelings and interests toward people and things in favor of preoccupation with one's own thoughts and fantasies.) It is often a quiet but deep and therefore sinister form of regression.

Another, but much less serious, type of withdrawal is one which has been properly called "strike reaction." It is illustrated by an unmarried young seaman of 23, who was sullen, resentful, depressed, anxious and irritable. He further complained of feeling tight inside, and particularly of being hardly able to eat or sleep, and of no longer being interested in women, friends, job or anything else. He also suffered from feelings of tension, startle reaction to sudden sounds, sweating and recurrent nightmares and battle dreams. These nightmares almost always consisted of a scene much like an actual experience, but not exactly the same. As is so often the case, this man's nightmares amplified the horrors of the reality by having all the naval craft around the patient blown up, a fate which, happily, they escaped in reality. It is already clear from the symptoms that the man was highly mobilized for fight or flight; and from the content of his repetitive nightmares, it was certain that he harbored terrific rage. Yet the patient himself denied that he had any idea of the causes of his condition.

It began, he said, after an invasion. He said that he was the youngest of seven children in a very pleasant and friendly family. As the baby of the seven, he was always especially well treated and well looked out for. Life in the Navy was for him a sudden and distressing change and a great contrast with his former existence as the protected baby of the family. For a whole month at the time of the first invasion, constant demands were made upon him; he was exposed to danger, saw a buddy killed and feared the same would happen to him and got but little sleep. Gradually, he began to reveal his true feelings, which in actual fact he never had connected with the symptoms. He bitterly resented the fact that he was not given all the solicitude and care he desired, which in his family he was accustomed to as his right, that he was restricted for minor infringements and that other men took things for themselves, leaving him to sweat alone for what he got.

As he spoke, his resentment mounted. Rather childish in appearance and attitudes, he complained about the childishness of the other men. He began to use the expression "fed up" and then told how he could not eat or sleep. His resentment was such that he no longer functioned. He had turned against work and friends, even sex. He admitted that he realized that the staff here had a real interest in him and was trying to help him, but said he was so fed up that he could not help but be angry at everyone. This resentment was expressed in his nightmares. The gist of his feeling was, "If I am not treated as I was at home, where I was the baby of the family, but instead am exposed to danger, hard work and lack of special consideration, to the devil with all of you; may you all be blown up, and, as for me, I just won't play at all any more."

The result was a psychophysiological sit-down strike. He was turning against life and consequently developing, in addition to his sullenness, a dangerous mood of depression, as if to say, "Not only won't I play anymore—I'm going into the garden and eat worms."

There was enough fighting spirit in him so that he showed pronounced improvement as time went on, apparently as a result of the doctor's interest as well as of the insight which he had gained into his childish demands and, because these were frustrated, his vengeful spite and his tendency to quit on life. He of course remained very sensitive to any frustrations or apparent withdrawals of interest, as when it was once necessary for me to postpone seeing him. However, here again, one could see the effect of insight and of feeling that he was understood.

INTERACTION OF FIGHT AND FLIGHT

Another patient demonstrates, in a simple form, the interaction of the tendencies to fight and to flight—both of these tendencies arising, as we conceive it, from the underlying psychophysiological mobilization for action against a threat, to escape from it or destroy it. This patient was a gunner's mate in his middle thirties, quiet, rather shy, alert, very pleasant and likable. He presented the usual combat-fatigue syndrome, in which the central symptom was a sense of anxiety without specific content—in other words, a feeling of fear without knowing what he was afraid of, and also the specific fear that he could lose control of himself and attack someone.

This fear of his own hostility stood in sharp contrast with his gentle personality. He had spent half a year on a subchaser, liked this duty and enjoyed the actions. In civil life, he had worked himself up to a good income. He was a steady worker, had put in long years with his company but had left his previous employer because of a sudden outburst of rage over a certain situation. His present anxiety developed after leaving his ship for a minor operation. Home on leave, he noticed in himself a hypersensitiveness, an irritability and a mounting fear that he might fly off the handle and strike one of his own children, toward whom he always had been most gentle and understanding. So great was this fear that he began to think seriously of returning to sea just to avoid such an episode, which he knew he would regret bitterly.

As an example of how this inner rage troubled him, one day he went into a cigar store and asked for a pack of cigarettes. The clerk told him abruptly to go to his post and get them. The patient was stunned by this harsh rebuff from a civilian obviously ignorant of what men in the service were going through, of the price they were paying in lost physical and mental health and of the incalculable debt he owed them. The patient's rage welled up, but instead of attacking the clerk, as was his first impulse—namely, to respond with fight—he suddenly felt acute anxiety and found himself running out of the door. Thus, fortunately for the clerk, this sudden overwhelming mobilization for action took the direction of flight, and the patient experienced it as anxiety and fear rather than as rage. Upon reaching home, the patient wept. Weeping is a wonderfully effective safety valve and was used freely by the men overseas.

Some days later, he sat down in a restaurant. The waiter harmlessly but suddenly dashed up behind the patient and asked rather explosively whether or not his order had been taken. Such was the state of the patient's psychological and physiological arousal to action that this sudden approach of the waiter caused not only a severe startle reaction, but, without realizing what he was doing, the patient let fly and floored the waiter with one blow. (Observations in civil life, as well as on patients with combat and operational fatigue, suggest that this is the essence of the startle reaction, namely, that the organism is already so aroused psychologically and physiologically for fight or flight that any sudden stimulus acts as a trigger release. Of course, other specific factors intervene, and men startle most easily to the sounds which for them were connected with the greatest danger or most distressing experience. Some jungle-shy marines startle violently at a barely audible footstep and not at loud noises.)

The patient was hardly conscious of hitting the waiter. He remembers that in a daze he dashed blindly across a busy street, mercifully missing the whirling traffic. He plunged into a shop and cowered, crying, in a corner. Again we see the first impulse to attack, followed instantly by flight, anxiety and weeping. The kind young woman clerk took him out on the street, where he felt such acute fear of men in uniform that he was unable to approach them. He was finally taken to the hospital.

As we have said, his chief symptoms remained his anxiety and his fear of attacking others. Since current pressures are apt to keep the condition going in these men, the patient was asked about anything in his *present* life that caused him emotional tension. He said that his home life was happy, that he was secure in prospects for a civilian job to which he could return and that all in all he enjoyed his Navy experience. But at this point he spontaneously complained of recent nightmares.

These had occurred a few nights before and consisted of a series of three dreams. In the first, he killed a child with a hammer. In the second, he was being investigated for this crime. In the third, he drove a locomotive into an elderly man, crushing him. He awoke from these dreams, as he usually did from nightmares, with a dull headache. As to the first dream, he quickly denied that he ever could do a thing like that, but then as he thought it over, he suddenly added with a sickly smile, "At least, I hope not. That is why I am so afraid." He then went on to relate his fear of being at home at all, because his irritability was so great that he dreaded lest a sudden act or the exhaustion of his patience might lead him impulsively to strike one of his own children.

The elderly man reminded the patient of one who had once made sexual advances to the patient's wife, which she had repulsed in no uncertain terms. The patient then said that one of his most distressing symptoms was an almost complete loss of sexual feeling and potency.

The sexual feelings often reflect this fight-flight reaction. While the man is very much aroused and this mobilization takes the direction of attacking, of overcoming obstacles and, in general, is lived out in some form in real life, however constructive or destructive, sexuality is often proportionately increased. Frequently, this increase is so great that the men are never gratified but feel so driven that instead of enjoying this exaggerated sexual urge, it causes them unrelievable distress, and they complain of it. Apparently, what happens is that the hostility reinforces sexual feelings and seeks expression in action through them. This is the usual, normal mechanism and is disturbed only because of the quantitative increase of the hostility and the consequent overexaggeration of the sexual urge. Sexuality drains other feelings as well as hostility. We are speaking only of this one point. In the case we are discussing, we observed the opposite effect. It seemed that the anxiety which accompanied every hostile act of the patient was so great that it inhibited the sexuality. In other words, instead of the fight reaction's increasing his desire and potency, the anxiety and flight reaction diminished it. The dream suggested that this sexual impairment caused him feelings of inadequacy and insecurity toward his wife and therefore was one source of continuing hurt masculinity and so of rage.

Speaking of the elderly man soon led him to talk of his father. Although his mother was a gentle person, like his wife, and he never had had the slightest difficulty with either of these women, his father was a man of great strictness, who whipped the children cruelly and with automatic promptness for any infringement or any act of aggression on their part. Thus, although the father trained them so harshly not to vent their own tendencies to attack, he himself served as a model for the opposite mode of behavior and vented his own anger in cruel attacks upon the children. Such a situation is bound to be very conflictful for the children, for children always tend to identify with their parents—to do what they do rather than what they say. Here, the *model* of the father gave them both the stimulus and the sanction to be violent themselves, but a strict *training* built up in them inexorable controls, inhibitions and counterreactions to any violence they expressed. It is like teasing an animal to anger it and then striking it on the nose when it tries to express its anger in any actual aggressive act.

Now, asked why a hammer was in the dream, the patient immediately recalled a time in childhood when his brother was given a toy which he refused to share with him. The patient's anger flared up, and, without thinking, he struck the brother on the head with the blunt end of a hammer severely enough to knock him out and leave the patient to enjoy the toy. For this the patient was thrashed by his father. A similar incident occurred a year or two later with another brother, and again the patient struck him impulsively with a hammer.

These incidents had occurred in the patient's early childhood. His father died when the patient was eight. It is readily understandable why, with his impulses to violence and with the certain knowledge of the punishment to follow, the patient should have lived in deathly fear of his father. He could never avoid aggressive acts and hence had to live in dread of the thrashing which would follow automatically. This is exactly the pattern he showed at this time— sudden aggressive acts, then fear and weeping, just as in childhood.

As the years passed, he became more and more friendly with his brothers and gradually established more and more control of his sudden temper and impulsive violence. It is interesting, and somewhat unusual that, as he stated, he did not seem to develop thoroughgoing and secure controls of his aggressive acts until his early twenties. When controls or, for that matter, any similar psychological reactions are developed so late, they are apt to be proportionately superficial. In general, the earlier reactions are established, the more deep-seated they usually are. As these controls developed, the patient became more and more popular, having many friends among both sexes.

As the patient began to see these emotional forces within himself, and how they operated, a great light seemed to dawn, and his expression became more animated. He saw that now, as in childhood, he was constantly tempted to attack others but then was overcome with fear of retaliation—that gradually over many years he had gained control over his temper, but that now it was aroused again by his Navy experience. Suddenly, he said that while on the subchaser he had become greatly excited when an enemy submarine was discovered, that he had found action against it fun and now for the first time he began to realize that actually he had *enjoyed* the kill. And now he said that just as when he struck his brother and feared the beating from his father, so, although he never had before made the connection, he had *enjoyed* the violence against the enemy, yet, however much this violence was justified, unconsciously he had feared a terrible punishment. This was the reaction of his own conscience, arising from his early training by his father, and this anticipated conditioned reaction to his own violence was the source of his continuing anxiety. No wonder, then, that he found combat duty so conflictful and became aroused by it and against it.

Here again, this single interview, obviously inadequate to re-solve a lifelong conflict, which, although once mastered, had erupted again as a result of combat, nevertheless produced radical improvement by transforming a mysterious, threatening anxiety into a realistic, comprehensible, practical problem. In this way it greatly reduced the secondary anxiety. No longer did this man fear losing all control, "blowing his top," "going crazy." Now he saw that he had a down-to-earth emotional problem, serious, difficult to master, but yet something that could be comprehended, grasped and wrestled with, and not the insidious mounting insanity he had dreaded. Under his emotional stress, this man, like most of those reported in this book, expressed motivations and achieved insights rarely reached in civil practice without many hours of work. His conflict was made conscious—at least the first steps were taken—and over the following weeks his progress continued with only occasional short talks with the psychiatrist.

(Two years later, he told me that his improvement had continued and he was again getting along excellently at his work and in his home. He was eager to have this episode of his life published "if it will teach even one parent that his hands do not belong at his child's head." This single heated remark shows that he grasped the *essence not only of his own problem but also of humanity's suffer-ing,* which is rooted in atrocious child-rearing—each generation tending to pass on to its children the treatment it received from its own parents.)

During and after World War I, one of the more dynamic general formulations of war neurosis described it as the outcome of a conflict between the sense of duty and the urge to flee because of fear. As we have seen, what went on in these men emotionally was usually much more complicated than this. However, this conflict is an important element. It is not always the sense of duty alone which urges the man to fight, but, in addition, one sees the results of his whole psychophysiological mobilization or fight and flight.

How this operates is demonstrated by a personable, intelligent young pilot of 24, who had been given the diagnosis of "effort syndrome." At the beginning of the interview, this young man stated that he was unable to define his symptoms or feelings clearly; his chief complaint was that he easily got "tensed up and wound up like a spring." He fatigued easily and on the slightest effort he experienced sweating, palpitations and fast heartbeat. He found sleep to be his only refuge from tension and fatigue.

He was highly intelligent, rather sophisticated and gave the impression of being quite understanding psychologically, but he denied having any idea of the cause of his condition. He had had several years of intensive training, repeatedly interrupted because of his symptoms, which kept him from any extensive combat experience, even though he had enlisted prior to the United States' entrance into the war. He had been grounded a year before and had been given an interesting executive job. However, he was unable to do it because of his tension and fatigue. For instance, some situation would develop, he would take care of it by giving certain orders, and then he would feel utterly exhausted. His emotional tension mounted so that he could not even sit quietly at a movie. He became so sensitive that he feared he might break down weeping in public. Pressed for a reason, he could only suggest that the cause might be too much aviation training.

Turning to his family history, nothing illuminating was elicited except that the family seemed to be made up of rather sensitive, artistic people and was very harmonious. The patient said that he had enlisted when he saw the war coming, because it seemed to be the normal, patriotic thing to do. Asked about his sleep and his dreams, he denied having any dreams whatever.

Remarkable as it may seem to one who is not on the lookout, *a person's relationship to his dreams,* the freedom with which he dreams and with which he is able to relate his dreams indicate that person's ability and willingness to express and face his own deeper feelings and motivations. It is rarely possible to understand thoroughly and clearly the major emotional forces which make up the personality in those persons who almost never dream or are unable or unwilling to reveal their dreams. The converse relationship, however, is not necessarily true. That is, a person may reveal his dreams and yet be hard to understand. Such being the case, this man's inability or refusal to recall or relate even a single dream boded ill for the possibility of understanding him—and without a good understanding of the emotions causing the symptoms, helping the man by whatever methods cannot be entirely rational or causal. For this reason, it is rarely so effective as when the therapist has this knowledge.

On the other hand, there is nothing in psychological work so difficult as discerning and eliciting the core of a personality, even when there is not a very strong conscious or unconscious resistance on the part of the patient against revealing himself. All other types of contact with the patient and all kinds of techniques and procedures are relatively easy for the psychiatrist, both intellectually and emotionally, when compared with sitting down with the man and understanding the emotional forces which make him the individual that he is. But *this is the very essence of psychiatry.* It produces rationally and causally based results, brings the whole problem into the light and yields the greatest satisfaction to the therapist who is interested in personality and in the solution of these emotional problems.

Hence, although the interview apparently had reached an impasse, it could not be given up until every effort to carry things further had been tried.

There are but rare situations in psychiatry in which honesty is not the only proper procedure. The patient was told frankly that there must be some cause for his symptoms, that this was probably very simple and comprehensible, but that he apparently refused, consciously or unconsciously, to face his own feelings. After some hesitation, the patient admitted that on one occasion he had been given sodium pentothal narcosis, and during this, so they told him later, he had talked about buddies of his who had been killed during training. He then was asked how he felt in reality about this. He replied that he had helped dig many of them out of wrecked planes. He was now almost the only one of this group left. But his only feeling, he said, was sorrow for the wives and the children of these young men. He, too, was married and had two young children.

He was told that no one becomes so upset as he was because of purely altruistic feelings and that he must have some reaction to the deaths of his buddies of which he felt ashamed or guilty—possibly only fear lest what happened to them might happen to him. "No," he said, "it could not be fear." He felt none. He was told that it was inconceivable, however, that he did not react with at least some fear, since obviously he might have been next. To this he replied that if he felt fear, it was unconscious. (This is a rather common form of response in patients who begin to admit their true feelings.) It was then pointed out that if it were unconscious, this was precisely because he was ashamed of it, yet it was a perfectly natural and unavoidable reaction and could be observed in any person or animal in similar danger. The patient still said "No."

We tried again. He was asked if it might be guilt rather than fear which troubled him—guilt perhaps not from anything he had done but only from the feeling of satisfaction that it was they and not he who were killed. With this question, the patient started and spoke with mounting excitement. He had never thought of the possibility of that, he said, but now he recognized that he was bothered for long periods by dreams, most of them nightmares, of a buddy of his. (Note that as we approached the core of his problem he spontaneously told dreams and was interested in their meaning, whereas he previously had denied having any.) These dreams came on after his buddy was lost on a mission. At that time, the patient was in the hospital with some minor symptoms; otherwise he might have been chosen for that mission himself, instead of his buddy. Now he admitted guilt and shame when he thought of all those men over the years killed in training or in battle, while he was still here, sound and whole and even frequenting night clubs. He should be in combat himself. He felt this so strongly, he said, that he refused a medical discharge when it was offered him. He *wanted* to stay in—duty was duty. "True," he was told, "but you also feel that if you do your duty you will be killed, as they were killed." Then the patient said he was beginning to realize what he never had known, namely, that perhaps he had had great fear without knowing it, and because of this perhaps he had unconsciously resisted going out to combat.

Without going into all the details of the interview, it can be said that, now the cat was out of the bag, the patient could talk freely of the fear which he had so long denied. It was clear that in reality he had tried his best. He had joined up before the war and had remained in when he could have accepted a medical discharge. He had forced himself to do his best. But, unconsciously, the fear exerted a power which dragged him back and inhibited all his activity. He was constantly mobilized for fight or flight—fast heart, elevated blood pressure, sweating, tension—all the signs of autonomic nervous activity. Consciously he wanted to fight, but unconsciously he wanted to flee. He responded with profound relief to being able to discuss openly and frankly what he had carried as a burdensome, guilty and shameful secret which was even largely repressed from consciousness. Now, he said, he saw that all this time he must have been suffering from tremendous fear without realizing it. On the contrary, he always had been proud of his composure. On one occasion, in an emergency, when he was copilot, he retained his presence of mind and saved the plane, while the senior officer yelled in panic. For, he said, it was deeply ingrained in him that he must not show fear. He was told that it was important to understand why this was; that we could already see one reason was that it hurt his pride, and that led him to hide it. He agreed with feeling and said that he often even forced himself into danger to prove that he was brave. He was shown that in this he was not acting rationally, like those men whose pride is not hurt by fear but who admit it freely and make no issue of it. Unlike them, he felt driven to danger by his pride and by his guilt toward his buddies. He even felt forced to volunteer for dangerous missions. He needed to deny the fear and to be looked up to by others, but now he had come to realize the powerful counterforce, so that when he exerted himself even a little, he felt the effort as tremendous and it left him exhausted.

This, then, seemed to be a form of flight, of withdrawal, of sit-down strike, of biological refusal of the organism to function. All his activity had to be accomplished in the face of this intense, unconscious, biological refusal. Hence, the slightest task required enormous effort to overcome this inner resistance and protest and left the patient disproportionately worn out. What part, if any, the guilt toward the buddies played in this case did not come out. It is known that guilt often causes feelings of depression. But whether or not this was a source of the fatigue in this case was not determined. However, there is another point of interest. This man was a pilot. Guilt toward buddies is what Grinker and Spiegel (1945) found so frequently to be the basic problem in the flying personnel in World War II, while the problems of the ground personnel seemed to be more like the various problems we have been describing, resulting from the long-continued strains of the service.

REFERENCES

Cannon, W. (1929): *Bodily Changes in Pain, Hunger, Fear and Rage.* New York: Appleton.
Grinker, R. and Spiegel, J. (1945): *Men Under Stress.* Philadelphia: Blakiston.
Saul, L. J. (1976): *Psychodynamics of Hostility.* New York: Jason Aronson.

15 | Court-Martial Cases

One's view of this group of patients with combat and operational fatigue comes into better perspective if one compares them not only with those men who have withstood the most dire trials of the war but also with two other groups of cases.

In the court-martial cases, the emotional problems and the stresses are very similar to those encountered in the men we have been discussing, but the outcome is different—for instead of controlling their feelings and developing symptoms, these men act out their impulses to fight or flee and hence become enmeshed in the disciplinary system.

The third group comprises those men who are not accepted for military service because of mental or emotional unbalance. The size of this group, totaling nearly a million in World War II alone, or almost 20 percent of all rejections, has opened the eyes of many persons to the nature and the extent of the problem of neurosis. This is helping to shift the focus of psychiatry from the psychoses, or insanities, which are only end results and extremes of breakdown, to the neuroses which represent the emotional problems of humanity and hold the key to human mental and emotional function. The psychiatrist in the training station has seen these men by the hundreds and the thousands, and here again he has seen how largely their weaknesses and eccentricities are *the results of unfortunate training and experiences during childhood.* And these childhood experiences are also the most important factor in causing hostility to self, as masochism, and hostility to others, as crime.

The ignorance of parents concerning the fundamentals of bringing up children is terrifying. The same parents who would raise flowers properly by providing them with suitable soil, moisture and sunshine, and then let them develop freely, will beat a six-month-old child for not eating properly, a year-old one for being messy with its food or a two-year-old for sometimes wetting in the daytime or at night. One child is beaten into submission, another cajoled into lifelong dependence, another forced prematurely out on its own. The emotional development becomes warped, and in adult life these children never outgrow these scars of childhood; they are insecure and anxious, often restless and striving, often giving up and becoming psychologically helpless, and, usually, out of their inner unhappiness and insecurity, they harbor a rage and a hostility which gnaw at their own souls, cause all kinds of physical symptoms, from headaches to heart trouble, and only too readily seek means of expression toward other persons in cruelty to family and children and even in criminality and political violence. *Irrational, pathological, hostile acting out is public health's most staggering but also most vital problem.*

However, we cannot consider the rejectees in detail. Let us return to the group of men who appear before a general court-martial in the service. These remarks are limited by the restrictions upon information permissible in court and by the strict discretion accepted by members of the court.

The personalities and the behavior seen in these cases form a striking series. The offenses are predominantly military in nature, most cases being tried for absence or desertion, which are not crimes in normal civil life. What is striking in the first place is something which is really well known, namely, that the same conflicts, problems and tensions that cause *psychological* symptoms, such as anxiety, inability to concentrate, loss of interest or amnesia (losing track of some hours or even days), or *"psychosomatic* symptoms," such as nervous headaches, stomach or heart disorders, are, in these court cases, *acted out* and so produce *behavior disorders,* including, as we keep emphasizing, hostility to self, as masochism, and to others, as violence-proneness of all sorts.

Let us recall that one of the common symptoms in combat fatigue is the hypersensitivity to taking orders and the fear of getting into trouble. Typically, a man fears that instead of merely suffering with his emotional tension and the symptoms that it causes, he will say or do something which will get him into trouble and will ruin his hitherto clear record, so he controls his speech and behavior, but his thinking and digestion are upset.

Of course, the great majority of cases, whether seen in hospital or court, reveal, on careful examination, some symptoms in all three spheres—thought and feeling, internal organs and behavior. This is to be expected since, under pressure of emotion, the whole physiology is mobilized; and both thought and bodily responses are in the service of action, even though this action may be inhibited and never carried out; and the thought of it, the feelings connected with it, and even to a considerable extent the visceral responses may be repressed to greater or lesser degree.

At any rate, the cases seen in court form an instructive complement to those well-behaved individuals who repress their dissatisfactions and inappropriate impulses and suffer from them only in the form of psychological or psychosomatic symptoms. Thus, one man exposed to combat develops an anxiety reaction with fears of injuring himself or others and perhaps with spells of amnesia. Another man shows little in the way of psychological disturbance but develops headaches, nausea and vomiting, cramps and diarrhea, perhaps with episodes of rapid heart beat. A third man, instead of developing these psychological or physiological symptoms, simply *acts* on his anxiety or hostility. He obeys the flight impulse, instead of inhibiting or repressing it, and goes absent without leave; or he obeys the fight impulse and harms himself (masochism) or attacks someone else (criminality). The motivating impulses cause a disorder of behavior rather than of thought, mood or visceral functioning.

Every person has his characteristic reactions to emotional tension, his particular combination of symptoms. These men seen in court were, in general, "acting-out" types, whatever other form their symptoms might take. Moreover, in most cases, their acting out always had been more or less neurotic, that is, unduly motivated by childhood impulses and unduly dominated by childhood attitudes and patterns at the expense of mature and realistic judgment. Although their present difficulties might be caused by the emotional rigors of life in the service, the majority of these men had developed these difficulties in life before. Such men have been termed "neurotic characters," "psychopathic personalities." The extreme, frankly pathological cases were screened out by the brig psychiatrists and did not come to trial.

Many of these particular neurotic personalities or behavior neuroses or "psychos," as they were known in vernacular, manifested faulty judgment, lack of realism and weakness of will and control, that is, they had "weak egos." This weakness of judgment, realism and control was perhaps one of the reasons why they acted out their impulses as they did. Not all "acting-out" types have such weaknesses. The men to whom we refer were recognized by naval justice as "weak brothers," dependent, immature, unrealistic persons, and psychiatrists were placed at strategic points in the whole court and prison system to try to understand and help them.

The most striking feature of these men was their tendency to get themselves into trouble. Their acting out took a form which resulted in their own suffering. The were "masochistic" characters, i.e., men with tendencies to make themselves suffer. The mishandling of their lives to their own detriment was a characteristic which went back through their lives to early childhood, and their experience in the service was usually just another example of the same self-defeating, self-punishing, self-tormenting pattern. Occasionally, this tendency was recognized by the man himself, but usually it operated unconsciously. There are some men who do deliberately choose prison to active duty and act accordingly, but we are speaking here only of those who get into trouble in spite of themselves, have always done so and are miserable because of it. Some of these men handled their whole lives, as well as their period in the service, as though they had deliberately figured out the best way to make trouble for themselves. That is, their neuroses came to expression in their handling of their lives and took a "masochistic," i.e., a self-tormenting, form. This is generally a result not only of weak ego and of dependence and immaturity but also of guilt, as described in Alexander's interesting paper comparing neurosis, psychosis, criminality and neurotic characters (1930). Among criminals only a certain (small) percentage get caught, and very often this is not only because of poor judgment but also because of the man's own unconscious slips, which, paradoxical as it may seem, represent a tendency to get punished (Alexander and Staub, 1931). The more fully "criminal" personality, in which guilt is a less potent force and judgment is better, is less apt to be apprehended. Criminal characters, as opposed to neurotic characters, were seen relatively rarely in the general military courts. Most of the men were neurotic characters of the immature, dependent and, above all, the masochistic type, as described above.

The general attitude of truly criminal characters, the impression one gets of them, and the "feel" of their personalities are different. Sometimes their hostility is so naked as to give a sense of their being evil rather than weak, foolish or peculiar. The criminal character accepts and acts out directly, consciously and willfully his hostile, cruel and even murderous feelings. In the neurotic acting out, these infantile, asocial impulses are rejected by the rest of the personality and so are acted out either in disguised form or else with great guilt and shame. If they harm other persons, it is only indirectly and unconsciously, not consciously and willfully. The man who goes absent without leave and repeats his offense harms primarily himself, and only secondarily and indirectly those near him. He may absent himself with only the conscious motive of helping a loved one and yet he handles himself so that he is punished and thereby only causes the loved one more, and not less, suffering. This is the nature of neurosis, that the motivation is rejected and in varying degree is not realized or appreciated by the man himself but is more or less unconscious in its intent.

The criminal character bears the same relation to neurotic acting out as neurosis bears to perversion. If a man has homosexual feelings which he rejects as intolerable, he may develop acute anxiety or even paranoia in the process of fighting off these feelings. That is, he develops a neurosis, the essense of which is a defense against these feelings which threaten his ideal, his masculinity and the rest of his personality. The symptoms are those of anxiety, hysteria or paranoia. The homosexuality is hidden by these symptoms both from the world and, where the neurosis is successful, from the man himself. But the man who has strong homosexual feelings and *accepts* them suffers, not from a "neurosis" in the classic sense of the term, but from what is technically called a "perversion." That is, the impulse is not defended against, repressed, distorted, rejected, to appear only in unrecognizable form, but is indulged more or less frankly and thereby influences the organization of the conscious part of the personality. So the neurotic personality typically has certain impulses, such as hate and hostility, which he cannot tolerate. He may not even feel the hate nor realize that he has it but may develop guilt because of it. He defends himself against expressing it toward his family and others but may live out a punishment for it upon himself.

That is why many of these men are so provocative and, even when they are smart enough to know much better, handle their affairs in ways sure to provoke punishment. It is easy for those in authority to react naively to this provocativeness, which is really a symptom, and oblige the man with the punishment he unconsciously provokes but consciously fears and detests. It is the duty of the psychiatrist to recognize *neurotic provocativeness* as a symptom and handle it as such.

The criminal personality, in contrast with the neurotic personality, accepts these impulses. The bad do what the good dream, as the saying goes. The conscious part of the personality of these men accepts the impulses and is corrupted by them. Such a man gives in to the impulses in greater degree. (All differences in the emotional life—normal, neurotic, psychotic, criminal—are, as has been emphasized, matters of degree.) He may even embrace these impulses as virtues. Taking hostility as an example, whereas the neurotic personality may not even be conscious of wishing to hurt anyone, deplores these impulses and primarily injures himself and only secondarily others, the criminal character may consciously wish to injure others and may extol violence, with the guilt and the self-injury ineffectual, secondary and in the background. The criminal does not inhibit the infantile, asocial impulses. He does what the neurotic only *dreams,* or transfers into symptoms.

As an example of behavior designed, consciously or unconsciously, to get the man into serious trouble, a young fellow remains absent over leave for a few days and is given very mild punishment. He soon repeats this offense. Then, while on authorized leave, he goes beyond the set limit of 75 miles from his station without permission, even though he could easily have obtained permission. By now he is acquainted with the system of justice and well knows the increasing severity with which repeated offenses are treated. Yet he now becomes disobedient in a situation in which this does not even serve any good purpose; and after that, he absents himself for a long period and this time is apprehended by civil authorities and turned over to the service, thereby assuring himself of trial by a general court-martial on the serious charge of desertion in time of war, with a correspondingly severe sentence.

Another type of patient seen frequently enough in court to merit recognition and special attention is the "schizoid" personality.

These men seem, even on superficial observation, to lack normal emotional relationships to other persons. They usually seem to be weak, and the typical schizoid emotional withdrawal, sometimes masked, may be readily apparent and may be a striking feature of the history. While absent, such a man may spend many months in his own home, or even rooming somewhere alone, having and seeing no friends, either male or female, taking part in no athletics, doing no work—an existence which a normal young man would find intolerable. One youth spent nearly a year in his home with his mother. Another older man spent as long a time with his wife and sister-in-law, supported by them, and literally doing nothing except sitting on a chair or lying in bed. These men have no frank neurotic or psychotic symptoms. If they are never under emotional stress and are left sheltered in their homes, or withdrawn and by themselves, no outspoken symptoms may appear. But exposed to too much reality, too many demands, too close human emotional contacts, or under other stress, such as danger or punishment, there may be risk of paranoia, suicide or overt schizophrenia, which is a more or less severe psychosis characterized by a withdrawal of normal emotional interest in people and things in favor of preoccupation with one's own fantasies, usually extreme infantile dependence and, in the severe cases, bizarre thinking, full-blown delusions and hallucinations. In other cases, however, the attachment of a person's strongest emotions to his own fantasies may help to make a fine artist or an eminent scientist.

The reasons or rationalizations given by the men brought to court-martial for their absence from the service were monotonously similar. One was that the man's wife or mother was ill or having other difficulties. Very often it was that the wife was unable to manage alone, especially when there were several children, and she either had no family to go to or else did go to live with her own family or in-laws and had run into difficulties with them. Suspicions of unfaithfulness were relatively infrequent but were usually extremely upsetting to the man when they did occur. At any rate, it was the relationship to a woman—mother, wife, or sweetheart—which was the most constant reason given by the men for their unauthorized absences. In many instances, even when the situation might be more or less distressing in reality, one got the impression that whereas the man might sincerely think of himself in a gallantly aiding role toward the woman, he was actually more like a small boy running to his mother or to a mothering wife. Certainly, in the long run, no real good accrued to the woman any more than to the man himself from such ill-advised action, which was part of an immature, masochistic pattern.

This does not mean that the family situation cannot be severely upsetting, even for the most stable and normal men. Taking a man out of his peacetime environment into the unusual life of the service in wartime necessitates in itself a difficult adjustment. Many of the men who made it satisfactorily so long as things went smoothly in their homes became seriously troubled, found their duties interfered with and even broke down in the face of broken engagements, unfaithfulness, illness, financial difficulties and the like. In many cases, men went through the horrors and the rigors of combat but developed symptoms or got into difficulties when things went wrong at home. Certainly, the role of the home, which is known to be of first importance in shaping the personality of the child and laying the foundation for future normality, neurosis or criminality, is also of the greatest importance in maintaining the morale of the man in the armed forces. The home situation, whether parental or marital home, as well as the strains of life in the service, can cause symptoms, neurotic behavior and even breakdown.

Sometimes the difficulties are indeed real and desperate, and, as the cases appeared, one saw the havoc wrought in so many homes by war. Here was a man in his thirties with a wife and four children, his income reduced, his wife not yet recuperated from a recent radical operation, one child on a special diet because of diabetes, no relatives to go to, no help available, and no money to spare for it, and the house in need of repairs with winter approaching. Here was a young man who already had three children. One of them had a spine ailment which prevented walking. The wife had developed stomach ulcers. They lived on a farm with no running water. Water had to be hauled, wood cut and other heavy chores done to maintain the household. Here was a boy whose father died, leaving his mother alone to care for four small children. One man's wife resented the burden of her three children, went out with other men, managed poorly and lost the home. And so on, one long procession. It is a tribute to many of these men that they served as well as they did in the face of such domestic tragedies and sometimes even the loss of all that they held dear in life. Small wonder that some of them temporarily lost their heads, went home, pitched in and helped and returned late. Such circumstances received due consideration by the service.

Many of the men who came into the service really belonged in the group rejected by the original psychiatric screening. The acting-out types and the schizoid personalities often put up good fronts and were difficult to detect by the very rapid, abbreviated techniques used. And when the question of competence to stand trial arose, the psychiatrist often found it difficult even to establish a clear-cut diagnosis of psychoneurosis. For their neuroses and psychoses, severe and even dangerous though they might be, were either "compensated," masked or latent, as in the schizoid personalities, or else appeared not as simple mental symptoms, such as compulsions or amnesias, or even as psychosomatic symptoms, such as stomach ulcers, but much more subtly and pervasively in the whole trajectory and behavior pattern of the man's life. So, when these cases were of borderline severity, the men found their way into the service—and inevitably into trouble and so into the courts. These were among the hardest cases with which the psychiatrist had to deal—to diagnose them and then to convince the layman that, although they may even be "bums," their deplorable outlook, attitude and behavior, if viewed psychiatrically and not moralistically, would be seen to be symptomatic of neurosis, emotional disorder, psychopathology (being a "bum," like being an addict or a criminal, is usually a form of behavior disorder) just as truly as the more clear-cut cases. In "pure" combat and operational fatigue, symptoms developed from emotional stresses powerful enough to break down relatively normal, stable men. But in the particular cases we are discussing, the neurotic outlooks, emotional relationships and behavior patterns were traceable less to *external* pressures than to the long operation of unfavorable emotional influences during the formative years of childhood. These influences impaired and warped the normal development to mature, stable emotional attitudes.

Another type of man, not too frequently seen, was the one who had been through considerable overseas experience and felt that this gave him some justification for taking the law into his own hands. If he felt he had sufficient reason for so doing, he simply absented himself for a certain, usually limited, period. Other men were not so deliberate but, under the pressure of domestic or other stress, "lost their heads" and then were overwhelmed with guilt, fear and remorse. Still others averred that their motivations were simply so strong as to be beyond their control. This was seen in some cases of homesickness in youths. The behavior of these cases was essentially "reactive," i.e., not a reflection of long-standing neurosis, but intelligible as the reaction which a relatively normal person might have to such stress and circumstances as the man had undergone.

REFERENCES

Alexander, F. (1961): *The Scope of Psychoanalysis*, ed. by T. French. New York: Basic Books, pp. 56–73.

_____ and Staub, H. (1931): *The Criminal, the Judge and the Public*. New York: Macmillan.

16 | The Use of Dreams

One of the most powerful aids in penetrating to the heart of a man's emotional problem is the dream. Every psychiatrist treating patients in military service has had Freud's experience: the patients force their dreams upon the physician. Nightmares were a central symptom. Astonishingly, many men *demanded* interpretations and insisted that there were explanations and that, if they could be found, it would relieve them. The dream, formed while one sleeps, while one is off guard, cuts through all the pretenses and defenses to the core of the problem. To him who learns its language it reveals what really troubles the man—what is central on his mind when not distracted by the occupations of the day. No other method even begins to approach dream analysis for speed and accuracy of understanding the essence of man's motivations and emotional forces. Although the mixture of conflicting forces may be so complex or defensively clouded that the dream is not intelligible, its main theme and main feeling tone are always revealing. Illustrations of how the dream can be used have been given in many of the cases quoted in preceding chapters.

Freud called dreams "the royal road to the unconscious." Although motivated more by superstition than by accurate interpretation, the pharaohs of Egypt, Alexander the Great, and many others among the world's most powerful leaders have treated the dream with the greatest respect and upon occasion allowed decisions upon which hung the fate of empires to be influenced by their dreams. Modern, civilized, sophisticated man has become supercilious and scornful about these remarkable creations which he forms while asleep but by so doing he has lost an important contact with the truth of human desires and motivations—a truth to which he is again beginning gradually to turn. A drop of blood is of little significance. Urine and feces are by-products and waste materials. But under laboratory analysis they reveal significant medical facts about a man's condition. Let us, then, not scorn to analyze another by-product—the dream especially when the patient himself insists that to understand his nightmares is to be able to help with his central problem.

That our understanding of the dream has been befogged by superstition is readily understandable, for the dream springs from our deepest feelings and tends to carry with it an uneasy sense of not quite comprehensible importance. However, the true significance of the dream has long been sensed and has been part of common knowledge, if not of science. That dreams have a meaning and, in general, what that meaning is, has been known to folk wisdom, philosophers and poets, long before Freud, long before a mechanistic phase in the development of the physical sciences tended through its influence to dehumanize the psychological and social sciences, and long before the Victorian world preferred blindness toward the nature of man to a scientific understanding of him. "The dog dreams of a bone, the chicken of corn." We all take it for granted that the lover dreams of his beloved, and we know that the poor often dream of wealth, and the weak of power. The dream, then, is an effort to satisfy by fantasy strong impulses and wishes.

If these impulses and wishes cause guilt and shame so that the dreamer cannot bear to acknowledge such feelings in his own nature, then the guilt and the shame tend to distort the dream and disguise the feelings which it strives to satisfy. That is why so many dreams seem on the surface to be "silly" or unintelligible (but let us not forget that when we are asleep, we believe them).

If one can penetrate beneath the surface, it is invariably found that "the dream is never concerned with trifles." In other words, it takes very strong feelings to form a dream. The significance of even "bad" dreams and nightmares is generally understood—as is shown by the saying that refers to them as unwelcome desires or as a bad conscience. The sound sleep is "the sleep of the just"—or of the adjusted. Literature abounds with examples of dreams of all kinds; Shakespeare gave the dream arising from the conscience immortal form in the sleep-walking scene of Lady Macbeth.

The nightmares which are so prominent a symptom of combat and operational fatigue seem to be no different in nature and origin from the nightmares and other dreams of civil life. It may be that there are true "traumatic" cases in which the man is overwhelmed by a sudden situation of danger and violence which he later tries gradually to digest by working it over in his mind, and that this working over is reflected in his dreams, in which the unbearable situation repeats itself again and again (French, 1939).

However, in the men who came for psychiatric help while in the armed services, the nightmares, no matter how faithful to reality, always selected only one particular terrifying scene out of many, and always altered this scene to some slight degree. This selection and slight alteration always revealed, on careful investigation, that the dream was formed by impulses of violence or guilt, or other unacceptable, rejected, threatening impulses within the man himself. The man's own hostile feelings or guilt feelings—or both—were aroused by his experiences, and it is these which continued to trouble his sleep. Examples of this have been given in the chapter on Hostility. (It was not clear whether fear was important in forming these nightmares. Theoretically, a man in danger dreams of being in safety, if his dream is to be considered completely successful. However, when actual fear continues to be so intense in sleep that it cannot be mentally escaped by such a dream, some fear permeates the dreams. Many men, aware that their combat obligations were completed, continued to experience the nightmares, while others, in acute danger—with normal, realistic fear of it—did not have these terrifying anxiety dreams.)

Even though it seems comprehensible to us that a man should be preoccupied with a terrifying experience to the extent of having terrifying dreams about it, let us not forget that the dream only arises from powerful feelings and wishes. Its essential nature is revealed in the simple wish-fulfillment dream, which can be considered the most "normal" dream. For example, one who is thirsty dreams of drinking, while one who is in danger dreams of safety.

A 22-year-old marine of the Third Division went through some of the worst combat of the war. At the end of the first day, only 29 men were left out of his entire company. Replacements came in, but three days later, only 22 were left. He himself was called upon not only to face incredible dangers, but also to do nasty close-in fighting. He had been through three major campaigns, and all his best friends had been killed. Yet he developed no combat-fatigue symptoms, no startle reaction, no nightmares; his appetite remained good, and he gained weight. During his whole time in the Marine Corps his dreams were only of being a civilian and doing the ordinary pleasant things of peacetime.

Here we see the true wish-fulfilling function of the dream; at night he could escape the carnage and enjoy, in fantasy, the pleasant days of peace. This showed an unusual degree of peace within himself, and actually he did not show the symptoms of combat fatigue. Had he had nightmares, we could be sure that there were conflictful impulses within himself; that he was troubled by impulses to violence, hatred, guilt or some other feelings which caused him anxiety.

There is a type of dream which, if it is not used to penetrate to the man's deepest feelings, yet leads very quickly to the life situation which is worrying him. Such was the dream of the young man we have discussed previously in which he was always weaponless against the enemy, which reflected his anxiety at feeling helpless in facing civil life.

Another example of this is the case of a man of 33, who developed the symptoms of combat fatigue after three years in the service, although he was exposed to relatively little combat. The symptoms had come on rather gradually but became worse after he narrowly escaped death when the man next to him was killed, and still worse after a naval engagement. He described his nightmares as "battle dreams" but upon pinning him down to an actual detailed example, we found that his usual dream was of hiding in a ditch alongside a railroad in an isolated place in fear of an approaching Japanese army. The out-of-the-way place reminded him both of the region which was his home and also of the out-of-the-way places to which he was sent in the service. The railroad recalled his love of travel but also the tens of thousands of miles he had been forced to travel against his will. Thus, a simple, enjoyable dream of being back home was distorted and vitiated by disturbing impulses. But the most striking feature of the dream was the Japanese army, for this man's duty had all been in the Atlantic. It was in talking about this element of the dream that we came to the heart of the problem.

He was 33 but had not yet completed his training as a lawyer; he was married but had not seen his wife for three years; she was struggling along on his lowered income and, like himself, was impatient to establish a home. His sister had run into serious financial troubles and would lose her business if he could not help her. Being a somewhat older, rather mature man, he did not fit in completely with the younger men aboard ship. Always used to traveling about in the open spaces, he suffered from the confinement of shipboard. And now, in the face of all these worries, he feared that if he went to duty in the Pacific he might be kept there on patrol duty for a year or two after the war ended and would not return home to begin his professional and domestic life until he was past his middle thirties. That was why he felt trapped by the Japanese in the dream. We did not go into the question of why his sleep was troubled by anxiety dreams rather than relieved by simple, wish-fulfilling dreams which would allow him to escape into fantasy from all the worries and anxieties of real life. Nevertheless, the few moments spent on this dream rewarded us by bringing into the open his central worries and anxieties in real life, which, in addition to the dangers of the service, caused his protest, his arousal to fight or flight, and his consequent symptoms.

Dream interpretation is only a means to an end. But it is invaluable for time-saving and for psychiatric accuracy. A man of 30 turned in some weeks after his ship underwent a near miss. He had been on a ladder when the bomb landed suddenly and unexpectedly. The blast lifted the ship half-way out of the water. Then he saw other ships hit and was petrified with the fear that his ship would suffer the same fate. Yet, when he turned in, his chief symptom was not fear but depression. He told very little which cast light upon his condition. But in going into his symptoms, he brought out the fact that he had no nightmares but did have many dreams of being reunited with his wife. Discussing this led him to tell that he had been married three years but had hardly ever seen his wife, and that his whole two years in the Navy had been spent on the same ship. They had operated in the Pacific for 18 months, during which time the greatest hardship for him was not seeing civilization. When they occasionally touched port, there was little to see but palm trees. He felt that he lacked those satisfactions which make life worthwhile. As time passed, the frustration became more and more unbearable. The near miss was the last straw. This, piled upon the frustration he had carried from long periods at sea, made him feel that life was no longer worth living and that he no longer cared "about anything at all or what happened." But his repetitive dream revealed clearly and frankly what could be only a powerful wish. Therefore, it was arranged for him to satisfy, in reality, what he strove, in his dreams, to satisfy in fantasy. In other words, he was given a leave to go home to his wife.

In this case, the satisfaction of this wish was so gratifying that his symptoms disappeared during the time that he was with her. After that, when back on duty and faced with the prospect of returning to sea, he became depressed. But, whenever he went home to the girl of his dreams, he felt his usual self.

Dream interpretation is the royal road to understanding the patient. And understanding the patient is the basis for all rational therapy and prevention (Saul, 1977).

REFERENCES

French, T. (1939): Insight and distortion in dreams, *International Journal of Psycho-analysis* 20:287.

Saul, L. J. (1977): *The Childhood Emotional Pattern*. New York: Van Nostrand Reinhold, pp. 49–58.

17 | General Formulation

Combat or operational fatigue appears to develop somewhat as follows:

1. Every man has certain emotional points in his make-up which are more vulnerable than others. These result from the way the patient was molded emotionally by influences during early childhood. Indeed, in most cases, the symptoms themselves were discernible in larval form during childhood or at some period prior to their full-blown eruption. This eruption was caused by the stresses to which the man was subjected.

2. In this particular series, these stresses were caused by life in the service. In civil life, they are caused by the stresses of peacetime living. These stresses irritate and threaten the man's particular emotional sensitivities.

3. When irritated and threatened, men and animals react with impulses to fight or flee.

4. These impulses themselves cause new problems and troubles. In the service neither fight nor flight can be acted upon. The man is ashamed and guilty about being short-tempered, irritable and combative. He is also guilty and ashamed of his tendencies to quit and extricate himself.

5. He tries to control himself and keep going, but the tensions mount, the protest increases, and sooner or later he breaks down.

6. Once symptoms develop, he reacts to them in many ways—minimizing, hiding, exaggerating, exploiting, and so on. His pride may be so hurt secondarily by the mere fact of his having symptoms that a new conflict develops. It is a question of how he handles his own reactions, how strong his forces of control, how sound his judgment, how firm his will.

How he controls his reactions and symptoms is also largely a matter of predisposition, being itself a result of early training and influences. For clarity of presentation, it is useful to discuss it as a separate factor. One man on an anti-aircraft gun shook so at the first airplane raid that he fell off his seat. He wept, vomited and lost control of his bladder and bowels. However, since he was the only man who could operate this radar-controlled gun, he stuck it out through 12 more raids.

The main steps can be condensed to the following formula:

Predisposition (conditioned during childhood) → Reaction to specific stress → Control of reaction.

The stresses to which the men were vulnerable, which precipitated the upsets, can be grouped roughly as follows: (1) combat and operational; (2) service conditions; (3) personal (family, career, financial, etc.); (4) mixed.

Of course, every man shows some degree of mixture. But in most, combat stresses, service conditions or personal troubles clearly predominate, and it is convenient to have a mixed group of those in whom there is no clear-cut predominance. In this volume we have presented mostly cases in which single factors were prominent, in order to illustrate the various points more clearly. The cases we have sketched as illustrative all reveal certain common emotional features. These features are primarily the same as those seen in the neuroses of civil life. This is an expected result, since again and again we see that neuroses are basically the result of *quantitative* shifts in emotion, so that there is no sharp line between the neurotic and the normal. And there is no sharp line between the stresses of war and peace. The emotional forces are the same in everyone, and the most nearly normal person still has many infantile tendencies and patterns, which can be mobilized if sufficient stress is applied to the vulnerable points.

The role of these external pressures in precipitating untoward emotional reactions, that is, neurosis in the broad sense of the term, can probably be seen in all stages and departments of a person's life. First, and most important, they can be seen in the home and in the young child, and even in the infant's reactions to the treatment it receives. It can be seen later in the schools, where physical and intellectual competition, social acceptance, and all kinds of interplay often cause serious problems for the students. In the world of business and the professions, one sees many neuroses arising from insecurity, from excessive competition, from difficulties in relation to superiors, and from all these problems which are inevitable in the struggle for existence in the midst of a complex society.

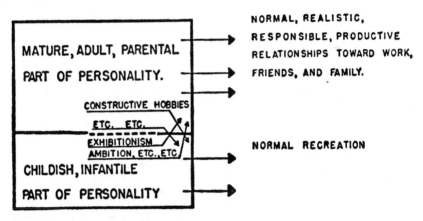

Figure 3   Schematic representation of a relatively normal personality.

In the service, one sees still other stresses. These are perhaps particularly difficult for men who have grown up in an adaptation to our civil life and suddenly find themselves in a military organization—one, moreover, whose goal is destruction, the very opposite of the goals of peacetime, with which they have been imbued. More stresses are engendered, and at the same time, freedom to deal with them is diminished.

That the difficulties engendered in war service persisted for short periods after the men's return to the States, can be accounted for in part by "emotional inertia." Men arriving at the stateside hospital were often highly keyed up, and it took several weeks before they began to relax noticeably. One of the most important reasons for this was not only the effect of *any* change of environment, but more specifically the *disruption of human emotional bonds*. It takes everyone a considerable period of time to adjust himself to breaking off old interests and friendships and establishing others. Every uprooting is painful. In civil life, the loss of those near to us may take months to digest. Mourning is not considered abnormal until it lasts for more than a year or two. Homesickness shows the strength of a man's emotional ties. It is often a wrench to leave even unhappy situations. Men who return from intense and absorbing overseas experiences and friendships do not easily relinquish these; nor are old emotional attachments quickly resumed or new ones formed after returning to the States; and a man in the service is not free to satisfy his desires in his own way. Almost every man coming to this combat fatigue unit showed some improvement merely on the basis of remaining here long enough to become acquainted and to establish relationships with other patients and with the staff. *The need for human contacts and acceptance is as essential to the proper functioning of the biological organism as is a proper diet.*

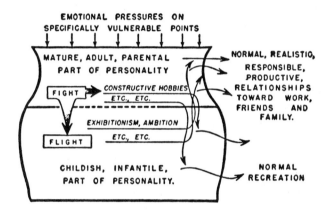

Figure 4 Effects of severe emotional stress. Increase in the infantile reactions causes distortions within the personality and the outside relationships.

A second reason why these men remained upset is the fact that although they were no longer actually in the situation of stress, they felt the threat of returning to it. As soon as it was possible to determine what the man's disposition would be in all probability, the psychiatrist could relieve his uncertainty and help him adjust to the anticipated disposition, whether this were return to full duty, duty within the continental limits or a medical discharge.

These men, because of their particular emotional make-up, and each for his own set of reasons, found their experiences intolerable—the restraints, the confinement, the routine, the regimentation, the demands, the din and confusion of battle, the shriek of dive bombers, the near misses, the blood and the carnage. They felt every fiber aroused against these experiences. They were still keyed up emotionally and physically. The least irritation caused belligerency; the least sound caused a jump. All their reactions were sensitized. And everything that reminded the man of the scenes he was aroused against caused a violent reaction. Hence, when it could truthfully be given, reassurance that he would not return was generally a tremendous relief. This did not cure everything. The revulsion persisted and was still aroused by even innocent reminders, but now desensitization became practicable. The man could be encouraged to face these memories and scenes, which he could now view in safety. Talking them over, writing them out, hypnosis and narcosis when necessary, carefully controlled motion pictures, and so on, now helped the man to digest these once intolerable experiences.

Emotional inertia, fear of being sent out again, and being "fed up" do not explain the persistence of the condition after discharge is assured and after leaving the service. This persistence may be explained by the fact that latent emotional problems were mobilized by the stress. Certain tendencies, previously not strong enough to cause symptoms, were so aroused that they become powerful enough to keep the man upset and to impair his adjustment to new situations. The insight gained into these motivations required a period of "working through" in a stabilized environment with access to the psychiatrist for brief periods, as needed.

Another reason often advanced is the system of disability compensation, which some authorities feel encourages disability. The series of cases seen at this hospital cast little light on this serious question.

18 | Treatment

Rational treatment depends upon understanding the person, the stresses upon him, and how he is reacting to them. Once these are understood, it is usually not too difficult to see what therapeutic steps are indicated. Sometimes it suffices merely to change the environment. In other cases, this is not possible, practicable or effective, but the patient improves through being won over to a change of attitude and a willingness to carry on in spite of his symptoms. In still other cases, these measures are insufficient, and the therapy must be directed to the person's main emotional reactions.

Whether or not changing the external situation relieves the emotional pressure and the symptoms depends not only upon the man's condition but also upon *how soon* the stress is relieved. For example, one young lieutenant did very well on little more than rest and relief from stress. This was certainly due largely to the fact that his commanding officer, upon noticing the first signs of jitteriness, instead of keeping him until these became worse, advised him to turn in immediately. Another lieutenant, in an important position, had been kept on duty even after he had developed nervousness, anxiety, insomnia and crying spells and was not turned in until he had suffered spells of amnesia, in which he would find himself somewhere on the ship with no memory of how he had got there or how long he had been there. By that time his condition was much more serious and more difficult to treat.

In some cases, breakdown occurs because of the suddenness and the kind of stress. In some, it seems to occur because of not being able to relieve the tension by action, whether fight or flight. For example one man who had always "fought like hell when he fought, and ran like hell when he ran," found himself under a flaming enemy plane as it catapulted toward earth. He was in a foxhole—he could not fight, he could not run, and because of the water, he could not even dig. Although scared many times, never

391

before was he totally unable to act—and at that point his anxiety developed.

In most cases, breakdown came only after a long, gradual process of attrition. Men usually bore the strain and resisted turning in. This refusal was very often a matter of pride. They felt that to do so was a sign of weakness. They did not wish to admit that anything had got them down. They insisted upon being considered "rugged"; but by doing so, they more often defeated their conscious purpose and gratified their unconscious one. By prolonging the strain they broke down into a condition which often led either to limited duty or discharge. If they had turned in earlier they might soon have been returned to full duty.

Getting along under strain is essentially a matter of *adaptation*. One of the most difficult situations to adapt to is uncertainty. This is obviously because the process of adjustment and adaptation cannot take place unless the organism knows and feels what it is adapting to. This is a fundamental biological principle. General observation indicates that most men prefer a longer tour of overseas duty if they only know with a reasonable degree of definiteness how long this tour will be, rather than a period which is indefinite, even though in the end it may be shorter. It seems even easier to adapt to the certain knowledge that one is overseas for a specific though prolonged period than to expect that one will return, in, say, 18 months, and then be kept on indefinitely. One large group of men was given the certainty of being returned to the States after 18 months overseas, and it was possible to carry this out faithfully. It is probably no mere coincidence that not a single breakdown occurred in this group.

However, it must be recognized that this group also had fair and interested leadership, a factor of the greatest importance. All people are children underneath, like the iceberg, five-sixths of which is submerged under water. Under stress and in danger, their childhood reactions, as we have seen in all the cases cited, are aroused. Fundamental among these is the need for interest and for being valued—the same need, showing throughout adult life, which the child had for love and attention from its parents. The sense of having a strong, capable, reliable father, or a substitute for him, interested in one's person and one's welfare, is a tremendous gratification and reassurance. It gives some men such a sense of security that with it they can endure dangers and hardships which they could not face alone. It is seen in many phases of adult life— in the need for leadership, for example, and outstanding leaders are often called "fathers" of their country, showing clearly that they stand in the position of the father to the child. Probably the same need plays a part in religion. The scope and completeness of childhood motivations is indicated by the paucity of real leaders.

A basic principle of psychiatric therapy is that the patient can only be won to new, more mature attitudes if these offer a decrease of suffering and an increase of enjoyment. This bit of human nature provides special difficulties for military psychiatry, especially in those cases in which cure means returning to unwelcome conditions. In many cases, however, striking improvement could be achieved by showing a man that he could gain what he desired through using mature, rather than infantile attitudes.

It was to be expected that the change of environment from the stresses of active duty to the status of patient in a convalescent hospital would alone produce considerable therapeutic effect. In reality, however, this change was usually less effective than might have been expected. The men we have described, and the concept of service fatigue to which study of them led, showed why this should be. The average man showed certain reactions under stress and returned to normal very quickly after the stress was relieved; but this was not the case in most of the patients seen here. With them, the stress had stirred up long-standing emotional reactions which previously had been under control. Now this continued, even though the stress was relieved, and the therapeutic task became one of enabling the man to regain control of these emotional reactions, or else somehow to assimilate them, to overcome them, or to integrate them into the normal part of his personality. Of course, the long-range stress is by no means entirely relieved, for recovery is apt to mean return to duty while failure to recover may mean the anticipation of life-long emotional difficulties and a sense of guilt or shame for a medical discharge.

Because the set-up of a convalescent hospital is not of itself sufficient to produce radical cures does not mean that it is not of the greatest importance for recovery. Without going into the whole matter in detail, it is possible to consider certain factors in the effectiveness of a convalescent hospital. In the first place, there are the physical factors. A quiet setting reduces external stimulation and gives an opportunity for gradually letting down the tension and relaxing. Sleeping conditions are of vital importance, as is to be expected from the fact that insomnia and nightmares are central symptoms. In a large ward of double bunks, there was constant difficulty and complaints. When patients were moved into a separate building with single beds, not more than six to a room, there was a tremendous lift in morale, certain rather despondent patients began to improve, attendance at various activities mounted sharply, and disciplinary problems fell off to a fraction of what they were.

As everyone knows, food provides more than calories and vitamins alone. A good meal, appetizingly set forth, satisfies not only the body but also something in the soul, symbolically recalling the mother's giving and care from the "oral phase" through all childhood feedings. Good food provides for most people a compensation for the cares of life, which, when not forthcoming, is often sought in less harmless and desirable ways. Quiet living and sleeping conditions and good food made a critical difference in the whole morale of the group.

These are a few of the simple essential physiological factors. However, sleep, food and quiet are not sufficiently effective for such men, because of the fact that the disorder is essentially one in the man's *feelings toward other persons* (*and also toward himself*). Although certain patients at first profit most by an almost complete withdrawal to little more than a vegetative existence, and do well with a complete rest and with relative absence from human society, for example, on farms or ranches, yet these men eventually, and the great majority from the beginning, need opportunities for readjusting their feelings toward others. They are filled with anger at people, fear of people, needs for giving and receiving love and other emotions toward human beings, which strive for outlets and must be adapted eventually to the requirements of social life. Scenery is no substitute. These men crave warmth and life. Hence, it is important for them not only to be quietly and pleasantly situated with adequate space for athletics and access to the countryside, but also near towns of sufficient size to follow their own bents and live their own lives during their liberties. Liberty is itself an important aspect of therapy.

Various activities in a hospital have great value in building the men up physically, which is often of basic importance in their emotional states and also in providing outlets for their interests and tensions and distractions from their worries. As an example of the latter, a photographer found marked relief by plunging into work in the darkroom. In these activities and in the educational facilities offered, many men find not only sublimated emotional outlets and hobbies but also develop occupational interests. This is of great importance, since for the average person life is much easier if he has some kind of concrete occupational goal and interest, and such goals are of inestimable therapeutic value. A genuine interest in one's *work* provides one of the greatest goals and is one of the most stabilizing forces in human life. Another great force is interest in *mating and family*. Together they form the two *great goals of life* and the *two main pillars of mental stability*. (Most people seem to desire wealth as a release from work, unapprised that restraint from work, for the mature person, is a terrible deprivation.)

Of great importance is the attitude of the entire staff. In general, the patients have expended too much emotional energy in their duties and in controlling their feelings. On the other hand, most of them have received much less emotional interest than they have been accustomed to. In other words, they have been living out of emotional balance—expending more than they have been taking in. Hence, their needs for interest, care and solicitude are heightened. And their self-esteem is sorely wounded by their breakdowns, their symptoms, their sense of failure and the necessity of being patients. Moreover, leaving the demands and the rigors of duty for the status of patient, they expect a certain amount of consideration and interest. By giving this, the staff is in a position to restore the emotional equilibrium and this can be done judiciously without causing so much regression to passivity and dependence that the way back to responsibility and duty is made harder.

Someone has said that some day it will be recognized that these requirements for attention and for being valued are just as important as the need for vitamins. This does not mean that it is necessary to coddle the patients or encourage regression, but only suggests that they be treated with interest, consideration and respect for their individual personalities, as good adults, and that an effort be made to restore the emotional equilibrium by putting in more and demanding less, for a time. Most of the men are quickly responsive to a little sincere human warmth and interest and attention to their personal problems. This is in line with remarks made concerning the vital childhood needs for reliable, accepting parents—an essential condition for normal emotional development. Men who have received ample interest from their leaders in the field are apparently much less apt to break down in the first place. *The overall task is to help the man to understand his problem and to help himself.*

In general, the set-up of the convalescent hospital, developed out of experience, serves to relieve the physical, intellectual and emotional stresses under which the men broke and to replace them by their opposites. It alters *external* factors in the man's environment. Meanwhile, the psychotherapy works with the *internal* factors, with the attitudes and the feelings within the man himself. The quintessential requirement remains one and the same thing: *to understand the patient.* Then whether altering the external environment or dealing with the patient's inner feelings, one works rationally. In the personal therapeutic interview the physician sees one man's underlying individual problem, and as he sees man after man, he gains a close-up, direct contact with the psychological features which these men have in common—anxiety, hostility, regression to childish patterns, hypersensitive egoism, needs for attention, support and guidance, the course of normal emotional development, the nature of maturity, and so on, and the relationships of these emotional forces to the symptoms. It is of some value to discuss these common features with small, selected, homogeneous *groups* of patients.

But without thorough understanding of the individual patient, one practices surgery without knowing anatomy. In military work such understanding is even more important than in civil life. For the emotions are highly mobilized, the tension great, acting out hazardous, and the time short. Everything depends upon penetrating insight, precision of understanding and accuracy of interpretation of the major emotions in a form that the patient can understand and digest. This is, above all, "aimed psychotherapy," and the rewards are proportionate to the marksmanship. The bull's-eye must be hit to ring the bell. Peripheral problems and side issues, however important, will be misleading and confusing. *The core of the emotional dynamics must be hit.* Then the man feels it, sees light and hope, begins to grasp it and is relieved. He starts on the way out of his jam. That is all one can do in one or two hours, but it is a great deal indeed, for such therapy, although very brief is *causal*, based upon understanding of what is going on emotionally in the patient. The first interview is almost invariably the crucial one, and it is best to make the major time investment then, even if it runs to two hours; later interviews may then be brief (Saul, 1972).

There must be insight, not merely into the fact that the patient has an emotional problem, but also into the underlying emotions which cause it. This insight results largely in turning a mysterious upset into a conscious, real, definite emotional problem that can be dealt with. For weeks and months thereafter, the patient uses the insight he has gained. He now sees the possibility, however difficult, of a solution and of working out of the distressing emotional situation by changes in his own attitudes, and this facilitates his emotional development. This process has been called "working through," and during it the psychiatrist can often be of considerable help with only brief interviews of about 15 minutes each. The "working through" is extremely important. Insight alone, often dramatically helpful in its effects, must be used again and again, worked with and consolidated, to be of value in effecting enduring shifts in the direction of development.

Insight almost always helps considerably, but it is by no means everything. For example, one man had served under a superior who frankly disliked him and tended to ride him. While on that station, this man had slight nausea and no appetite, but these symptoms disappeared completely when he was away. The man knew he could not eat while on the station because of his emotional tension in relation to this superior, but this knowledge alone did not restore his appetite. It did help, however, and would have been more effective if the man could have been guided to new attitudes.

The effectiveness of such carefully aimed therapy depends, of course, upon the selection of cases—upon the nature, the severity and the duration of the symptoms, the health of the rest of the personality, the capacity for insight, the emotional accessibility, and also upon the man's intelligence, and his position, opportunities and goals in life, in a word, on his psychodynamics.

Some of the men showed rather deep-seated personality disorders, being infantile, schizoid, and so on. When these were developed to such a point that the men were unable to carry on in military service, the procedures described above, although of some value, were not sufficiently thoroughgoing to effect the personality reorientation called for.

In some cases, as in civil life, it was even dangerous to make interpretations. For example, it is not well to push depressed or very guilty patients with interpretations or investigations except with the greatest care. Judgment must also be carefully exercised, too, with schizoid personalities—some respond very well, others should be left alone. Some have too much insight already, although very few of these are seen here. Nor does one interpret with impunity very conflictful and untreatable trends, like latent homosexuality. In the particular series of cases we are discussing, roughly one-third were helped radically, another third considerably, and the rest relatively little. However, very few did not derive at least some benefit.

In many cases, because of the unusual stresses to which the man had been subjected, the most important emotional trends and conflicts in his make-up were mobilized and came right out in the open; now the solution of his *immediate* problem was identical with the solution of his *fundamental* emotional problems; and by treating his immediate problems his basic personality problem was helped and his emotional development reopened. What one accomplished in from one to three hours is a miniature psychoanalysis, a blitz-analysis, with the main features of the major procedure, except the analysis of the transference.*

---

* Since the question may arise as to the relationship of insight and dreams to psychoanalysis, it may be well to include a passing note on this subject, as it is shrouded in a fog of misconceptions. The term "psychoanalysis" has three meanings. It signifies: (1) a body of knowledge covering the motivations and the processes of man's mind and emotional life, (2) a method of investigation and research and (3) a method of treatment.

As treatment, its essence is this: Emotional disturbances are primarily disturbances in feelings toward other persons—at any rate probably only cases of this sort are suitable for psychoanalytic help. This treatment consists in providing, through the relationship to the analyst, a sample of the patient's feelings toward other persons. The patient should not be emotionally involved with the analyst prior to treatment, for if he is not, it is possible for him, with the insights furnished by the physician, to observe the development of his feelings

In certain cases it was well to maintain contact with the men, by letter, if necessary, to continue the transference and to help them with their "working through" of the insights they had gained and along the path of reopened development. We have discussed a man who, when the mirror was held up to him, was able to work out of his neurosis and save his marriage and career. As he gradually learned that he could handle life situations, his confidence was regained—a "corrective emotional experience" (Alexander and French, 1946).

As understanding of these men increased, it expanded the rational, scientific basis for treatment, including accessory methods, and laid down the basic knowledge for *prevention*.

REFERENCES

Alexander, F. and French, T. (1946): *Psychoanalytic Therapy*, Chap. 8. New York: Ronald.
Saul, L. J. (1972): *Psychodynamically Based Psychotherapy*. New York: Science House, pp. 136–150.

---

and reactions toward the physician in this controlled sample situation. In vaccination the patient learns to control the relatively harmless dose of the germs and their poisons, and thus become resistant to real, virulent infection. So in the office of the analyst, he learns to handle, work out and mature his feelings toward the analyst and thus becomes able to do so outside of the office toward other persons in life. The analysis of the "transference," that is, of the laboratory sample of the patient's emotional reactions to other persons, is the essence of the psychoanalytic procedure. This is one reason why this procedure is very time-consuming and is indicated only in carefully selected cases. Although classic psychoanalysis as a method of treatment was out of the question in the service, yet psychoanalytic *knowledge* as well as certain features of the technique were indispensable in understanding, handling and treating the men by brief procedures.

19 | Conclusions

SOME EFFECTS OF THE SERVICE EXPERIENCE ON RETURNING VETERANS

From the men we have described it is clear that "combat fatigue" and "operational fatigue" are not simple problems. Most popular ideas about them are misconceptions and oversimplifications. The men who returned with diagnosis of "combat fatigue" were by no means all the same. Like all the returning veterans, they were individuals of widely differing personalities.

Some of the men seemed to be almost untouched, or to show little more change than might have been wrought by the experiences of civil life during a similar period. These men were not always the best-balanced ones. Some even had serious personality problems and long-standing neuroses with which they had wrestled and suffered, which they continued to carry with them, often causing them more anxiety and distress than any experience in the service. Yet many such men, as well as those of very healthy, stable make-up, seemed to come through unscathed.

Other men seemed to be broadened by their experiences. They had been thrown out into life and had absorbed a knowledge of the world and its realities which many years as a civilian would scarcely have yielded. Outside the protecting walls of home and school and the pursuits of peace, they had learned something which was not to be found in books, something which was of far greater importance for living than purely intellectual knowledge. They had learned the truth of the human emotions, the bases of the human spirit, the forces which, at bottom, underlie love and hate, egotism and vanity, accomplishment and war. The human experiences and the fires through which alone they gleaned this knowledge, the sacrifices, the comradeships, the demands, the dangers, the trials, the pettinesses and the greatnesses—all tempered and matured them. Their stability, judgment and self-confidence increased.

They were more at ease with jobs, with people of all stations and with themselves. They had developed and broadened and were the better for all they had gone through. War, like other life experiences, can cure and mature; make as well as break.

For other men, the experiences were too much. They had forced upon the man a maturity beyond his years. The doses of reality were too large and too sudden to be digested. The man had learned too rapidly and too harshly how different the world is from the concepts of it he had formed in home and school and had built up all during his past life. Nor could he adapt to this stern reality and the unexpected pressures of all kinds. His preconceptions were too rudely shattered. He was disillusioned. But if his reaction was at all constructive there was hope in this. However disappointed, depressed, embittered he might be, yet he was now closer to reality, and the problems of the world, no less than to those of his own little life, much of which can be solved on the basis of illusions, but only through firm grasp of reality—which even at best is not easy to comprehend accurately.

In some of these men the strain was so great that they began to develop symptoms. In the fortunate cases these were caught in time while the emotional tensions they had built up could still be controlled and while the whole process was still reversible.

In others, the tension mounted to such a pitch that major emotional upsets occurred with long-standing changes in mood, and apparently with shifts in outlook and personality.

In the most extreme cases one got the impression of permanent changes, as though the man had so far given in to childish patterns of reaction that he could no longer climb out and up to mature, controlled attitudes, feelings and behavior. However, it is questionable whether this ever occurs in men who were previously mature and stable. It is probably a matter of the *degree of vulnerability* and then of the *degree of regression* of the rest of the personality. In some extreme cases one could even think of organic changes—as though the long, severe emotional tensions broke through over new conducting pathways in the brain. This is, of course, only speculation.

Even in many of the serious cases, the outlook with proper treatment was good. In fact, some of these men, with the insights they had gained, were even better men than if they had not broken down. This was true of some of the men who have been reported on in this book. In these, the underlying tensions and problems were brought into the light by the pressures of the service. Had they not been, these underlying tendencies, ruthless egotism, pervasive guilt, childish dependence, latent anger, and so on, would have continued to exert their influences, quietly but steadily, over the years, to cause increasing anxiety and inferiority, impaired efficiency, deteriorating marriages, and the insidious growth of unhappiness, tension and even full-blown neuroses, internal or acting-out. But the service had brought the emotional problems into the open, where the man was forced to see and recognize them, to appreciate their reality and power, and so to be able to come to grips with them and move toward solving them. By tackling the emotional problems which caused his "combat fatigue," he dealt with the fundamental emotional issues upon which depended his adaptation, his inner peace and his satisfaction in life. His emotional development was reopened, and he was a better man for the insight his breakdown had given him. But this was only true if, through proper psychiatric help (or otherwise), he achieved such insight.

In this particular, selected group, we dealt with men in whom specific, definite, serious emotional reactions had been aroused. Their need was for expert psychiatric help. But sometimes an understanding friend or an experienced pastor is able to discern the core of a person's problem. Perhaps this will most often be true where the problem is largely external, as where a man faces a jeopardized or shattered career. In other cases, skilled psychiatric help is necessary. Much harm can be done in this field if the man is not *accurately* understood and properly handled. It is no light matter to deal with a man's deepest and most powerful feelings and motivations—those which determine his happiness and misery, his cruelty and kindness, his success and failure, his mental health or mental disorder, even homicide and suicide. *Primum non nocere*—the first task is to do no harm.

Thus we are confronted with a grave situation, for there is a serious shortage of psychiatrists competent to deal with the strongest emotions and adequately trained in *understanding* and in treating *causally* and *rationally* the problems to which these passions give rise. How this need might be met is a huge problem of treatment, training, education and organization. The ultimate goal must be prevention.

We have been focusing our attention upon the emotional problems arising in military life, but let us now remind ourselves that *such disturbances occur quite as frequently among civilians*. The more seriously neurotic individuals were kept out of the service by the psychiatric screening examinations. At the same time, these examinations brought to light the enormous extent of emotional disturbances in the population as a whole. No doubt Freud's remark is true that everyone is at least a little neurotic. But the extent of the severe disturbances in civil life, enough to handicap a man's life and to make him unfit for military service, was not appreciated. According to the Surgeon General's office: "during approximately five years of United States' participation in the Second World War, 1,850,000 men were rejected at induction stations because of neuropsychiatric disorders. There were 1,000,000 admissions of psychiatric patients to Army hospitals, and 545,000 men were separated from the service for the same cause. Rejections alone amounted to 23 percent of the entire strength of the United States Army, at home and abroad, on V-E Day. They represented 12 percent of all men examined by the Selective Service system and 38 percent of all rejections for all causes." * Eight out of ten rejections were for simple emotional disturbances in the form of personality disorders and neurotic symptoms. Many breakdowns under the stresses and dislocations of the war years have occurred in the civilian population. There is no more reason to look askance at the serviceman than at anyone else, man or woman.

NATURE OF NEUROSIS

A tentative formulation of the emotional dynamics of combat fatigue has been advanced in previous chapters. In all cases, what causes the symptoms is the emotional tension generated by the four factors: (1) specific emotional vulnerability, (2) specific stress, (3) intensity and extent of reaction, (4) forces of control and integration. *In what forms the tension manifests itself,* whether disturbed

* John M. McCullough: *Today* (Philadelphia Inquirer, January 21, 1947).

digestion, palpitations, fear, anger, depression, agitation, compulsive thinking, alcoholism, sleeplessness, or in hostile acting-out against self or others, *reveals nothing of the cause.* The essence is the basic psychology—the interplay of the underlying emotional forces (described in Chaps. 2–9) in a word, the "dynamics," or more precisely the "pathodynamics"—the dynamics of the psychopathology.

This formulation helps to clarify our concept of "neurosis." This term, so widely used and abused, is of as much interest to the laity as to the psychiatrist. No satisfactory and generally accepted definition has been advanced. However, certain features are apparent. In the first place, as we have repeatedly emphasized, neurosis is *a way of reacting* which follows disturbed earlier childhood or infantile patterns. Secondly, since everyone has some emotional problem, everyone has some of these ways of reacting. Indeed, the amount of headache, anxiety, nervous stomach, superstition, violence-proneness, individual, organized and political crime, and other sick reactions in the population is apparent to the most casual observation and is eloquently indicated by the extent and the success of the advertising of all kinds of products for the relief of the functional organic complaints from headache to constipation. Thirdly, the label "neurosis" is used for at least two different conditions: (1) failure in adaptation to the various stresses of life, external and internal, including those in one's parental family, to one's sex, to growing up, to the menopause and aging, etc.; and (2) internalized problems and aberrations of development. In all cases, one must bear in mind the fact that "neurosis" is a purely functional concept. It denotes how the person thinks, feels and behaves.

In the war neuroses which we have been discussing, the central feature has been adaptation to unusual external stress. This highlights the difficulty in distinguishing between "normal" and "neurotic." Try to select normals and neurotics, and one may pick a man who is "normal" only because he is in a situation which he *fits,* while if subjected to what these men endured, he might have broken far sooner than they.

Everyone has his particular emotional make-up with his particular weak points. These vulnerabilities may be within normal limits, and no difficulties may develop unless unusual stresses bear down specifically upon them. Only then do tensions mount and childhood reactions appear.

In other cases, the stresses to which the individual reacts are not the current pressures of life outside his family, but they arise within the parental home itself. Some men with parental problems improved in the service: they could adapt better to the service than to their parents.

Unfortunately, long-continued, undesirable emotional influences, even though exerted by the best-intentioned parents, soon produce permanent internal disturbances. Spoiling or deprivation leave insatiable hungers for love and attention. Domination usually produces intolerable submissiveness; harsh treatment results in antisocial truculence, etc. These attitudes, shaped by the upbringing, often conflict with what the individual himself wants to be like, make him feel unbearable to himself and guilty and ashamed before society. Externally, they may impair his functioning, if they do not work in the social group. These disturbances in development may persist long after the parents are dead and the individual has aged. For example, one man, the last of a long line of children, felt the fact that he was unwanted by his parents as a terrible wound to his self-confidence and self-regard. He reacted with a rage that caused him intense inner anxiety and with a sense of depression at being unloved even by his own parents, which kept him on the verge of suicide. In addition, he suffered from certain compulsive symptoms, in particular, the necessity for arranging all his clothes and personal possessions in precise and meticulous order. Despite his severe *private* neurosis, this man had a highly successful military career. He went in a captain, discharged his duties admirably, and came out a lieutenant colonel. When I saw him after discharge, his private neurosis, so far as could be seen, remained entirely unchanged. He provides a good illustration of the *internalized* neurosis, for both his parents had been dead for many years. Apparently, the experience of being unloved and unwanted by his own parents completely overshadowed any adverse experiences in the service.

The term "neurosis" (always herein used broadly to mean emotional disorders of all sorts, eventuating in psychosomatic, psychological or acting-out symptoms) implies, as we have seen, two concepts: a failure of adaptation and a disturbance of the patient's emotional development. A man is extremely dependent upon his indulgent mother and never weans himself from her sufficiently to enjoy an independent life. If this situation causes acute conflict, then he is not well-adapted to his life situation and develops tensions which may lead to neurotic symptoms. Suppose, however, that he enjoys this type of life and does not develop unusual tensions because of it, that is, that he is adequately adapted to it. Then he is not neurotic by the standard of adaptation; but by the standard of full emotional development, of normal maturity for his age, he has a "mother fixation" and in the broad sense of the term is a neurotic personality of the dependent type, at least so far as his relationship to his mother goes. Perhaps he is quite mature in other ways.

In general, the more normal the emotional development to maturity, the less are the general and specific emotional vulnerabilities, certainly the less the tendency to regress to childhood ways of reacting. However, we have seen that there are situations in which the mature individual labors under greater strain than the man who can drift with the tide. We also saw a man who did not fear death until he married and his wife became pregnant, and only then, knowing what it would mean to them, did he become fearful for his own safety. The more childish, self-centered man, pursuing his own pleasure with little concern for his family and no excess of effort in assuming or discharging responsibilities, might adapt more harmoniously and sustain far less strain. Mature functioning may not *fit* a given situation so well as immature patterns and so may expose the better developed adult to greater strain. But if a man were *sufficiently* mature, then presumably he would not exceed his tolerance and would sustain these frustrations and those of the underlying, more childish needs without breakdown. A man of 40 had lost, one after another, his beloved wife and six children. But he did not break down or give up. He rallied from these shocks and truly began life at 40 by remarrying and again rearing a family of five children through whom he is now many times a grandfather.

The nature of neurosis is reaction to stress upon vulnerable points and fight-flight reactions along the lines of childhood patterns.

The essence of neurosis is the undue predominance of untoward childhood reactions. These may be caused by failures in the emotional development (fixations, internalized reactions) or, in well-matured persons, by failures in adaptation to specific stresses (regression); under sufficiently severe and prolonged stresses, even nonspecific for the person, probably everyone shows these reactions in some degree. The critical factor remains *the undue preponderance of untoward childhood reactions, whether persisting from earlier years or mobilized by and reactive to emotional stress.*

How we define a term is less important than the realities we endeavor to comprehend through it. Whether in attempting to formulate the meaning of the term "neurosis" one emphasizes the failure of adaptation, the external stresses, the emotional vulnerabilities, the make-up of the man, or the form of the pathological reaction which determines it, study of these processes leads to a better understanding of human adaptation and also of the course of human emotional development. Apart from the relationships of adaptation, maturity and regression to neurosis, the concept of *emotional development to maturity emerges as a standard of mental and emotional normality.*

PART FOUR

The Dynamics of Personality

20 | Determinants of Personality

The study of man's emotional life is beset with certain difficulties. In the first place, emotions, although they motivate our lives, cannot be perceived directly as can the brain or behavior. Like electricity, they are essentially "forces," which must be studied through their effects. Since the observer has been trained to certain moral standards, it is difficult for him to suspend these entirely and see all parts of the emotional life objectively, in the way the physician learns to examine all parts of the body without repugnance. Then, too, powerful feelings in others, even when repressed, stir up thoughts and emotions in the observer which impair his objectivity, and he tends to be either blind or hypersensitive to those things in others which he has repressed within himself. Some people fight in others tendencies which they find intolerable in themselves.

Man even "projects" full-blown his own repressed drives upon other persons and upon nature, peopling the world with a range of good and evil spirits, as varied as his own hates, hopes, fears and lusts. The Western world no longer burns witches and sorcerers but sees these unfortunates as the victims of their persecutors' fantasies, of man's readiness to accuse others and believe of them evils which are within the accuser. Yet to a large extent the witches of old are merely replaced by minority and majority groups which serve as screens for projection—whites to blacks and blacks to whites, radicals to "establishment" and "establishment" to radicals, and nations to nations. Although all advances in knowledge meet initial powerful opposition, it seems that man can face the truths about the physical world, his own body or his own intellectual processes far more easily than he can face his own emotional nature. Furthermore, to understand others a certain capacity for feeling and identification is needed, a certain relationship to one's own drives, and also that experience in life without which the

411

reality of deeper emotions cannot be grasped. That is why the man on the street who has struggled among men and whose livelihood depends in no small part upon his understanding of people often has more realistic appreciation of the emotional life than does a secluded professor, however brilliant his capacity for abstraction, logic and intellectualization.

But scientific knowledge differs from that of the man on the street and from that of the philosophers and the poets. It is part of the great cathedral of exact, systematized and classified fact and theory which grows through the painstaking work of thousands of researchers and provides the firm and permanent foundation of human understanding and control of nature. To be made accessible in this way, the insights of the great "Menschenkenner" need to be absorbed into the body of organized scientific knowledge. Appreciation of this knowledge necessitates a *feeling* for people, a psychological capacity.

Not only are there many determinants for human emotions and behavior, but even those which are known have not yet been fully integrated with one another. The fact that this book is about *certain* of these determinants implies no underestimation of the importance of the others which lie outside its scope. Some of these will be surveyed briefly here.

It seems quite certain that heredity, for example, cannot influence the whole body and its performance without also influencing one's intellect, talents and emotional development. It probably affects not only the *rate* of maturing but also the *degree* of maturity reached by the various parts and functions. As we have said, however, there is no evidence that heredity is of any major importance in psychopathology, with the possible exception of certain psychoses (Kety and Rosenthal, 1968). Systematic studies of development have been made by Gesell and his associates (1972).

Illustrative of thinking as to the unity of the organism and the reflection of apparently constitutional physical characteristics in the emotional life is the work of Sheldon and Stevens (1942). As these authors put it, psychoanalysis begins with the psychological manifestations and goes down as far as it can into the deepest biological motivations, while, conversely, these authors begin with the biological germ layers and go up as far as they can in tracing their influence upon the higher psychological functions. They estimate this aspect of constitution in terms of the three basic tissues or layers of the embryo which form the body: the entoderm, which becomes the gut and its related organs; the mesoderm, which forms the muscles and the blood vessels; and the ectoderm, which forms the skin, the sense organs and the nervous system. Predominance of the gut layer leads to Falstaffian individuals, who love food, drink and self-indulgence—the so-called "oral characters" long recognized by the psychoanalysts. Predominance of the bone— blood-muscle layer, the mesoderm, leads to powerful muscular types, who have a tendency to find their greatest satisfactions in action. When ectodermal development, or skin and brain, over-balances the development of the other two layers, there results the slender, hypersensitive individual, whose chief outlet is in the life of fantasy and of the intellect. By estimating in a given person, from many physical measurements, the proportional influence of the three germ layers, the authors can make surprisingly accurate predictions as to many of his traits of personality and temperament. This is represented with the light poetic touch by Charles Wadsworth, with whose kind permission the following is included:

An Introduction to Somatotyping
or
Typing Made Easy

Oh, I'm a little endomorph
Asittin' in the sun.
I dote on beer and skittles;
And I like my bit of fun.
I'm just a trifle lardy,
Just a trifle fat,
I may be somewhat tardy,
But I like to be like that.

Oh, I'm a busy mesomorph
Encased in gorgeous muscle.
My thinking is a trifle short,
I'm long on vim and hustle.
I'm a certified go-getter;
I'm the boy who will succeed
(Minus reason even better)
Perspiration is my creed.

Oh, I'm a spectral ectomorph,
Full of ratiocination
The mind's my happy hunting-ground
And I loathe participation.
Lonelier than any cloud
I'm always quite superior
To the mouthings of the motley crowd
And the grunts of the inferior.
                    Charles Wadsworth, 1945

That the proportional development of the layers is possibly influenced by early training and experience is suggested by work such as that of Stunkard (1975) and others (Collipp, 1975) on obesity. Bruch and Touraine (1940) found that in a series of 65 obesity cases, there was regularly severe restriction of activity in childhood, so that eating became the one freely permitted form of pleasure. In the study of personality one can never be satisfied with a single causal factor. Multiplicity and interaction are the rule. Much disagreement arises from overemphasis upon certain factors, however important, at the expense of failing to recognize or appreciate others.

Not very much is known of congenital factors, present at birth although not hereditary. "Prenatal influence" has long enjoyed popular esteem but usually in a superstitious way. The development of the fetus is known to be impaired by certain diseases of the mother, such as syphilis and of course by drugs, probably including alcohol and tobacco. It is no doubt affected by other more subtle conditions during pregnancy, such as lowering of the general physical health and vigor, and perhaps through physiological disturbances which are caused by emotional upsets, such as depressions or anxiety states. That intense prolonged emotion in the mother could affect the fetus might be expected, since transient and relatively minor emotional upsets can disturb the female physiology enough to disorder menstruation. Recent experimental work lends preliminary confirmation that the sporadic births of mongolian idiots into families with long lines of intellectual forebears may result from the parents' being on the borderline of fertility. This implies that if each parent had married a more fertile partner, the level of fertility of the pair would have been raised, and only normal offspring would have issued. Certainly age, condition and emotional as well as the physical state of the parents at conception and of the mother during pregnancy and any other possible influences on the fetus are factors which cannot be neglected in evaluating the potentialities of the infant and its later development.

Hereditary and congenital factors are not in conflict with environmental influences but are complementary to them and interact with them. Every person is the product of his constitution—the potentialities he is born with—interacting with environmental forces and experiences. A visit to the nursery of a maternity hospital, where one can see a dozen or more newborn babies, reveals dramatically the differences in temperament and personality. One is placid, another more reactive; one quite mature, another not. Each is born with an individual personality, and once one observes them there is no difficulty in recognizing them on subsequent visits. But these personalities at birth have been influenced for nine months, prenatally, by the health and emotional state of the mother, by the drugs she may have taken, and by other factors. Too much sedation before childbirth may inhibit the baby's starting to breathe and thereby indirectly cause damage to the brain from insufficient oxygen. But how many of the newborn will be allowed to develop in their own ways? In most cases, all sorts of pressures will be brought to bear—some will be forced to eat, others forced prematurely to control their excretions; some will be only tolerated and emotionally rejected, others will be smothered with love and made forever dependent; some will be doted on and then driven into a fury of jealousy by the transfer of all this feeling to a new baby. A weakling whose development is facilitated may turn out better than a lusty infant who is intimidated into submission or irritated into rages. The development of the child is influenced from the very moment of conception, both in the womb and after birth. Each starts with many potentialities; how these develop, which are brought out, which repressed, and how they are transformed depend upon the strength of the hereditary forces and upon the influences which bear upon them.

These influences, impersonal and personal, are manifold. There are the effects of organic diseases in childhood, both upon the physical and the emotional development. Severe illnesses sometimes retard teething, walking, talking and the like; and protracted illnesses, even if they leave no permanent structural alterations, may affect the emotional outlook in various ways.

The human influences to which the child is exposed and subjected from birth on are both personal and cultural (including economic). The particular personalities of the parents and of others into whose care fate brings the child, the accidents which break up homes, the chance which makes the child the first, the last, the middle, the only one, or whatever—all these conditions of the immediate family have an importance which is only gradually coming to be appreciated. The cultural and the economic forces operate to a large extent through the parents and their substitutes, who bring up the child in certain ways because these are the accepted methods of the particular culture into which he is born. They also operate more directly through schools, religious training, the press, prevailing ideologies, and so on. In a complex society like ours, there are many backgrounds and great cultural and economic contrasts—poverty-stricken sharecroppers, wealthy "coupon-clippers," manual workers, university professors, "tycoons," "hillbillies," slum dwellers, "solid citizens," communal families, and so on. The child's outlook is molded both by his position in the family and by his position in society, but mostly by the personalities of those close to him and responsible for him.

What kind of person the child develops into determines to a considerable extent the position he will make for himself in society. His place in the world is largely a result of his own make-up, his total personality, his childhood emotional pattern, his central dynamics. The forces of personality are chiefly unconscious, so this does not mean that each person can freely and fully choose his position. Far from it. Indeed, as we shall see, some men struggle doggedly toward their chosen goals, only to be defeated by what on careful examination turn out to be such factors as inadequate intelligence, neurotically impaired reality sense, poor human relations, or contrary, self-obstructing tendencies within themselves, which make them their own worst enemies.

A man's reactions at any given time, and even the course of his life, are also determined by the current external circumstances, regardless of the extent to which these are or are not of his own making. At present we are anxious about pollution of all sorts, which through drugs in food, e.g., insecticides or mercury from industrial waste in rivers entering meat and fish, through impeding the penetration of the ozone layer of the earth's atmosphere by sunlight, through radioactive fall-out, especially strontium 90, may affect the germ plasm which may warp the bodies of children not yet conceived. The number "0–6" should be vividly engraved upon the consciousness and the conscience of every human being. *For "0–6" signifies the most formative age of the human young—the period when the future character of the individual is most critically shaped and thereby the whole future character of human living on this planet.*

Some alterations in personality can be observed even in adult life, but in general the younger the organism, the more readily is its development affected. Adults change—but only a little—once their fundamental reaction patterns are established, which is usually by about six years of age—and altering them is difficult.

The process of maturing and then of aging and decline not only influences the individual's reactions but is itself a changing condition to which he must adjust (Erikson, 1964; Lidz, 1968).

We have skimmed over several of the factors which affect human development and behavior: hereditary and congenital factors, intellectual capacities and talents, organic disease, relationships with the intimate family group, cultural and socioeconomic factors, and the current physical and mental condition, age and life situation. There are other factors as well, such as climate and diet.

Our interest is primarily in the emotional forces. We are endeavoring to present, for the mind, a rough equivalent of the gross anatomy and physiology of the body. Man is a biological organism. What we label "mind" or "psychological" as distant from "physical," really means the activity of the highest levels of the brain, which we perceive and experience as our thoughts and feelings and express in psychological terms. The impulses to action and to the control of action, as well as thought, memory, judgment and all the sensations, passions and gradations of feeling, wherever these arise in the organism, whether from responses to stimuli in the outside world or from the relatively autonomous secretions of internal glands, whether from pain or from hunger, from love or from hate, seem to be mediated through the central nervous system, above all through that great computer, sifter, coordinator and integrator, the brain. Little is known of the intimate details of operation of the brain in terms of correlating our subjective emotional lives with neurophysiology. But what urges and impulses it is dealing with, and what it will do with them, this we unconsciously sense and can consciously estimate every time we are in contact with another person—or an animal. Animals sense the attitudes and the motives of men and of other animals—trusting some, suspicious of others until proved to be friend or foe. Whatever the subtleties of thought, however fine the wisps of dream or fantasy, however much a person or a people is influenced by cultural forces, it is always a biological organism which is behaving, reacting and striving. The psychodynamic study of this biological activity leads in each case to a deeper understanding of the development of the personality. It shows which forces favor this healthy maturing, which impair it and which warp it to neurosis, psychosis, neurotic or criminal character. Thereby it leads to an understanding of what normal development is, how to achieve it and how to avoid the pitfalls which beset it. Whatever is accomplished in this direction is a step toward overcoming the personal and social aberrations of the emotional life—mental disturbances, criminality, disruptions, violence, revolutions and wars. The base must be a healthier emotional period for every child, from conception through his and her most tender years, that is, *0 to 6*. There is no other way. Changing a social or economic system will not do it; for every society, however organized or anarchic, can only reflect the emotional health and maturity and the psychopathology of its individual members.

REFERENCES

Bruch, H. and Touraine, G. (1940): Obesity in childhood, *Psychosomatic Medicine* 2:141.

Collipp, P., ed. (1975): *Childhood Obesity.* Acton, Mass.: Publishing Sciences Group.

Erikson, E. (1964): *Insight and Responsibility.* New York: Norton.

Gesell, A. (1972): *The Embryology of Behavior: The Beginnings of the Human Mind.* (1945) Westport, Conn.: Greenwood Press.

Kety, S. and Rosenthal, D., eds. (1968): *The Transmission of Schizophrenia,* Proceedings of the Second Research Conference of the Foundations' Fund for Research in Psychiatry, 26 June–1 July 1967. New York: Pergamon Press.

Lidz, T. (1968): *The Person.* New York: Basic Books.

Sheldon, W. and Stevens, S. (1942): *The Varieties of Temperament.* New York: Harper.

Stunkard, A. (1975): From explanation to action in psychosomatic medicine: the case of obesity, *Psychosomatic Medicine* 37(3):195–236.

21 | The Operation of the Mind

Psychodynamics is to the mind what physiology is to the body. Physiology is the study of how the body works. Psychodynamics is the study of how the mind works. It deals with the interplay of the feelings and desires and reactions which form the mainsprings of our lives and make us feel and think and act in the many ways we do. Psychodynamics studies the interplay of the emotional forces which motivate us. Perhaps some day neurophysiology will reveal the detailed activities in the brain which we experience subjectively and understand in others as emotional forces.

In foregoing chapters we have discussed various interrelated emotional forces. Certain of these are readily represented in the following diagram.

MAJOR MOTIVATIONS

ANXIETY

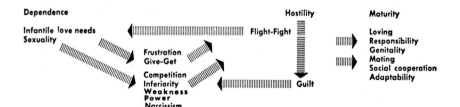

Two great poles in the emotional life are Dependence and Hostility. These are basically important in probably all emotional problems and therefore in every analysis. Dependence, originally that of the young child on the parent, if persisting too strongly, produces (1) inevitable frustration and (2) inferiority feelings with hurt to egotism, self-esteem, narcissism. Both of these stimulate hostility. The erotic side of dependence is seen in the child's needs not for physical care alone but also for affection. Hence, we can use the broader term "dependent love needs," including therein the infantile sexuality. Hostility is part of the universal fight-flight reaction of adaptation. Flight, usually impossible in reality, tends to take the form of psychological regression to infantile patterns. Hostility regularly leads to guilt, which also contributes to inferiority. Anxiety is a danger signal, produced by any of these motivations which involves a threat. Other motivations such as curiosity, however essential to life, are secondary. For example, curiosity, as content, is a pathway for other feelings, that is, the sexual drive makes curiosity about sex; hunger curiosity is directed toward finding food and so on.

Two central infantile libidinal forces in everyone are (1) the give-get balance, which becomes an issue when there is too much infantile demand and protest against responsibility and giving and (2) feelings of weakness and inferiority emphasizing strivings for prestige, esteem and power; the competition can be fed by the needs to receive and by the prestige wishes.

The progressive, developmental drives are toward outgrowing these motivations in favor of maturity in sexual mating and in social cooperation. Not that the infantile is ever fully outgrown, but in health the mature predominates, so that the *adult enjoys both* the exercise of his mature functions and also the infantile ones in a sense of play and zest, as part of his responsible activities or as socially acceptable recreation. However, if the child is badly reared, so that certain of his infantile motivations are warped, intensified and fixated, then these form motivational patterns which lead to every kind of neurotic (i.e., persisting, excessive, warped infantile) symptom: *internal* psychosomatic and classic neuroses (as hysteria, compulsions, minor depressions), psychoses (as paranoia) and *acting-out* against self (as in addictions and other forms of self defeat) and against others (as cruelty to intimates—

family, co-workers and others—and to non-intimates—as anti-social behavior or as individual, or organized violence and political criminality) leading to turmoil, revolution, tyranny and war. However convincingly these personal motivations are rationalized as nobly devoted to good causes, they are actually neurotic behavioral patterns.

It is not so surprising that only a relatively *few basic biological motivations seem to underly the infinite variety of personalities* and emotional disorders. Children are so differently raised, are so conditionable superego-wise, so many *combinations* of these motivations occur, and the ego is capable of so many forms of defense—hence, one sees such an endless spectrum of outcomes. (Just as a few features make up all of the different faces, no two alike any more than two snowflakes, three primary colors make all of the rest, and only a few more than 100 elements make every substance known to man.)

The above description of the major forces in the mind is presented here in highly condensed form only as a suggestive beginning and to emphasize the importance of distinguishing the fundamentals, exclusive of the complex detailed interpersonal constellations and the reactions and the defenses of the ego.

It will now be well to further condense and organize these observations into a general formulation of the dynamics of personality, using an individual case as a basis.

A young, attractive, married lawyer of 35 seeks help because of general feelings of depression and anxiety. It soon becomes apparent that his suave manner covers feelings of insecurity in his profession and among people, and to some extent in his marriage. Although his smooth manner belies it, he finds life a struggle. In reality, able and in a good professional and social position, with superior intelligence and a charming personality, rather than enjoying life he feels inadequate, frustrated and in danger of losing his position. He also feels vaguely inadequate toward his wife. It soon comes out that his desires to be supported by others and to relinquish the daily responsibilities and demands which he carried were much stronger than he had realized. Moreover, he set far greater store by prestige and was far more envious of and depreciatory toward other men than he had ever dared admit even to himself.

These feelings had a history. His yearnings to shuffle off the burdens of responsibility in favor of some sort of dependence dated back to the over-indulgence and overprotection which he enjoyed throughout his upbringing by his mother. As sometimes happens, his mother had none too high an opinion of his father but set all her hopes and ambitions upon her son. She hovered watchfully over him and nothing was too good for this future champion, who was to gratify all her own ambitions for success. At the same time, consciously or unconsciously, she imparted to him her depreciative attitude toward the father. Thus, the boy grew up basking in his mother's favor, and this lent warmth and confidence to his personality. But, ingrained with it, was the sense that to keep this love, he must achieve success and prestige and certainly surpass his inadequate (in his mother's eyes) father. Thus, his natural ambition was heightened. So also was his sense of guilt toward his father who was always very good to him. At the same time, his attachment to his mother's apron strings, wittingly or unwittingly fostered by her, impaired his initiative, masculinity and independence. He continued to feel in adult life as he had felt in childhood that he must win love by achieving prestige and by surpassing male rivals, but at the same time his need to have a strong, protecting mother to lean on made him feel inadequate to this task. Moreover, insofar as he did defeat his rivals, he was overwhelmed with guilt. (Competition is often felt unconsciously as very aggressive, even as a death wish; defeating a rival may be equated with killing him off.) He achieved success as his mother had bid him and external fortune smiled upon him; but because of his own motivations, he felt inadequate, guilty, insecure and frustrated, and from these feelings sprang his sense of anxiety and depression.

STRUCTURE OF THE MIND

The major emotional forces within the patient interacted in certain typical ways with one another, which can be grouped together. Such grouping has led through clinical experience to the emergence of a conception of a structure of the mind. Just as in the body we observe certain systems such as the gastro-intestinal, the cardiovascular, the respiratory, the genito-urinary, the skeleto-muscular, and the like, so the activities of the mind fall logically into certain systems.

This structure reflects the function and the purpose of the mind.

The mind is our subjective sense, our experience in psychological terms, of the activity of the brain. It coordinates the activities and the desires of the organism and seeks to satisfy them in the outer world in accordance with the conditioning of the conscience. The ego is the mediator between (1) the desires (id), (2) the conscience (superego), and (3) inner and outer reality. The lawyer wants security, prestige, the elimination of certain rivals. These are his "id" impulses. But he does not rob a bank or kill a competitor, although he might have such impulses. His ego is too realistic, and his judgment would not let him risk his career in this way; and even if he thought he could get away with it, his conscience would not allow

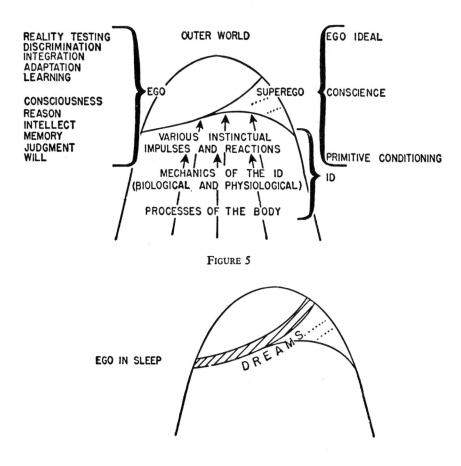

FIGURE 5

Figure 6

it. Thus, he tries to get what he wants by other methods which his ego and superego can accept, for example, by charming people and by pleasing his superiors, methods which worked with his mother when he was a child. Insofar as he can satisfy his desires in the real world and remain in harmony with his conscience, he is well-adjusted and has peace of mind. What he is trying to do is not different from what the amoeba does, except that, so far as we know, the amoeba has no superego. And because his organism is so large, he needs a central nervous system to integrate its behavior.

The structure of the mind can be diagrammed purely schematically and with no relation to actual anatomy (see Figure 5).

Certain major emotional forces which are of universal importance have been dealt with in previous chapters. Although each individual seeks his satisfactions in somewhat different ways, yet we can distinguish the basic craving for love and protection, the fight and flight reactions, the genital-sexual drives, the mature impulses toward productivity and responsibility, and the effects of conditioning and training. These impulses and functions can now be added to our purely schematic diagram as shown in Figure 7.

INTERPLAY AND CONFLICT BETWEEN
EMOTIONAL FORCES

Two interrelated major motivations (one almost says "purposes") in life are: (1) psychological development and fulfillment of the life course, and (2) adaptation. The organism throughout its life cycle, as it grows, matures and declines, tries to adapt to these inner changes and to the external world. This adaptation to changing internal and external conditions requires the learning of new attitudes and adjustments. Disturbances in development and in adaptation cause the various difficulties in functioning which we call neurotic, emotionally disordered, sick, pathological. No one is fully mature emotionally or in perfect harmony with his desires, his conscience and the outer world about him. This discrepancy between the desire and the fulfillment is expressed in the degree of unhappiness, emotional tension and "neurosis" which everyone sustains.

Reflected in Figure 7 is the obvious fact that the mind of man, as we see it today, is not made for harmonious operation but has

SCHEMA REPRESENTING CERTAIN
FUNDAMENTAL BIOLOGICAL FORCES

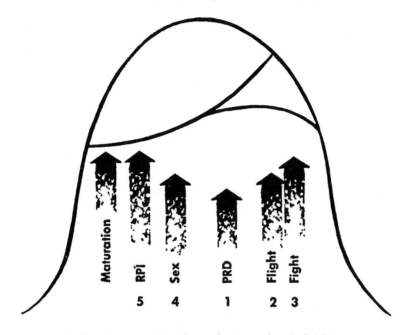

1. Passive-receptive-dependent needs of child toward parents. (PRD)

2. Flight-fight reaction.

3. Flight-fight reaction.

4. Genital-sexual drives. Responsible, loving mating.

5. Various impulses toward mature, adult functioning, both sexual and nonsexual, "object interest," responsibility productivity independence,
   etc. (RPI).

Figure 7

conflict built in. This may not be all to the bad. To it we must
attribute perhaps in part the development of man's intelligence
over that of the other animals. Nor is man necessarily doomed to
the degree of inner turmoil which he now sustains, since it is
primarily a result of atrocious childrearing.

SCHEMATIC REPRESENTATION OF CERTAIN OF THE
MAIN CONFLICTS IN ILLUSTRATIVE CASE

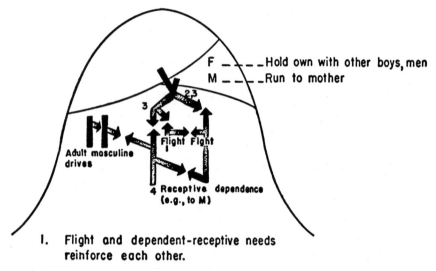

I. Flight and dependent-receptive needs reinforce each other.

2. Guilt.

3. Shame.

4. Fear of loss of protection, etc.

Figure 8

The man we have described exemplified a variety of these conflicts. Let us consider a few of them as illustrations. They are schematically represented in Figure 8. In the first place, he was in part torn and confused by two sets of ideals. His mother considered the boys of the neighborhood to be tough and dirty and exerted a constant pressure upon him to shun them, remain close to her, and devote himself to more cultural interests. She encouraged him to run to her with his every problem. On the other hand, his father, as well as the social group itself, set for him a standard of self-reliance and expected him to stand his ground, fight his own battles and be a "regular feller." Throughout life he continued to feel a difference between himself and other men. This conflict between the standards of his mother and those of his father must be considered as taking place between two ego ideals, two opposing conditionings, within his superego. Of course, it had further results in his development and his later personality functioning.

The intensification and the prolongation of his dependence upon his mother conflicted with the masculine ideals of self-reliance set him by his father and by the community. Therefore, he felt ashamed and inadequate for not living up to his masculine idea. Here the conflict is between the superego ideal and the instinctual impulse, namely, the dependence.

The attachment to mother's apron strings not only ran counter to certain ideals learned from his father and from other persons in the outside world, but it also conflicted with his natural biological drives toward independence from the parents. Here the conflict is between two instincts. On the one hand, the impulse is toward masculine independence and, on the other, toward the exaggerated need for mother's protecting wing, which he sensed as a babyish and feminizing influence and hence felt as shame.

Being gently reared, his impulses to violence were quickly checked and, like all civilized persons, he was made by his parents and others to feel guilty about tendencies to be angry or cruel. This is another superego conflict, felt as guilt rather than as shame. The hostile impulses arose mostly from feelings of inadequacy and were directed largely against his mother in a sort of blind, unconcious, instinctual rebellion and fight for emancipation from her. But here they conflicted with a still stronger instinctual desire, namely, his dependence upon her and upon her adoring love. The fear of jeopardizing this forced him to control his angry rebellion.

MECHANISMS OF DEFENSE

If all our unacceptable impulses, such as greed, indiscriminate sex, laziness, wishes to attack, wishes to run away, and the like, were only controlled by conscious effort, no doubt we would use up most of our energies in this continuous exertion of will. But our inhibitions, built in by training and experience, operate automatically and unconsciously to free us from this strain. When we go into a social group, we know that we will behave in a civilized fashion. If we have confidence that our superego, with its checks upon instincts, can be counted upon, that our psychological "brakes" are good, we can all the more freely "let ourselves go." These checks upon instinct are called defenses. They are achieved through various mechanisms. These defense mechanisms comprise some of the most interesting activities of the mind. They result from training, experience and conflicts.

It is while the child is small and weak, not only physically but also in will and experience, that he must learn to forego pleasures, endure anxieties, control his impulses and try to conform to the pressures of civilized thinking and behavior. Hence, he resorts very readily to "putting out of mind" or "repressing" impulses which he would find too painful or which he could not otherwise control. It appears to be out of this wrestling with the instincts and fears of childhood that the defense mechanisms develop. Once developed, they are never lost, and once an urge is gratified and yields pleasure, it is never abandoned fully, no matter how infantile.

Let us remember that the patient whom we have been discussing was by no means a patient so far as his family, friends, associates and clients were concerned. On the contrary, to the world he was very much the cultured, successful young man his mother had reared him to be. The interplay of feelings which we have described took place, for the most part, beneath the surface, that is, he recognized some of these feelings but easily controlled them and consciously put them out of his mind. This is called "suppression." Other reactions he dimly sensed, and, of still others he was quite unconscious. Like everyone else, he had developed automatic checks upon his animal impulses.

Driven by the standards of society, the example of his father, and his own biological, developmental and masculine drives, he strove to achieve self-reliance, and he put out of his mind yearnings to run to mother and be cared for and supported by her. When an impulse is banished from consciousness and cannot be recalled like an ordinary memory, it is called "unconscious," and the process is called "repression," as opposed to conscious control or "suppression."

The patient felt inferior and inadequate but did not know why this was. He did not realize that it stemmed largely from his childhood wishes for a mother's care, incompatible as these were with his independent, successful, adult, marital, professional and social life—an "isolation" of two related tendencies.

He could discuss dependence as an idea without appreciating the power of this drive and the intensity of feeling which it evoked within him. Nevertheless, he unconsciously reacted against it, striving to deny this source of his inferiority and inadequacy through demonstrations of his superiority and masculinity. This overemphasis or "overcompensation" revealed these efforts as partly "reaction formations." Shame and disgust are common reaction formations against infantile interests, for example, in excretions or in sex.

When he did visit his mother, he always attributed his motives to altruism and to her need for him. As he unconsciously strove for prestige, he thought his motivation was only a wish to provide well for his wife. Advancing the good reasons, he failed to see the real reason. This is "rationalization."

In part, he denied his feelings of inferiority through thinking of himself as a superior person, thus denying a more unpleasant reality by a form of "reversal."

The constant anger which he felt because of his unconquerable feelings of inferiority, his envy of others and his failure to achieve unachievable, childish goals was, as we have said, pent up within him. Raised to be over-gentle by a mother who had a horror of any roughness, his normal boyish aggression was overstrongly inhibited. It was inhibited through taking into himself the precepts, the training and the example of his mother. This is called "introjection." (Its importance in the formation of the superego is obvious.)

He could not admit even to himself that he harbored any hatred of more masculine and more successful men, although competitiveness, resentment and need to defeat them burned within him. Missing the beam in his own eye, he saw the mote in others' and was quick to recognize the slightest negative feelings of others toward himself. This "projection" of his own repressed impulses to others helped him to feel like a white knight in a hostile world, but feeling this hostility as directed toward himself, of course, increased his anxiety. On the other hand, feeling an "identification with the aggressor" serves as a defense against fear.

His exaggerated gentleness and pity were in part "overcompensations" for impulses to cruelty. If he ever unwittingly caused hurt to anyone, he was overwhelmed with guilt, thus "turning against himself" his hostile aggression and flaying himself for his behavior.

This self-attack is an important element in depressions, in much the same way that projection is in paranoia. It is a form of "displacement," taking out an impulse on someone other than the original object.

There were certain indirect ways in which the patient obtained some unconscious satisfaction for his repressed hostile feelings. One of these was his legal work with criminals, with whom he partially "identified" himself. As a hobby he wrote short murder mysteries. He thus "displaced" some of his hostile feelings and "sublimated" them by transforming them into socially useful activities. If an event occurred which injured the patient's pride, such as an award to a rival, he would have an impulse to ignore or "undo" the painful occurrence. Not infrequently, when especially frustrated, his sexual desires would be heightened and his feelings would find considerable satisfaction through sexual relations. In other words, his hostile, aggressive impulses were partly "erotized" and satisfied unconsciously under the guise of sexuality by virtue of being part of the natural aggressiveness which enters into the male sexual drive and "fuses" with it.

In the preceding section of this book, "The Nature of Neuroses," we saw how flight can take the form of "regression" to childhood patterns. An example was given of a man in military service who defended himself against the pain of his buddies' deaths by not letting himself get close to them as friends and eliminating all personal feelings. This is a form of "depersonalization." It is not infrequently felt toward onself—not feeling real, not feeling like oneself. It is a defense in situations involving great physical danger and is also a defense against inner anxieties.

Humor, which represents many things, can also be used as a defense. An illustration is the story of the man mounting the scaffold saying: "This will sure teach me a lesson." Another example was the case of a distraught young man who came for help because of his anxious impulses to kill his mother. He could not help laughing uproariously about this impulse and dealing humorously with the related material as though it were all a great joke and the impulses in no wise real.

There are still other mechanisms by which we defend ourselves against conflictful feelings and impulses; various emotional forces can be used in this way, for example, hostility as a defense against dependence. Those we have mentioned demonstrate briefly the

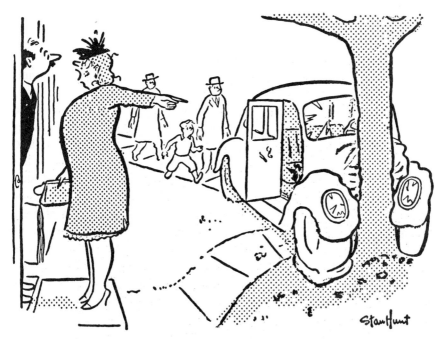

"Is that your darn fool tree out there?"

Figure 9

most common mental processes of this type without attempting to
be exhaustive or to make a significant classification of them. They
show that a given emotional impulse can be handled in many different ways. We have seen that one young man reacted against his
hostile impulses by suppressing them, by repressing them from
consciousness and dealing with them through overcompensatory
kindness, projecting them to others, sublimating them into constructive work with criminals, turning them upon himself with feelings of depression, displacing them from their original objects,
draining them sexually, and so on. We have also mentioned isolation, reaction-formations, rationalization, reversal, introjection,
identification, depersonalization, humor and regression. All sorts
of other impulses, such as dependence or sexuality, are also experienced, reacted to, fused with different urges, diffused and altered as to aim and object in a similar variety of ways. Figure 9
shows how useful a defense mechanism can be in protecting the

ego and keeping it comfortable (A. Freud, 1937; Laughlin, 1970). In this case the lady is using "projection."

FUNDAMENTAL EMOTIONAL MECHANISMS AND CAUSAL CHAINS

Man's motivating impulses apparently arise in a relatively unrelated and chaotic fashion out of the biological functioning of the body, yet there is a certain logic in the way the emotions operate. Certain relationships, patterns, syllogisms, complexes or constellations of impulses and feelings form and become recognizable. Some of these are encountered so regularly, perhaps so universally, that they warrant the term "fundamental emotional mechanisms."

For an example let us turn again to the patient who shows a mechanism with which we are already familiar. His mother, restricting his normal, independent, masculine activities and cultivating his dependence upon her, intensified and prolonged his needs for dependence to such an extent that they persisted in exaggerated form in adult life. Because one cannot satisfy in adult life the child's needs for maternal solicitude, these needs were doomed to frustration. Unconsciously, the patient hoped for the same indulgence from his employers that he had enjoyed in childhood at the hands of his mother. Frustration was therefore inevitable and, as a result of it, bitterness and anger. But even if these childishly intense demands could have been satisfied, as a 35-year-old adult, a husband, a father, and a man in a responsible position, the hurt to his mature masculine drives and ideals would have made unacceptable the role of a little child toward his parent. He never could sink to this infantile relationship to his employer. But the tendency to do so was there and, although he did not fully recognize it, it irked him. It caused a hostile, rebellious attitude as a defense against being dependent, and the feeling of inadequacy engendered an impotent rage. Thus his passive-receptive-dependent-love needs toward his mother had shaped a childish attitude toward other persons, and these childish, dependent needs were a source of anger through frustration, as a defense and because of hurt pride.

This mechanism is often part of a vicious circle which is extremely common—at least in our culture. The anger pent up within causes anxiety. If this man expressed his rage, he not only would be overwhelmed with guilt because of his own conscience but would be justified in the real fear that he would arouse retaliatory antagonisms from others. He would thereby lose the approbation and the help that he deeply craved and would jeopardize his security with his friends and colleagues. On the other hand, pent-up hostility through the mechanisms of projection and turning against the self, causes anxiety and depression. But now the anxiety resulting from the hostility increases the needs for help and thus augments the very dependent desires which, through hurting the pride and causing frustration, generated the anger in the first place. This well-known constellation can be diagrammed as follows:

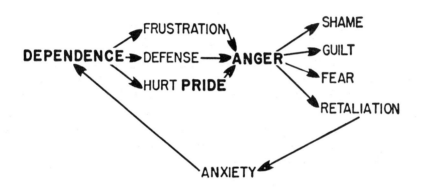

Figure 10

As an example of simple "emotional logic" involving receptive frustration, let us consider the case of a young woman who had been rejected as a child and starved for love, although her parents had freely given her material things. As an adult, she never outgrew her intense childhood demands for attention and for material proof and demonstrations from others that they valued and esteemed her. This young woman felt ashamed and guilty at the vastness of her demands upon others. She reacted with two common emotional syllogisms: "Because I want to take so much, I must constantly give" and "Because I want to so much from others, I deserve to have nothing." Thus, in life she was extreme in her giving and mothering toward others and she lived in dread of losing her friends

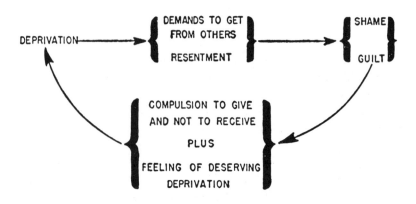

Figure 11

and possessions. The essential dynamics in her case are common and are represented schematically in Figure 11.

Joyless, compulsive overwork can be motivated in many ways. In some cases, it is part of a rather simple vicious circle in which the person, because he feels driven, resents his work and wishes to escape it altogether, but then feels guilty and undeserving of recreation and respite and hence is again driven to keep his or her nose to the grindstone. This can be schematized as follows:

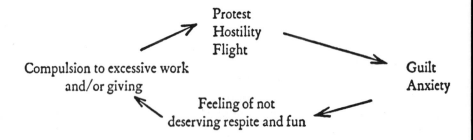

Figure 12

This constellation arises in different ways. Frequently, it is seen in housewives who, perhaps deprived or spoiled in childhood, resent more than they know the demands of home and still dream, if only unconsciously, of escape to adventure, romance and fun. But they then feel guilty toward husband and children, cut themselves off from what respite and enjoyment they could and should have, and make themselves slaves to the mop and the kitchen. Sometimes the wife blames her husband for deprivations which are generated by her own dynamics. Many men are caught in the same reactions to their own work, for these as well as for other reasons.

Another type of vicious circle is seen in situations of envy. Here one individual often envies another and, because of this, feels guilty. The guilt results in self-depreciation and in idealization of the person who is envied. The more the person feels depreciated and the more he idealizes the other, the greater the envy. This can be diagrammed schematically as follows:

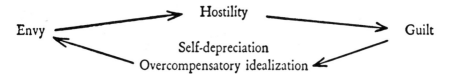

Figure 13

There are also vicious cycles between people. For example, one becomes slightly irritable; because of this the other becomes a little angry; the first reacts to the increasing irritability of the other, and then the second, in turn, reacts to the mounting anger of the first. The relationship is "functional," i.e., the anger of each person increases the anger of the other. One must be ever on the watch for these reciprocal relationships in observing the emotional life. They are of special importance in marriage. If one of the partners learns not to react, it may make the relationship much easier, and in some cases may even prevent a breakup.

These diagrams are schematized and oversimplified, but for every case the main features can be represented. Typical, fundamental mechanisms are seen again and again and deserve cataloguing and explicit study. They are important for treatment as well as for understanding, since every improvement in one tendency is reflected in the others because of the functional relationship between them.

Two further fundamental mechanisms, possibly of slightly different nature, are "The Punishment Fits the Source" and "Out From Under."

A man envies another for his money and, out of guilt for the envy, has repeated dreams of being poor and actually handles his finances badly. Another man, an overambitious young instructor, is hostile to the older, experienced lecturers and, when he is assigned some lectures, he dreams of being embarrassed before a group and in reality develops considerable stage fright which impairs his lecturing well. A young wife was deprived emotionally as a child, being insufficiently loved; now she is bitter against her husband because whatever he does she *feels* insufficiently loved by him, but the guilt for her hostility to him makes her feel that she does not deserve to be loved; she dreams of being deserted by him and in life cannot help provoking him against her. Guilty for anger because of frustrated wishes for love, she punishes herself unconsciously, specifically by denying herself love. Thus in every instance that desire (for money, recognition, love) which, frustrated, is the particular *source of the hostility,* also *determines the form of the punishment.* Conversely, if a person is masochistic, i.e., unconsciously self-punishing in a certain way, it is more than likely that the form of punishment is a clue to what wishes, frustrated, produced the anger and the guilt (Saul, 1976).

"Out from under" refers to the tendency to reverse a situation in which a person is unhappy through feeling weak, dependent, submissive. A man suffered in childhood under a strong dominating mother. He grew up unable to tolerate any situation in which anyone had control over him and developed the characteristic of being independent and dominating himself. This mechanism is related to "identification with the aggressor" but is broader and not confined to aggression. A charming young woman, much indulged by her parents and overly dependent upon them, surprised her friends in her choice of a husband. They thought that she would marry a stable, secure, solid citizen who would care for her as her parents had. Instead she chose a weak, clinging, dependent, inadequate, semi-opportunistic youngster. She saw these characteristics but was impelled out of her own feelings of being under her parents' aegis, guidance and power into the reverse situation in which someone weaker than herself looked up to her, needed her, was dependent upon her, in which she could feel herself to be the stronger.

MENTAL HEALTH AND THE DYNAMIC DIAGNOSIS

We have noted that "normal" in the sense of "average" bears little if any relation to normal in the sense of mental and emotional health. There is still much confusion on this score, including the question of normal criminals. A view of the development of personality contributes considerable clarification. Going directly to the point, mental and emotional health is the adequate achievement of emotional maturity which means the growth from helplessness and needs for love to the capacity to love, to be a good, responsible spouse, parent and citizen; and this depends upon good human relations in the earliest years, for the pattern of these feelings and relationships continues on through adult life. If a person grows up hurt, anxious and frustrated and therefore hostile, he will be incapable of sufficient mature, unselfish, responsible love to carry the responsibilities of spouse, children and citizenship.

This seems to be a broad statement, but I think that it holds up to all tests. For brevity, let us oversimplify somewhat, restrict our focus to the hostility and the reactions of the superego to it, and condense what we have already referred to frequently. If the superego is strong, and the frustrations and the hostility well controlled, yet the repressed regularly returns in some form; perhaps the person will be a good, productive spouse, parent and citizen but have an internal *psychosomatic* symptom such as headache or asthma or high blood pressure. Here the person himself suffers and does not take out his resentments upon others—directly. However, the symptom itself impairs effective mature functioning, and the repressed tensions may produce primarily *psychological* symptoms of classic neurosis or psychosis, with their *indirect* effects, imposed mostly upon intimates. The tensions may be *acted out* mostly *against the self* masochistically, i.e., as addictions or wrecked careers, indirectly injuring others. Bitterness often comes out in *direct action against others.* If it is within the family, it may be overlooked by society, but if directed outside of the family, it is *antisocial* and ranges from psychopathic behavior of all sorts to naked crime (individual, organized and political). The expression of the bitterness depends upon the amount of maturity, the kind and the extent of the superego ideals and controls.

The essential point is that irrationality or any psychotic manifestations are only one of the many effects of disturbance in human relations which begin often with birth and impair mature feelings and behavior in adult life. This dispels much of the confusion over "normal criminality." It is not a matter of irrationality or psychosis being associated with criminal behavior. If it is, we have mental illness, and a hospital is indicated; if not, then trial and punishment. *Both* irrationality *and* criminal behavior are merely different *forms* of emotional disorders, of disturbed human relations, of impaired maturity. It is by no means uncommon for a person to have one or two acute psychotic episodes and then have the hostility erupt in a criminal act. In fact, there is much unrealistic thinking in narrow, artificial categories. Actually, every human being is a mixture, and it is rare to see a person with only a single symptom—a person with headaches can be depressed, a paranoid can kill, lions can be good family men, pacifists can beat their wives—the balance of forces can, and usually does, produce a variety of symptoms in different people and in the same person.

DIAGNOSIS AND PROGNOSIS—WHAT IS KNOWN AND NOT KNOWN

Psychiatrists are often expected, in connection with the law and otherwise, to give authoritative "diagnoses" and reliable prognoses, for example, on questions of parole, as to whether or not a man will repeat a criminal act. Actually, it is difficult in the extreme for a psychiatrist to learn much about the deeper motivations of any human being unless that person is powerfully motivated to reveal himself, as to a physician, for relief of suffering. Even then, special techniques are required and often much time (Saul, 1972); and while the main forces in the psychopathology may be seen, the actual quantitative balance, especially under unforeseeable future situations in life, can rarely, with present knowledge, be evaluated quantitatively or predicted with any certainty. No one, psychiatrist included, really knows anyone from behavior and talk in life, not even his best friends or his own wife or children, not all the impulses and potentialities which move in the heterogeneous mixture that constitutes the personality. The psychiatrist can see what he sees and evaluate it, but he can be sure that he never sees *all* that there is in anyone. I will not give examples of surprises. Let the reader look for these within himself so far as he can and at his own life and those of others he knows. Sometimes the surprises are for the best, often not. But no one, from what he knows of a person, can know what there is that he does not know.

REFERENCES

Alexander, F. (1942): *Our Age of Unreason*. Philadelphia: Lippincott.
Freud, A. (1937): *Ego and the Mechanisms of Defence*. London: Hogarth.
Laughlin, H. (1970): *The Ego and Its Defenses*. New York: Appleton-Century-Crofts.
Saul, L. J. (1972): *Psychodynamically Based Psychotherapy*. New York: Science House.
_____ (1976): *Psychodynamics of Hostility*. New York: Jason Aronson.

22 | Genesis of Emotional Disturbances

DEVELOPMENT AND REGRESSION

The lawyer's problems in adult life (Chap. 21) arose because whole patterns of functioning formed in his childhood carried on into his adulthood. Dependence on his mother, the ambitions for prestige and success which inbued the rivalry with his father and the depreciatory attitude toward him, the failure to identify with other men, the whole constellation continued on, still potent, although, for the most part, unconscious, automatic and resistant to conscious efforts to change. The rest of his personality developed adequately in the direction of those attitudes, feelings and ways of functioning which we are beginning to recognize as mature. In general, it is the persisting childhood attitudes, orientations, desires and reactions which form an important part of the core of the personality and also the predisposition to emotional difficulties.

In dreams we see these impulses and also the defense mechanisms against them and the devious ways in which they strive for expression and satisfaction. But if reality becomes too difficult and too frustrating, then we see that people tend to return in their waking life also to desires, interests and psychological mechanisms and patterns which obtained and worked more or less satisfactorily in childhood. This return is called "regression." It is the key to psychological understanding of the functional neuroses and psychoses.

THE DYNAMICS OF NEUROSIS

Pathological physiology readily demonstrates that the body reacts in a highly coordinated fashion to every sort of disease or insult. Psychodynamics has shown that the mind does the same. Its reac-

440

tions to stress and strain are by no means random, are no senseless disintegrations. When we call behavior "crazy," this term is only a confession of our own ignorance and failure to understand it. Pathological mental processes follow as strict laws as do pathological physical processes or, indeed, any other phenomenon of nature.

The central feature of psychopathology and the key to the neuroses and the psychoses is the tendency in everyone to *regress* under stress to earlier childhood ways of thinking and reacting, to those childhood patterns which, as we have seen, lie if only latent at the unconscious core of every personality (Freud, 1916). In nearly every functional neurosis or psychosis, the history reveals that the patient reached some form of adjustment, and that, under inner or outer stress, broke down with symptoms which become intelligible as partial returns to emotional reactions of childhood (Alexander, 1961).

The hysterical emotional displays over minor matters reflect the labile shifts of the small child from tears to laughter. The phobic's refusal to go out alone duplicates the fears of the small child. We laugh at the child's indecisions, for example, over which candy to choose, or we are amused by his passing phase of insisting that everything must be just so before he can go to sleep. In the doubts and the ceremonials of compulsion neurosis one sees exaggerations of these same tendencies. The psychopath is dominated by his impulses, like the child who acts out his urges because his ego is still weak and he lacks judgment and control. The paranoid feels watched, like a guilty child. The sexual perversions were among the very first reactions to be recognized as infantile expressions of sensual feelings which have not matured into normal heterosexuality. Depression reflects the child's spiteful withdrawal in the face of frustrations, as though saying, "Then I won't play any more. I'll go eat worms." The hallucinations and the delusions of schizophrenia, as well as the frequent apathy and fecal incontinence and smearing, recall early infancy before the grasp of reality is well developed and before disgust appears. These similarities of the neuroses and the psychoses to reactions of childhood and infancy are by no means merely superficial resemblances. They reflect a true organic relationship. Faced with the difficulties of life, there is a partial return to the emotional patterns of childhood. The greater the disturbance in the emotional development to maturity, the greater the "fixation" to these patterns because of traumatic influences during childhood, the greater the tendency to relinquish adult functioning and to return to them. In other words, the greater is the emotional vulnerability and the predisposition to neurotic reactions.

As an especially clear example, a boy of 19 had been overprotected and overrestricted during his early years, chiefly because of the death of the two older children. He apparently matured normally and went away to college. Here he suffered a sudden and unexpected rebuff at the hands of a group of young men whom he had counted his friends. He returned home, feared to go out or even sleep alone and only felt secure in his mother's bed. For a week he remained in bed, fed like a small child. He then forced himself to get up but feared to leave the house unless his father or mother accompanied him. He would not retire at night unless the door and the objects on his bureau were just so and unless he were repeatedly assured that he would not die in his sleep. His anxiety continued in his sleep as nightmares of animals attacking him. He lost all interest in studies, friends and even in girls. With treatment, he gradually came to tolerate being alone without calling anxiously for mother. Then he became able to go out by himself so long as he could see the house or one of his parents. Later he could go to town, first accompanied by his mother or father, then all alone. Under pressure he became able to see friends and even venture a date—and so, gradually, he returned from the anxious behavior of the overprotected little child to the orientations, the interests and the independence appropriate to his age. The flight reaction led him literally to the infant's dependence upon mother; the fight was "projected" and experienced as fear and anxiety—as the dangerous animals of his nightmares.

The genesis of emotional disturbances can be reduced with some oversimplification to the following steps:

1. Childhood emotional influences interact with the infant's congenital (heredity plus the physical and emotional forces acting upon sperm and egg, prior to conception and until birth) endowment and developmental forces, the child being most formative up to the age of about six.

2. These influences facilitate, retard or warp the development and cause emotional patterns which persist, mostly unconsciously, in later life.

3. These "nuclear patterns" contain certain vulnerable emotional points; everyone has specific emotional vulnerabilities.

4. The environment exerts certain demands, pressures and frustrations.

5. The individual endeavors to harmonize the conflicting impulses within himself and to adjust himself to his environment.

6. In general, the more mature the individual is, the more stably and flexibly he adjusts; but when the pressures impinge upon his emotional vulnerabilities, he reacts with mobilization for fight or flight.

7. The fear and the flight and the anger and hostile aggression tend to be handled as they were in childhood, with partial return to childhood forms of satisfaction, thinking and behavior.

8. These regressive reactions constitute and produce symptoms which can be grouped as above: 1) *Inner* (a) psychosomatic, (b) neurotic, (c) psychotic, and 2) *Acting-out* (a) masochistic, (b) destructive social behavior, (c) criminal.

9. The ego reacts secondarily to the tensions and the symptoms over a range, from denying to exploiting them.

The study of the emotional life is now emerging as a descriptive science, at present comparable with anatomy. Yet it deals with an interplay of forces with intensities and quantities. The science would make great strides if methods of measurement existed. Those that are available at present are crude and depend chiefly upon the setting up of scales ranging from one extreme of whatever is being studied to the other, as for example, degrees of dependence (Saul and Sheppard, 1956). No doubt, these will be greatly refined over the next years or decades. It is premature to formulate in mathematical terms any of the dynamics described above, yet an attempt to do so, although crude, naive and qualitative, will at least express a hope. Although of no precise or quantitative validity, the general relationships which lead to neurotic symptoms of whatever form might be expressed as a first approximation in the following formula:

$$V_s \times S_s \propto \frac{Ad}{F} \times \frac{R}{P} \propto \frac{T}{E} \propto N$$

V_s = Specific emotional vulnerability.

S_s = External stresses, especially in relation to specific emotional vulnerability.

Ad = Difficulty of adjustment, internal and external.

F = Flexibility, adaptability, including capacity for temporary and partial regression.

R = Regressive forces, including fixation (toward childish dependence or infantile attitudes or reactions).

P = Progressive forces (toward independence, responsibility, productivity, maturity).

T = Emotional tension.

E = Ego strength (especially control and integrative capacity).

N = Degree of neurosis, psychopathology.

VARIETIES OF OUTCOME

Emotionally determined symptoms can be grouped as follows: (1) psychotic reactions in which the regression is so great that the perception of reality is seriously impaired and the control and the judgment (the ego) so influenced that the individual is unable to maintain his social adjustment or else does so only precariously. These grade into (2) the neuroses. This term can be used broadly to include perversions, alcoholism and similar disorders. Here the repressed emotions generate tensions which cause disturbances in thinking, feeling and behavior but in which the ego is sufficiently strong and intact for the person to carry on. No one is entirely free of such tensions. (3) "Psychosomatic" symptoms, in the narrow sense of the term, are the physiological disturbances caused *in part* by emotional states. Such symptoms (which, of course, have other causes as well) are high blood pressure, nervous stomach and even ulcers, asthma, and so on. (4) When impulses, especially hostile aggressive ones, are directly lived out, the result is *behavior disorders,* with damage to self or others including criminal behavior. (5) But the commonest expression of these childhood emotional patterns and the tensions they generate is not in the frank psychotic, neurotic or bodily symptoms or in obvious behavior disorders but in what might be called "social symptoms," that is, in the behavior of men. It is here, in man's inability to handle the affairs of the world because of his emotional immaturity, that he causes himself and others the greatest share of the misery which humanity endures. Frank psychoses, neuroses, psychosomatic symptoms, neurotic characters and criminality are all usually recognizable as pathological or abnormal behavior, at least in the sense of deviating from the average. But the "social symptoms" are masked (often as political activity or as devotion to laudable goals) and difficult to distinguish—and, hence, all the more dangerous. They may even be condoned by a prevailing ideology and may pass as average behavior, appearing as immature or neurotic only by comparison with man's potential for full emotional development.

The same elementary drives and desires can cause any of these six types of reaction and any combination of them. The lawyer handled his anger by remaining gentle and turning it upon himself to cause neurotic anxiety and depression. The psychosomatic concomitants of this were tachycardia and mild essential hypertension. Another man with a much weaker ego may react to frustrations and anger by relinquishing his position in life and regressing to paranoid, schizophrenic psychosis. Yet another, deficient in social training, sheds his veneer of moral restraint and resorts to unlawful practices in his pursuit of success and expressions of hostility. And, finally, another man conducts himself in a socially approved fashion and yet sometimes, without himself or others realizing it, contributes materially to human suffering. Those who stay within the law but whose behavior supports criminal behavior and contributes to human suffering may appropriately be called "criminoid."

What determines the outcome of the drives in one or another of these categories of symptoms is the as yet unsolved problem of the "choice of neurosis." Certainly, the strength and the intactness of the ego and the relationship to the superego, that is, to the training and the conscience (in other words, the man's "character") are critical factors. The strength and the degree of the fixations and of the tendencies to regression are another factor. *The choice of outcome* is determined, in large part, by the *quantitative relations between many emotional forces*—the nature of the drive or the desire, the effects of other needs and of the treatment, the training, and the gratifications during childhood, the whole complex "nuclear emotional constellation" and the constitutional make-up. Some of the factors are represented schematically in Figure 14.

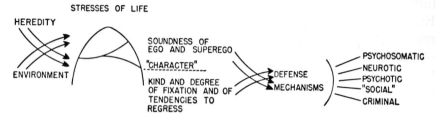

Figure 14

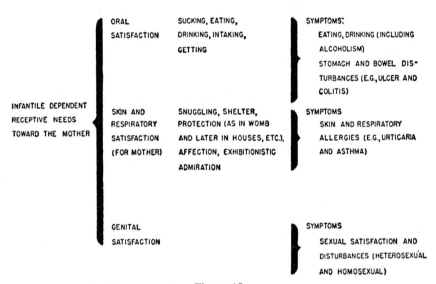

Figure 15

Even within each category of symptoms, the drive, the desire or the emotional tendency can find expression in a variety of different ways. It may be that when the wish is chiefly for getting, the tendency is to affect the stomach; when the wish is rather to be protected and sheltered, it affects the skin and the respiratory system; but when, for some reason, perhaps demonstrativeness or fondling in childhood, the desire become erotized, then it seeks satisfaction in sexual form, and so on (Saul, 1950). This is represented in part in Figure 15.

All neurotic and psychotic symptoms and behavior disorders are *ways of reacting, which are more or less infantile* and reflect disturbed reactions at different stages of the emotional development. Everyone has, and to some degree uses, all of these ways of reacting—the weeping of hysteria, the doubts and the compulsions of obsessionals, the feelings of depression and the withdrawal to fantasies of schizophrenia. There are no disease entities. It is only the *quantitative amounts and degrees of these ways of reacting* which determine whether or not the condition oversteps the bounds of normal, and what diagnostic label can be used. It is also a matter of prominence of one symptom over others. If a man has full blown delusions of persecution, we are apt to diagnose "paranoia," although he may also have headaches, upset digestion, anxiety and phobias.

Psychiatric diagnosis began with description and classification of symptoms. Medical diagnosis has progressed from this to categories based upon understanding the underlying process. This same tendency is observable in psychiatry. Someday our diagnostic terms probably will indicate not only the outcome in symptoms but also the main dynamics underlying them. The following will serve as an example of the idea.

THE DEPENDENT-HOSTILE MAN

A certain pattern of behavior in men comes under one's observation so frequently both in the office and in life that one is justified in calling these men a "type" and perhaps grouping them together diagnostically as "the dependent-hostile man." The basic dynamics are no doubt known to all analysts: there is a prominent, pervasive wish to be the dependent, cared for, admired child; this creates feelings of inferiority and often actual inadequacies with efforts at overcompensation by glittering promise of great accomplishments. The emotional influences in childhood which shaped this constellation of motivation in the adult vary from person to person. The connections between these conditioning influences of childhood and the present personality are probably most simple and seen most clearly in these men who were overly protected all during their early years. This overdoing of tender care during childhood produces many different outcomes, depending upon the quantitative relationships between these and other forces; but in the type of man we are describing, the result is a rather direct continuation into adult life of the childhood attitudes fostered by this treatment at the parents' hands.

Typically, the man of whom we are speaking is so obsessed with gaining personal success and applause for himself that he is not genuinely realistic and considerate in his relations with others, especially with those dependent upon him. He is apt to have in mind grandiose undertakings, such as a great novel, painting, scientific study or community project. However, usually, these do not materialize. Years may pass, and the creation is never finished, or else the project is never completed because, before it can be, the man's enthusiasm has turned to another one.

Sometimes the man burns himself out in these strivings for greatness, usually without accomplishing much in reality. He may develop all sorts of psychological and physiological disorders as a result of his unremitting strivings.

In other cases there is no such shiny promise and ambition. The man simply works along, sometimes appearing to be a pillar of society but actually, to the closer observer, dissatisfied, unhappy and holding his position in the world only precariously. Not infrequently, this insecure grip is lost, and the man relinquishes his work or sinks to a much lower level of accomplishment. This lower level is apt to be a great blow to his self-esteem and so causes increased rage and regressive behavior and even breakdown.

One such man had an extremely overprotective mother who could not let her children go. In spite of his superior ability, handsome appearance and impressive warm personality, he reverted, when in his early forties, to the playboy life of his adolescence. His marriage ended in divorce, and he withdrew from his responsible position in a large company.

Another man with this pattern was constantly on the verge of losing his position; he finally did so and went from job to job. The greater his inadequacy became (because of his emotional orientation and not at all because of any limitation of intellectual ability or physical strength) the more he became enraged. He took to dressing in Western fashion in an effort to emphasize his masculinity but included in this hobby guns and knives with which he began to threaten his wife. His passive, receptive and dependent desires increased toward her, and as they did so his hostility did also—until she felt her person to be in actual danger, and the marriage terminated in divorce.

This relationship to the wife is also typical. The man often repeats toward his wife the desires for a childish kind of love, devotion and helpless dependence which he enjoyed all too well in relation, usually, to his mother. He is apt to feel that his wife is responsible for him in the same sense that his mother was when he was a small child. His wife must make the decisions, but if she makes the wrong ones or if they do not turn out well, then he is furious at her. Whatever is wrong with him or in his life, he tends to blame his wife: If she would do more housework herself or cook different foods or do or not do any number of other things, then all would be more harmonious within himself and between them. The dependency is often most naive. The man may simply expect his wife to put on a meal for unexpected guests almost without notice; or to meet him when and where he wants, adjusting her life to his as though she had none of her own; and the same for the children. In childhood the household revolved about him, and in marriage he expects this to continue. It is his own needs which are paramount. His internally determined dissatisfactions with his wife often lead, logically, to his involvement with another woman who is to him his true love. Unconsciously he merely hopes that she will be a better "mother" to him. Conversely, one man left his wife because she was, in his mind, so much like his mother, although in reality she was not comparable.

He rationalizes these in part by never forgetting that he is the breadwinner for the family. Underneath he unconsciously but bitterly resents this. He longs to be the little child he once was, with everything provided and adoration too. Now as an adult he finds that he cannot play all day, he cannot freely indulge in every wish, he no longer has an all-giving, all-loving mother to hover over him. Instead, he must be the giving adult himself. It is he who must support his family and give out emotional interest to them. Often this is more than he can tolerate. He may worship his wife and his children but inwardly rebel against any real responsibility for them beyond supporting them. As we have pointed out previously, the converse is also seen, the man being most devoted toward his wife and children but notably inadequate in taking any financial responsibility for them. The passive, receptive, dependent (PRD) needs to be supported and taken care of and to be free of responsibility are so strong in one man that he is able to contribute financially but not with real emotional responsibility; while another man gives the kindness but does not contribute financially. There is just not enough capacity for giving out emotionally to do both. It is those men who can do neither who are apt to fail in their responsible, productive independence (RPI) in work, marriage or both. For a discussion of the dynamics of marriage, including typical examples, see Saul, L. J., 1979.

The strength of the dependence upon the wife or, before marriage, upon other women, usually creates a powerful potential jealousy. This is not the mature, sexual jealousy of the emotionally well-developed male toward his mate. It is rather the child's jealousy of its mother, so intense because of the child's helpless dependence. In these cases the mother has been too exclusive a source of gratification (or else there has been deprivation or other trauma), and the child has not learned to find pleasures in more self-reliant, independent ways in its own activities and in relation to other persons and interests.

This wish to be passive, in the sense of being freed from responsibilities and to be dependent and admired, exerts itself not only in marriage but also in the man's occupation. Very often the man was perferred to his brothers and sisters or was actually an only child or treated as one during his formative years. This adds to his needs a quality of exclusiveness and special preference. Sometimes the dependent love needs are so strong because of the opposite, because they were deprived from 0–6. The man can realistically demand somewhat more exclusive attention and regard from his wife than he usually can in his occupation. Whatever his work, there are usually others who rate as much attention, recognition and emotional support as himself, but this may be hard for him to tolerate. If so, troubles develop toward his superiors or his peers or both.

Perhaps the most sinister feature of this psychodynamic pattern is the hostility which it generates. This hostility may be quite subtle and only appear in a negative way through the man's failures and neglects. These may be with or without benefit of alcohol. With alcohol the destructive components toward himself and toward others may be more evident.

Usually, however, the hostility is apparent. The man's child is sick, but he simply does not have the time or the energy to do much about it. He initiates a project and then unloads it onto others.

Often the hostility is not only overt but direct. There are unrestrained temper tantrums and scenes. Sometimes there are dire threats. The hostility may mount to such an extent as to cause psychotic formations such as depression, paranoia, or schizophrenic symptoms; and, of course, it may come out as criminal or "criminoid" behavior (Saul, 1976). Many men, weak because of their infantile passive, receptive, dependent needs and frustrated desires for praise, become evil (i.e., hostile) men; and these dynamics operate with but little regard to socioeconomic status. A wealthy man or the son of a wealthy family may have such a motivational make-up and, like any person in any economic position, may vent his hostilities in a wrecked marriage and in behavior which is destructive for his intimates and society. Economic status can be an important factor, especially in the ways in which this pattern is lived out. However, it is not usually a primary factor.

Neither is marital status a primary factor. Some of these men never marry. They go from girl to girl and from woman to woman, changing swiftly or only after long periods, or else they marry and change wives frequently or do not remarry at all. They constitute a special problem for women; since their spoiling or deprivation has usually been by their mothers, they are apt to be attracted with exaggerated intensity toward women. They seek, unconsciously and with great intensity, to reestablish what was during childhood the emotional relationship of highest pitch for them, namely that toward the mother. Women are apt to feel the intensity of this emotional reaction and to be flattered by it and aroused by it. The girl or woman also senses how powerfully the man needs her. If she is somewhat experienced in the world, she may recognize the compulsive pathological quality in this need, but if she is young and naive, she may interpret it as a reaction to her own charms; she will not perceive the neurotic, that is, the warped infantile, elements. Difficulties may develop. She may notice that in spite of these obviously deep, all pervasive feelings, the man does not always show her great interest and consideration. Sometimes he is easily distracted by other women or other persons or interests. Nevertheless, the girl may not see that, underneath, the greatest force is the man's infantile egocentric needs for the satisfaction of his own dependence, praise and acceptance and his hostility. If she cools off and he cannot stand it, she is apt to attribute his anguish to his love for her, failing to distinguish sharply between *true love* which is a form of thoroughgoing interest in her own welfare, as opposed to the man's own selfish childish needs *for* her love, which are totally different. If she continues the relationship, she may learn painfully that the interest he shows is only a means to the end of getting what he wants. However charming he may be, however excellent the rest of his character, the forces which make him use a relationship primarily for his own benefit will assert themselves over the mature capacity to enjoy responsibility for her, for children, for job. She will find that what she has is too much a child-man, a man with the characteristic pattern which we set out at the beginning to describe.

This pattern of dependence and hostility is not confined to men. It is seen in women also. Very often women whose own childish, dependent needs are great marry men of this same type for that very reason. At first it brings them together. However, later, as these reactions emerge toward each other from identification to object-relation, they create such difficulties as we have endeavored to depict.

The constellation of childish dependence and hostility which we have described probably occurs in some degree in everyone. Therefore, it is only through its *quantitative* features that an individual might be designated as belonging to the type which we here separate for explicit study.

Of course, the therapeutic problem in each patient varies with that balance of forces in the personality and with the life situation. Some of these men respond most gratifyingly to even a little insight. They have felt handicapped and inferior without knowing the reasons for this, and there is a great reopening of emotional development as soon as they see what the block is. Some, though, cannot stand any insight whatever, and it may be impossible to hold them in analysis. They will not allow their rosy picture of themselves to be disturbed by unpleasant realities. Still others continue in analysis only so long as the analyst sympathizes deeply with the dependent needs and the hostility, identifying himself very closely with the patient who sees his difficulties as the fault of others. It may take great technical skill to keep the patient in analysis and then hold him as he begins to see the nature of what is really going on. Often it is not the matter of hurt pride alone; it is the sense that to be cured involves becoming mature, relinquishing his dependent attitudes and having responsibility as well as consideration for others. The threat to the dependence may prove to be well-nigh intolerable, especially in the schizoid personalities.

In still other cases the response to treatment is too good in the sense that to save his narcissism and win love the patient feels that he must relinquish his passive-receptive-dependent attitudes too rapidly and thoroughly. He may plunge into excessive activities and responsibilities with a compulsiveness which must in turn be analyzed, so that he becomes able to achieve a well-balanced life, enjoying both mature responsibility and legitimate forms of recreation and relaxation.

In sum, these men are, unconsciously, too much the children they once were—dependent, hostile, *child-men*. This is a type commonly seen and very significant for difficulties in marriage and occupation, and probably for society. Typically, there is much show, much promise but little accomplishment and much damage.

Biologically, human history appears as the story of man's struggle to domesticate himself to social life. This task is difficult for many reasons. We have touched upon three of these which seem to be of special importance. First, man's hostile aggression is so quick and brutal that it is the most difficult part of his nature to socialize. Second, his protracted childhood with its long years of dependence upon the parents is, no doubt, a condition of his intellectual development beyond the other animals and provides greater opportunity for civilizing influences, as well as other advantages. But it also involves fixations in childhood patterns, so long indulged as never to be overcome, which create manifold problems and irritants in adult life. And third, the whole process of rearing and civilizing the young has been based on the feelings and instincts of mostly neurotic parents without sound scientific knowledge. Of course, this would be better biologically if only these feelings of the parents were predominantly mature feelings and not so regularly warped by their own childhood patterns. Great religious contributions like the Ten Commandments and the teachings of Jesus have formulated the major social and psychological goals. The means toward these goals are in the hands of major religious groups, the State, law, education, family, and other great human institutions. Psychodynamics should help materially by providing a scientific base of knowledge and understanding of the main psychological forces and issues. Meanwhile, it is some consolation that out of this struggle of man with his instincts come sublimations and projections in art, science and thought—as well as his fears, devastations and agony.

The struggle itself represents the essential adventure of the human spirit. Man's present misery is a direct index to his failure in biological adaptation. His irrational hostility and cruelty threaten always and operate insidiously, breaking through individually as crime and erupting socially in war and revolutions. It is this problem, under the shadow of which we all live, that beyond any others should be the primary concern of science and of all of us. We must improve childrearing, particularly from conception to about age six, in order to diminish the infantile motivations, especially the hostile ones, and to free the mature forces if we are to improve human living and even perhaps to survive.

REFERENCES

Alexander, F. (1961): *The Scope of Psychoanalysis,* ed. by T. French. New York: Basic Books, pp. 116–128.

Freud, S. (1916): Introductory lectures on psychoanalysis, Lecture 22, some thoughts on development and regression, *S.E.* 16, pp. 339.

Saul, L. J. (1950): Physiological systems and emotional development, *Psychoanalytic Quarterly* 19:158.

———— (1976): *Psychodynamics of Hostility.* New York: Jason Aronson.

———— (1979): *The Childhood Emotional Pattern in Marriage.* New York: Van Nostrand Reinhold.

———— and Sheppard, E. (1956): An attempt to quantify emotional forces using manifest dreams—a preliminary study, *Journal of the American Psychoanalytic Association* 4 (3):July.

PART FIVE

On Psychodynamics

23 | General Concepts and Terms

Psychiatry, alone in medical practice, has as yet no basic science for a foundation. However, psychoanalysis represents both therapy and the beginnings of a basic science. This basic science will have to draw upon and cross-fertilize with other behavioral sciences in order to establish itself upon confirmed observations and proved conclusions. Thus are the foundations of psychodynamic therapy being laid.

The use of the term "force" has been questioned by some but seems to be fully justified if one considers that what impels biological organisms is at least analogous to, but probably similar or identical with, what is called force in physics and chemistry. There is no hesitation in conceiving of force as that which produces manifest changes and effects. Force in mechanics is what produces a change in the motion of a body. (Force = Mass × Acceleration.) We speak freely of gravitional forces and chemical forces. Psychic forces are, so far as we know scientifically, the reflections in our minds—what we are able to perceive subjectively—of the operation of chemical forces in our bodies. These chemical forces generate hunger, sexual urges, reactions of fear and attack, mature drives, and so on—and that by which we are impelled we rightly call "forces."

Here psychodynamics borders upon chemistry, physiology and biology and must work with them if these problems are to be clarified.

As a simple illustration, Hughlings Jackson's concept of "levels of integration" of the nervous system is invaluable in psychological and biological thinking. Love and hate are not opposed to indigestion in affecting a person's thinking, feeling and behavior—they are only on a different "level." Like all matter, we are a grouping of electrons and other atomic particles. Hence, it is essential in scientific thinking about biological behavior and its reflection in the mind to be able to move with the greatest ease from one level to another, especially in studying humans, who can have hemorrhoids and a virus infection while composing a soaring symphony and trying to support a family.

Psychodynamics deals with all the forces of feeling and motivation which are on the "psychological levels." By this is meant all those urges, impulses and feelings which possibly can be perceived in our minds. Even though such a force, for example fear, may be thoroughly repressed and not at all conscious to a person, yet if its nature is such that it has the potentiality, the possibility of being perceived in the mind, then it is a psychological force—as opposed to the subpsychological forces which raise our temperature when we have a fever and never can be made conscious.

These forces on the psychological level are for the most part, if not altogether, those motivating the entire organism as a *unit,* what makes a person or other animal behave as he does, rather than what makes the heart or the liver behave as it does (Saul, 1972).

The term "psychodynamics" is comprehensive and includes *all* of the psychic forces. There seem to be no valid reasons to restrict its meaning either (1) to the central pattern of gross, primitive motivations at the core of each personality in contrast with the highly refined activities of the ego such as esthetic sensitivity, or (2) to the disordered infantile complexes of motivation which produce neurosis, psychosis, violence and other aberrations; for these pathogenic forces differ only *quantitatively* from those which produce healthy, mature functioning.

The term "emotional forces" is not semantically unimpeachable. "Motivational forces" is more nearly correct. However, the motivational forces arouse in us intense feelings. Frustrated, dependent needs can cause painful sensations which we call loneliness. Mating impulses we feel as romantic love. Danger arouses an impulse to attack or to flee, and with these are associated feelings of fear and rage. Hence, the term "emotional forces" conveys very well a sense of forces which are biological and also that we experience these forces subjectively.

In each person the quantities, and hence the balance, of the emotional forces are specific and characteristic of him as a unique individual; and what he is conscious, partly conscious or totally unconscious of varies widely in proportion to the forces of repression; so does the fixity of each force and of the whole constellation. Thus one man is quite conscious of his dependence and relatively unconcerned in his acceptance of it, while another man reacts against it so violently that almost his whole life is an assertion of his independence, which he feels that he must perennially prove to others and to himself. One person is conscious of his sexual drives but not of his hostile feelings, while in another this is the other way around. So too for objects. One man sees his hostility to everyone except to his brother, where it originated. Another sees it toward his brother, but not its displacements to others.

The effects of awareness of motivation vary in individuals. Some patients immediately make use of every insight, while others see all, understand all (or rather *nearly* all, for something is usually lacking in these instances) and yet can only say, "So what?" Taking an extremely simple little example, one man was irritated in the extreme with his wife every night because she insisted that he open the windows. It soon turned out that his mother had done this for him during his childhood, whereas the wife's father had done it for her. He quickly learned to accept this little chore as his responsibility. However, he could not adjust to his wife's coming to bed long after himself and was unable to sleep until she retired, even though he came to realize that this carried on a pattern of his childhood when, put to bed on the third floor of a large house, he lay in rage and fear, unable to sleep until at long last his parents came up to turn in, for this connected with deeper roots than the window opening.

REFERENCE

Saul, L. J. (1972): *Bases of Human Behavior.* (1951) Westport, Conn.: Greenwood Press.

24 | The Main Emotional Forces—General Characteristics

The interplay of emotional forces covered by the term "psychodynamics" can be grouped around the three major goals, kinds or purposes: (1) the developmental and the regressive, (2) the conditioned and (3) the adaptational.

1. The developmental forces are those which impel the organism, from the fertilization of the egg cell, toward growth and maturity. These forces are opposed by the regressive ones which tend to reestablish earlier patterns. These id forces are neither all unconscious or all infantile—mature drives toward mating, parenthood, care of the young, and toward social living (hives, flocks, herds, etc.) are also id forces and are reflected in the interplay of motivation in the mind. Birds' building of nests, their care and the feeding of their young, are assuredly expressions of id forces and certainly mature. So is their social cooperation, e.g., crows, with their sentinels. This social cooperation can be considered properly the kernel of the superego. This is consistent with Freud's view that at birth the organism is all id, and the ego and the superego develop out of it.

2. A second group of emotional forces can be designated as "conditioned," meaning by this all the motivations which result from emotional influences and experiences of all kinds—the motivations which are "learned," through training, imitation, identifications and through all sorts of necessities and experiences, bitter and happy. These influences shape and mold the feeling, the thinking and the behavior.

The primitive, unconditioned instinctual impulses are inhibited, exaggerated, deflected and otherwise influenced and affected by conditioning experiences. The harsh parent, the teasing brother or sister, the loving aunt, all shape or condition the child's motivations, molding them by precept and example, for better or for worse, as the child grows. The superego, in this light, includes that whole group of mental activities which we properly can call conditioned. Cultural anthropology demonstrates the conditioning effects of cultures and customs.

The motivational patterns conditioned by living through infancy and childhood in a particular family persist, as we have seen, in the social living of the adult in marital home, work and society.

3. A third cluster of emotional forces can be called "adaptational." These encompass the many mechanisms of survival and adjustment. On the physiological level, the interrelated field in physiology and the term introduced by Walter Cannon for the body's tendency to maintain equilibrium is "homeostasis." Hans Selye's studies of physiological responses to stress have led to the concept of "diseases of adaptation" which is of obvious significance in the field of psychosomatic or comprehensive medicine.

On the ego level, the adaptational reactions are related to learning theory in psychology (Hilgard, 1956). They represent all of the individual's mechanisms of adaptation, on all levels, to the realities of the world and of his own body and mind.

REFERENCE

Hilgard, E. (1956): *Theories of Learning*. New York: Appleton-Century-Crofts.

25 | The Basic Dynamics of Personality

This chapter is meant to add no new material but rather to synthesize a more comprehensive formulation of the major motivations. Therefore, it will serve as a review and a summary of much that we have discussed.

There is a basic physiology for all human beings, and the fundamentals are close to those of lower animals. Individual men and women may vary enormously in size, shape, color of skin, etc., but the principles of their anatomy and of the workings of their organs and bodies are so closely alike that a physician or a surgeon can use his knowledge, gained mostly from animal experiments, to treat people all over the world. Is there a similar anatomy and physiology of the mind—an essential design in the interplay of motivations which underlies the enormous variety of individual personalities? There are basic physiological principles of operation for the digestion, for the heart and the circulation, and for the other organ systems. Are there also principles for the operation of the mind which hold for everyone? If so, they must be somewhat complex, and we must formulate them in abstract terms. Because of these difficulties, let us develop the picture in stages.

In the psychoanalytic study of human motivation, a person is apt to find himself lost in a jungle of mental and emotional details and complexities unless he discerns the *major* forces and discriminates the *fundamentals* from the *details,* the *essentials* from the *incidentals,* the *central* from the *peripheral,* the gross from the minutiae.

There are three elemental forces seen in every analysand—three poles to guide by. One is the person's hunger for dependence and love, the core of which is the remainder of his childhood's need for parents. In the healthy adult these needs are satisfied by family, friends, business associates, membership in organizations, being part of society, and so on—but, as we have seen, the dependent

462

needs for love may be exaggerated or warped to make serious emotional troubles. The second pole is hostility. Dependence and hostility are the basic forces in every case. They interact with a third great force, the superego, which term we have used to include certain mature forces toward social behavior as well as the effects of early conditioning. The main interactions are depicted schematically in Figure 16. Of course there is a fourth great force; *sex,* and this is always a bearcat of a problem; but how it is dealt with is determined by these first three.

As we have seen, the child's needs for dependence and love cannot be satisfied in an adult. Because of these needs, everyone wants love and care in some form—but few there are to *give* it. Hence, these needs are doomed to frustration, and the reaction to frustration is rage, hostility. Moreover, these needs themselves are probably the greatest single source of hurt vanity, self-esteem and of feelings of inferiority. Typically, a person wants to be dependent and loved like a child; therefore, without realizing it, he feels like a child toward others and puts himself in the position of a child toward others as though they were parents upon whom he could depend, who would freely give the love he wants. Feeling like a child, he feels weak and inferior; but he only senses something wrong without understanding what it is that enrages him. His feelings of weakness and inferiority hurt his vanity and cause a sense of impotent helplessness. His childish desires for dependent love conflict with his adult needs to feel mature. The result is bafflement, shame and rage.

However, no one can be filled with rage and hate without acting out some of this hostility against others, and this generates guilt. Guilt and a sense that one should be punished are the usual reactions of the conscience against hostility to others, the reactions, in other words, of the mature superego's standards for considerate social behavior toward other human beings; but the superego which should be mature, can be infantile or corrupt.

Anxiety results from all of these forces, probably most often and directly from the hostility and guilt; and anxiety in turn makes people seek all the more for help, care, emotional support and love. This closes the vicious circle, which is schematized in the following chart.

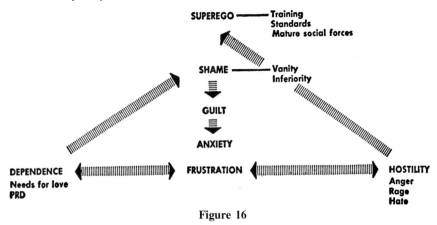

Figure 16

A person's mind is bounded by the motivations and the feelings welling into it from within and the outside world externally which impinges upon it through the senses.

As we have noted hitherto, two major directions are seen in human motivation—the *progressive* and the *regressive*. The progressive forces toward responsibility, productivity and independence (RPI) lead to the mature functioning of the adult human biological organism. Expressed in a few words, this is the capacity to enjoy responsible loving and working; the ability to have a true interest in the welfare of others for their own sake and without thought of personal return or gain. This is the sort of loving interest that parents are expected to have in their children and also toward each other, which in maturity is extended to include friends and other persons in the world, their society and even humanity at large. The regressive trend is back to the infant's passivity, receptivity and dependence toward its mother (PRD) and the rage and violence proneness associated with this.

The standards and the ideals are the result partly of progressive forces in the personality but also are formed from training by and identification with sufficiently mature parents and other emotionally important persons during the earliest formative years of childhood. Insofar as they reflect the child's training, they show the enormous *conditionability* of the human mind. People go through life reacting very much in accordance with the ways in which they were conditioned during their earliest years.

The *flight-fight* reaction is one of the great mechanisms of *adap-*

tation. The tendency to *fight,* especially if carried out as open hostility against others, usually produces a fear of retaliation. The standards and the ideals, the effects of the progressive, mature forces toward love and the conditioning by training against violence, all produce a force in the opposite direction, a force toward inhibiting the hostility. This usually takes the form of feeling that one deserves punishment and it is experienced to some extent as guilt and anxiety.

Just as hostility and attack generate *guilt* through the counter-reaction of the mature standards and the ideals, so flight, whether actual or psychological, tends to create a feeling of weakness and shame.

Flight often takes place psychologically in the form of regression to attitudes and reactions of childhood, especially back to the infant's dependence and needs for love, which once gave assurance of security.

The contrast between the infant's intense needs for the mother and, on the other hand, the good mother's (and of course father's) outpouring of love and energy in caring for the child, provides a pattern for the immature versus the mature attitudes.

No one completely overcomes his childhood attitudes and needs; everyone *wants* love, attention and help from others, but few people are mature enough to *give* it. Obviously, if most of the world want it and few can give it, there is bound to be widespread frustration, and many human troubles result. The "give-get" equilibrium is so often not maintained.

The goal is not to overcome all that is infantile, which is impossible, but rather to have what is infantile *healthy* in its nature and satisfactorily *balanced* and blended with what is mature. Schematically, one might consider the goal to be at least 51 percent maturity with healthy, infantile needs providing recreation and a balanced life.

Expressed another way, the major gratification in life lies in *loving and being loved.*

Certain features of the mind are so outstanding as to warrant repeating in summary form.

1. The interaction of two basic trends which are seen in every personality, the progressive motivations toward development and maturity, to become the responsible parent, worker and citizen

THE MAJOR EMOTIONAL FORCES — CONCENTRATED REPRESENTATION

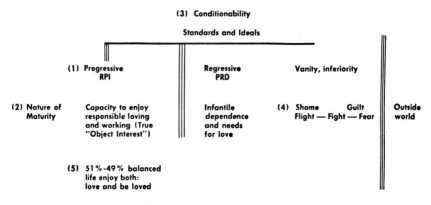

Figure 17

versus the regressive tendency to return to the child's position of being cared for and dependent upon adults who take responsibility *for* him.

2. The nature of maturity, the capacities of the adult to enjoy responsible, independent, productive loving and work.

3. The enormous "conditionability" of the mind.

4. The fight-flight adaptational reaction of such fateful import for our life on earth.

5. The ideal solution, the balanced life, in which the mature, progressive drives are enjoyed in mating, child rearing and in occupation, friendship, humanitarianism—and the regressive wishes are also enjoyed in recreational, nonhostile, socially acceptable form.

We are now in a position to attempt a comprehensive, although highly condensed, description of the major emotional forces and something of the interrelationships and the basic principles of their operation in the mind.

The outside world, external reality, especially other human beings affect a person in two major ways: (1) through their early conditioning influences upon the child from the very beginning of its development (conception) and especially during the first few hours, days, weeks, months and years of life when it is most tender and formative; and (2) the current pressures, stresses and strains of life under which everyone lives and which must be handled; these may in turn be (a) long range and (b) sudden, unusual pressures such as occur in time of war or economic crisis or unusual misfortunes with a family.

The various human motivations have been so grouped as to be intelligible as three main mental agencies: the id, the impersonal biological organism with its progressive and regressive drives; the superego representing the mature social motivations and also the effects of early conditioning and learning; and the ego—the part nearest to consciousness with which we (a) perceive the external world and our needs, urges and impulses from within, (b) integrate these, and (c) direct urges and behavior and endeavor to handle the world around us. One of the important functions of the ego is that of comprehending reality, both inner and outer. The ego integrates urges and reactions from the id and the superego with memory and experience and with its perception and comprehension of the outside world and acts as executive agency.

We have referred to the progressive forces as "developmental." The motivations of the organism arising from its biological nature, that is from the id, can for the most part be divided into (1) the mature and (2) the immature. The model for the mature is the attitude of the good parent to a loved child. The model for the healthy immature motivations is that of the wholesome child toward its parents. This division between mature and immature runs through both the supergo and the id. It divides the superego also because, if a person has had infantile parents, then he is apt to have been conditioned by identification with them and by training, at least in part, in an infantile way, so that his resulting capacity for love and social cooperation and his standards and ideals are apt to be largely immature.

Further facts can now be filled in concerning the progressive and the regressive forces in the id. The relationship of the good mother to the healthy baby shows (1) the contrast between mature independence and normal infantile dependence, between the capacity for productive loving and working and the infantile needs for love, attention and care; and (2) the mature capacity for interest in others and social cooperation as contrasted with the child's egotism, needs for adulation and for measuring itself against others and competing with them—out of its sense of insecurity and needs to assure itself that it will be loved and therefore cared for by adults; and (3) the mature use of sexuality for mating, reproduction of the species, making of a home, and rearing of the young in contrast with the child's interest in sex (a) only as play (b) with its attachment to the members of the family rather than to those outside of it (Saul, 1979).

Of the adaptational forces the flight-fight reaction can now be elaborated with further details—the biological arousal to fight appears psychologically as hostility and produces fear of retaliation. Internally, through the reaction of the superego with its conditioning to social standards, the hostility generates guilt and expectation of punishment, or actually self-punishment. On the other hand, the automatic tendency to solve problems by flight produces attempts at (1) actual flight; (2) psychological flight through the use of alcohol or other drugs; (3) what might be called biological flight by "withdrawal," with depression of the biological functioning, slowed activity, loss of appetite and of sexual interest, constipation, and so on—a sort of shutting down, rather analogous to the opossum's "playing dead"; but the most common form of psychological flight is through (4) regression to those attitudes of childhood which proved to be useful in achieving some degree of security and satisfaction in those days.

This whole combination of forms of fight and flight and the reactions of guilt and shame toward them combine in various ways and degrees to produce the many forms of disorders of thinking, feeling and behavior. The cause is mostly internal, the result of faulty upbringing which has warped the personality, but in some cases the fight-flight reaction is mobilized chiefly by unavoidable pressures from the external world in the immediate family or in such situations as wars or economic depressions or other seriously threatening crises.

The overall *goal* of the organism for which it strives through all these reactions and adjustments is the *completion of its life cycle,* including reproduction and the rearing of the young. To do this, it seeks to achieve a *balanced life* in which the healthy infantile wishes fuse with and balance off the mature, so that the individual can enjoy *both* the mature and the infantile—his work and responsibility and the use of his powers, and also his needs for legitimate self-indulgence, recreation and rest. Any interference with the completion of the life cycle is probably the basic threat to the organism which arouses the fight-flight response. Conversely, the

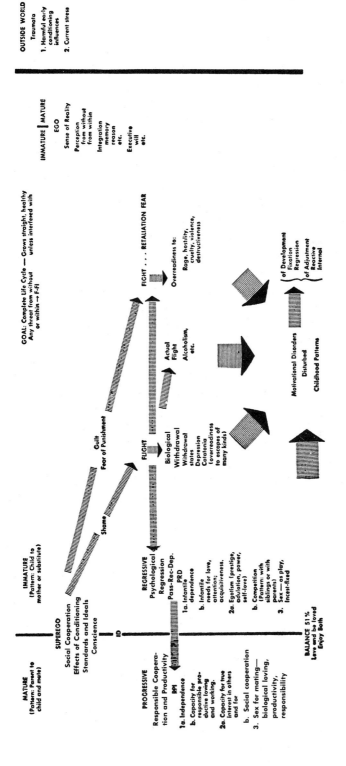

Figure 18

most fundamental significance of anxiety and hostility is this: they are signs of a threat to the individual's fulfillment of his life cycle.

This is cast in diagrammatic form in Figure 18. Some people do not like charts, but they can be helpful to those who can read them in synthesizing the concepts and in clarifying the interrelationships. This chart is, I believe, a distillation and a condensation of a considerable amount of knowledge of basic psychodynamics, which underlie healthy motivation and functioning and, when disordered, underlie all of psychopathology, of emotional aberrations.

REFERENCE

Saul, L. J. (1979): *The Childhood Emotional Pattern in Marriage*. New York: Van Nostrand Reinhold, pp. 465–486.

Epilogue

The fight-flight reaction is a deepseated physiological, primitive animal reaction, first explored and described in both humans and animals by a physiologist, Walter Cannon. The ways in which this reaction, rooted in our animal nature, impinges on our psychological life have been extensively described in the preceding chapters and the consequences can be readily seen in all of history and daily living. Human beings are animals, called upon by the necessities of living together in large numbers to control their instincts, especially the sex instinct and the fight-flight reaction with its impulses to hostility and escape. They must live in a "culture" or "civilization" with myriad rules that prevent men from destroying each other, rules that have grown into morality and ethics, into religions and government and legal systems. But despite all these efforts at restraints, especially of sex and hostility, the visitor from Mars would readily see man's animal nature in his mostly uncontrolled sexual behavior with its prostitution, infidelities, promiscuity and mounting divorce rates, and his brutality to his fellows in wars and revolutions, as well as violent crimes enacted during times of peace, making our civilized cities no longer safe in which to live or walk. At any given time, war exists or threatens all over the world, such as now in the Middle East and in several parts of Africa, to say nothing of the bloodshed in Southeast Asia and also Northern Ireland between two of the outstanding religious exponents of peace on earth. Indeed man—men and women—human beings—are animals struggling to live together without destroying each other, whether indirectly by overpopulation, pollution and exhaustion of the earth's resources or directly by nuclear weapons. For the present, we human animals suffer in the struggles to control our sex drives and hostility to our fellows and report the occurrence of these in the news media and write literature to amuse ourselves with these trangressions and animal outcroppings. If one of our kind succeeds in fully controlling his or her sexual and hostile impulses, the others are apt to dub him "saint" and in some mixture to admire him, deride him, and like as not, kill him.

It is almost unknown among other species of animals to be as destructive of their own kind as humans are to one another. Is the hostility of man to man much stronger than that of other species to each other? Or is man's hostility the result of a pathologically exaggerated congestion of population in societies, societies formed out of need for cooperation for survival in optimal numbers? It all remains a relatively unexplored field for study.

In the long-range historical, archeological perspective, humans seem to have made but little progress over the millenia of their existence in substituting the gratifications of social life and loving for the pleasures of hostility and killing. Now it seems to be a race between the pro-social, pro-human forces and the employment of man's nuclear weapons which are no longer in the future but ready now. Is there no realistic hope then for the survival of *homo sapiens?* I think a ray can be detected. This ray is psychodynamics, which is an epochal development. It holds the promise of an upturn in the potential of humans for realizing their mature, social nature through the formation of wholesome childhood emotional patterns during the earliest hours, days, weeks, months and years of every child's life, from conception to age about six.

Humans are animals trying to adapt to social life for their own self-preservation and survival on this planet. But there is truth as well as hope in the saying which we paraphrase as: "If we had one generation of properly reared children, raised with love, patience, understanding and respect for their personalities from birth, with good, easy harmonious relations with their parents, we might have Utopia itself." Let us study and strike not merely the branches but the roots of the problem of man's inhumanity to man, with all its evil consequences in sadism, masochism and other mental and emotional disorders.

Difficult though it may be to raise children properly, we can hope that increasing knowledge will generate all the necessary sympathy, sensitivity, patience and love that are required. The following poem shows it can be done.

A CHRISTMAS POEM TO MOTHER AND DAD
By Meg
December 1978

Merry Christmas, Mom and Dad,
  you're the greatest parents I could have had.
As I thought about what we could give to you
  I realized perhaps a poem would do;
One that expresses how we feel
  about your love and support, both in spirit, and real.
I think back over my growing up years
  when you saw me though illness, joy and tears.
When I sat on your knees as a little tyke
  when I was six and you bought me my first 2-wheel bike.
How you loved me no matter what I did
  when even-tempered and when I flipped my lid.
And through those rebellious teenage years
  you were there when I needed comfort and cheer.
You put up with my many high school days:
  the parties, the dances, the overnight stays.
Remember "Teddy," my only horse
  who threw me off? You sold him, of course.
Then came the days of learning to drive.
  I'm surprised you got through all that alive!
I failed the first time I took the test
  but practiced til I could do my best.
Then after college Dad bought me a car
  and I drove it to North Carolina afar.
That little jetfire Oldsmobile made me feel
  like a queen behind the wheel.
Two years later was my wedding day
  and you gained a son in a very fine way.
The apron strings were finally broken
  the day our marriage vows were spoken.
Then off we went to Wisconsin to live
  our love and support to our own children to give.
Now you are grandparents, the best we could know
  and we just want to tell you, we love you so.
And tho' we've moved from coast to coast
  it's you we think of most.

You are in our thoughts many times each day
remembered in the most loving way.
So at this blessed Christmas time
we thank our Lord for words that rhyme.
So I could write this gift to you
and you must know each word is true.
Merry Christmas, Mom and Dad,
to the "bestest" folks I could have had.

All our love,
Meg, Carl,
David and Carla

INDEX

INDEX

475